"*The Mindfulness and Acceptance Workbook for Anxiety* is so much more than the sum of its title. It's a way to live, a way of being, and a way of bringing kindness and compassion to our lives and to the lives of those around us. In short, this is one of the most beautiful guidebooks toward life, and living a more heart-centered, kind, and compassion way, that I've ever seen. Take your time going through it, and do the homework, and see yourself shine! We all have magic inside, just waiting beneath our worries and concerns. This workbook helps you move those aside—or technically befriend them, which is pretty amazing—to unlock the magic and help you shine bright. Much more than a workbook, this is a kind and compassionate guide to life! I cannot recommend this book enough. It's a life-changer!"

—**Michael Sandler**, host of the Inspire Nation Show, and author of *Barefoot Running*

"You have in your hands a wise and healing workbook that is based on a radical premise: fighting or resisting anxiety adds fuel to the fire; learning how to relate to it with mindful presence and compassion leads to true well-being. Filled with accessible, well-researched exercises and practices, this guide can free you to live from your full aliveness, heart, and potential."

—**Tara Brach, PhD**, author of *Radical Acceptance* and *True Refuge*

"*The Mindfulness and Acceptance Workbook for Anxiety* combines the accumulated wisdom of the ages with up-to-date, cutting-edge developments in scientific psychology. In an easy-to-read and fun format, those suffering from anxiety in all of its guises will find the keys to breaking loose from its shackles. By emphasizing acceptance of toxic emotions (and illustrating ways to accomplish this) rather than struggling to overcome them, the person inside you may finally emerge to set your life on a new, productive, and valued course. Highly recommended for all those struggling with worry, anxiety, and fear."

—**David H. Barlow, PhD**, founder and director emeritus of the Center for Anxiety
and Related Disorders, professor of psychology and psychiatry at Boston University,
and author of *Anxiety and Its Disorders*

"This book presents a tried-and-true approach to turning your life in a new direction. If you want to stop running, hiding, struggling, or just waiting for your life to start, this book will help show you how to start living, now. Clear guidance, beautifully presented. Highly recommended."

—**Steven C. Hayes, PhD**, codeveloper of acceptance and commitment therapy (ACT),
and author of *Get Out of Your Mind and Into Your Life*

"In this fully updated and expanded edition of their best-selling workbook, Forsyth and Eifert show how giving up your attempts to control anxiety and fear will help you to leave your anxiety problems behind and get on with your life. In the years since the first edition, a number of studies have demonstrated the benefits of the approach described in this practical and clearly written book. I recommend this new edition for anyone who struggles with anxiety."

—**Martin M. Antony, PhD, ABPP**, professor of psychology at Ryerson University, Canada, and coauthor of *The Shyness and Social Anxiety Workbook*

"This is the definitive handbook for how to reduce the suffering that stems from anxiety-related problems. More importantly, the authors offer readers a perfect blend of lucidity, kindness, research-based knowledge, and concrete strategies such that readers walk away with the skills to live a successful life."

—**Todd B. Kashdan, PhD**, professor of psychology at George Mason University, and coauthor of *The Upside of Your Dark Side*

"Steeped in the rich tradition of psychological theory, *The Mindfulness and Acceptance Workbook for Anxiety* by Forsyth and Eifert represents a major advance for the practical treatment of anxiety and related conditions. This book will assist clinicians and patients in constructing a treatment plan that insures progress in overcoming the many obstacles associated with conquering fears. A major contribution to clinical care, this workbook will contribute to the growing knowledge base on acceptance and commitment therapy (ACT), joining other evidence-based approaches as a major tool for treating the disabling symptoms that accompany anxiety. This reference book belongs in every clinician's library."

—**Terence M. Keane, PhD**, director of the behavioral science division of the National Center for PTSD, and professor of psychiatry and assistant dean for research at Boston University School of Medicine

"If you suffer with anxiety, Forsyth and Eifert have given you a gift. It is not a structured manual for how to get over your anxiety as much as it is a book of wisdom. They raise the inevitable truth that anxiety is a part of all of us, and they show us the way—through willingness, compassion, mindfulness, and acceptance of ourselves and others—to live a life worth living, to understand our important values and to live in concert with them. This is a book well worth the reading, and its message is worth keeping close to your heart."

> **—Richard G. Heimberg, PhD**, professor of psychology and director of the Adult
> Anxiety Clinic of Temple

"The second edition of *The Mindfulness and Acceptance Workbook for Anxiety* is like great software. It has proven to be simple and intuitive to use but powerful and effective for people all over the world. This workbook also gives clinicians interested in acceptance and commitment therapy (ACT) a powerful, elegant approach and set of tools to use in their mental health practice."

> **—David Schaffer, MSW, LICSW, PLLC**

"Most 'how-to' self-help books try to teach people ways to improve and optimize their problem solving or fight their deficits. This book is different, as it encourages people to let things be and give up efforts to control those problems which they cannot change. An intriguing, inspiring, and deeply humane approach—one which was shown by one of our studies to even be successful for people who did not benefit from a previous psychotherapy. Firmly grounded in basic psychological science, the book tells the reader more about approach than about avoidance goals—easy to read and an ideal recommendation for anyone with anxiety problems."

> **—Jürgen Hoyer, PhD**, professor for behavioral psychotherapy and director of outpatient
> clinical services at Technische Universität Dresden, Germany

The
Mindfulness & Acceptance
Workbook for Anxiety

—————— SECOND EDITION ——————

A Guide to Breaking Free from Anxiety, Phobias &
Worry Using Acceptance & Commitment Therapy

JOHN P. FORSYTH, PhD
GEORG H. EIFERT, PhD

New Harbinger Publications, Inc.

Distributed in Canada by Raincoast Books

Copyright © 2016 by John P. Forsyth and Georg H. Eifert
      New Harbinger Publications, Inc.
      5674 Shattuck Avenue
      Oakland, CA 94609
      www.newharbinger.com

Cover design by Amy Shoup

Acquired by Catharine Meyers

Edited by Rona Bernstein

Library of Congress Cataloging-in-Publication Data on file

Printed in the United States of America

19   18   17

10   9   8   7   6   5   4   3

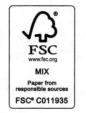
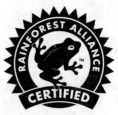

To our good friendship and support. With gratitude for fifteen years of collaboration, fun, sharing, and learning from each other. Writing this book together was a pure joy!

—JPF and GHE

I approached a dark tunnel with a bright light at the end. For years I feared taking a step inside, knowing that it would be long, uncertain, and difficult. But you came along and held my hand, and for the first time I knew that it would be okay to step, and step again. And so I did, and I am forever changed because of it. I am eternally grateful for you, Jamie, my love and my wife, for always being there to hold my hand in my moments of darkness and light. I now know what love means.

—JPF

To my mother, Margarete, who taught me kindness and compassion through the way she treated me and others—and by continuing to act with loving-kindness regardless of what her mind was telling her.

And to my wife, Diana: I am grateful and truly blessed that we can share our paths toward fulfillment with love, humor, and happiness—it is all within us.

—GHE

Contents

Acknowledgments

About eight years ago, we wrote the first edition of this workbook with a deep and abiding intention to help. At the time, we had no idea whether this workbook would be helpful and for whom. Now we know. We know because of the courageous efforts of readers like you.

We are grateful for the thousands of readers who took a chance on the first edition of the workbook, including those who offered us feedback and testimonials about the difference the workbook made in their lives. We also wish to convey a heartfelt thank you to the 700 people, spanning twenty-five countries, who took part in two controlled research studies we conducted to find out if our workbook works as well as we had hoped it would. You can take a peek at the prologue to find out what we learned from our research with people like you, but for now we simply want to thank each one of you.

Of course, it wouldn't have been possible to write this second edition without the kind and generous support of many other people, beginning with John's lovely wife, Jamie, and Georg's dear wife, Diana. Both Jamie and Diana offered us loving support, sage advice, and encouragement as we revised this workbook. They also reminded us of the value of this effort, and our intention to help people who, perhaps like you, are seeking freedom from fear and anxiety *and* the space to live life fully and in ways that matter. We couldn't have done it without them.

The ideas and inspiration behind this book are not just ours—they belong to a broader group. This group, of which we are proud to be a part, is working diligently on the problem of human suffering and its alleviation in a way that honors the pain and difficulties we all face as we attempt to create a life that matters to us. This collective body is the engine behind a rapidly growing approach to psychological health and wellness known as acceptance and commitment therapy (ACT, said as one word). This group has touched and inspired us with its research-supported practical skills; its wisdom, generosity, and kindness; and its plain old hard work.

We are particularly grateful to Steven C. Hayes and the broader ACT community. Steve's personal and professional odyssey, coupled with his wit, wisdom, and energy, sparked the beginnings of ACT. And in 1999 he, along with his colleagues Kirk Strosahl and Kelly Wilson, published the first full-length book on ACT—*Acceptance and Commitment Therapy: An Experiential Approach to Behavior Change*, now in its second edition. Several of the exercises we adapted for use with anxiety-related difficulties first appeared in that book. Since then, ACT has mushroomed into a treatment with broad scope and solid research support. This new knowledge has guided us in writing this revised and expanded second edition of the workbook.

We've also been touched and influenced by people outside the ACT community. Pema Chödrön, an American Buddhist nun, has written widely about the wisdom of meeting the strong energy of emotions, such as fear and anger, with patience, compassion, acceptance, and forgiveness. Her words— and those of Jon Kabat-Zinn, Jeffrey Brantley, Zindel Segal, Tara Brach, Sharon Salzberg, and many others—are simple and clear and mirror the central message of this book: that learning skills to let go of the ongoing struggle with anxiety and fear enables us to show up to life with the intention to do what matters. This message embodies the ACT approach that we'll be sharing with you here. We are forever grateful for their willingness to share their astute knowledge and practical wisdom.

Joseph Ciarrochi, David Mercer, and Sara Christian contributed the wonderful hand-drawn sketches that you'll see throughout the book. We would like to thank each of them for kindly giving us permission to reproduce their work.

We're also grateful to Kelly Wilson and our Swedish friends, JoAnne Dahl and Tobias Lundgren, for sharing with us their work on values, which includes assessment tools, illustrations, and useful activities, with additional thanks to Joanne Dahl and Tobias Lundgren for providing inspiration for the Life Compass that we adapted from their work (Dahl & Lundgren, 2006). Thanks also to our British colleague Peter Thorne, who shared with us the "Anxiety News Radio" and "Just So Radio" metaphors.

Special thanks also go out to the many professionals, students, and colleagues who have helped shape our thinking, and particularly to David Barlow for his groundbreaking contributions over the years on the nature and treatment of anxiety disorders. All this generous sharing of ideas and materials by our ACT colleagues has occurred in the spirit of "spreading what is good and what works," which unfortunately is not the norm in the competitive world of science.

New Harbinger is a major outlet for the dissemination of newer third-generation behavior therapies such as ACT. We are grateful to Matthew McKay and all the New Harbinger staff for seeing the value of this work and its potential to alleviate a wide range of human suffering. We also owe a debt of gratitude and heartfelt appreciation to Catharine Meyers of New Harbinger for her tireless energy, encouragement, and kind support with this project, and to Rona Bernstein for her masterful, diligent editing and attention to detail.

Finally, we would like to thank the countless people who have sought our assistance because they believed that we could help them heal their anxious pain and reclaim their lives. They, like you, are suffering with anxiety problems that are getting in the way of doing what matters. We have learned much from them. Their courageous spirit on the path out of suffering and into wholeness is present everywhere in this book. This book is a testament to their willingness to risk doing something new to get something new in their lives.

We sincerely hope you'll benefit from reading this book as much as we have from revising and updating it. It has profoundly and deeply changed how we view and approach the emotional pain and suffering of the people we encounter (our clients, colleagues, family, and friends), as well as our own pain and suffering, in ways that keep all of us moving in directions we value. We know that you can have that too.

—John P. Forsyth, PhD   —Georg H. Eifert, PhD
University at Albany, SUNY   Chapman University
Albany, New York   Orange, California

Prologue—Does This Workbook Really Work?

Research is the process of going up alleys to see if they are blind.

—Marston Bates

There are many self-help books out there for anxiety problems. Most are written with the guiding intention to offer something that may be helpful. This was our intention in writing this book too.

Still, we know that good intentions do not always translate into good outcomes. You know this yourself as well. You may intend to help someone but lack the skills or resources to make a difference. In the same way, writing a wonderful book is no guarantee that it will actually enrich the lives of those who read it.

The only way to really find out is to test the book by doing systematic research. And there are only three possible outcomes: (a) the book helps, and the lives of readers significantly improve; (b) the book hurts, and people get worse; or (c) the book doesn't make one bit of difference, and people are no better off after finishing it than when they started.

Of course, most authors would love to hear that their book was helpful, but to know that, they need to be willing to find out if they were wrong. The only way to find out in an unbiased way is test the book itself using sound research methods. We did just that with the book you have in your hands.

Here, we'd like to share what we learned and what it means for you.

WORKBOOK STUDY

The focus of this study was to see if this workbook is, in fact, helpful and in what ways. So, we designed a study to see if the workbook makes a difference in the lives of people just like you (Ritzert, Forsyth, Berghoff, Boswell, & Eifert, in press).

We recruited an international sample of 503 people who reported struggling with severe anxiety and depression. Our research team then randomly assigned them, by flip of a coin, to either begin using the workbook right away for a period of twelve weeks, or to be on a wait-list for twelve weeks. After the twelve weeks, we offered the workbook to those who were initially on the wait-list, who then used the workbook for a period of twelve weeks too. We then followed everyone to see how they were doing six and nine months later.

You should also know that we had no contact with any readers in the study, so there was no coaching or therapist guidance. All we asked was that participants read and work with the material in the workbook on their own. That's it!

Improvements in Skills to Disarm Anxiety and Fear

As you will find out, this workbook teaches many skills to help foster a different kind of relationship with anxiety and fear. These skills include being less avoidant and less tangled up with difficult thoughts, and more present, flexible, compassionate, kind with yourself, and accepting of your internal experiences just as they are. In this study, we measured these facets of peace and genuine happiness at the beginning of the study, after twelve weeks, and six and nine months later.

The good news is the results strongly support the benefits we mention throughout the workbook. Readers who used the workbook reported significant and meaningful improvements in mindfulness, self-compassion, and the ability to detach from unpleasant thoughts; they also became less avoidant and more accepting of anxiety, fear, and other unpleasant emotions. These changes coincided with using the workbook. Those on the wait-list showed these benefits once they started working with the workbook, but not before. Most importantly, readers maintained their improvements at the six- and nine-month check in.

So, the bottom line here is one of justified hope. The results show that the workbook radically changes the relationship people have with their anxious minds and bodies. Moreover, the results also show that—in line with its strong focus on values and doing what matters—the workbook improves the quality of people's lives.

What About Anxiety and Fear?

As you read the workbook, you will find that we don't focus much on anxiety and fear reduction. The reason is that it's not the absence of anxiety but the presence of a high quality of valued living that brings us more genuine happiness and peace. That's why we focus on improving your quality of life by helping you move toward your values. Still, we did look at what happened to the anxiety and fear in this large study of people from all over the world. What we found will be good news to you.

Readers who worked with the workbook reported significant reductions in their anxiety, fear, worry, and depression. You may wonder how that might be. How could a book that doesn't focus explicitly on anxiety reduction end up decreasing anxiety, fear, and worry as well as depression?

To get the answer, we reanalyzed the data using sophisticated statistical analysis (called multiple mediation, in case you're interested). We will walk you through what we found in the section below.

What Accounts for the Good Outcomes?

Using mediation analyses, we looked to see if the skills we emphasize in the workbook have anything to do with the reductions we found in anxiety and depression and the improvements in quality of life. It turns out that they do (Sheppard & Forsyth, 2009).

In fact, when you focus on learning the skills and cultivating a kinder and gentler relationship with your anxious mind and body, you will feel better. It is the skills that lead to anxiety lessening, depression lifting, and quality of life improving. It doesn't work the other way around. Working to be less depressed and anxious does not lead to learning to be more skillful or having a better life. Let this sink in, and linger with it a bit.

Reductions in anxiety and fear did not happen by going after anxiety and fear directly. It was just the opposite. By first focusing on the skills needed to live a more valued life, readers then experienced a decline in their anxiety, fears, and depression, and ultimate improvements in their lives. This is an important message—one that supports the approach we offer in this workbook.

Above all, these findings mean that you should spend time focusing on the skills, for each will help you cultivate a new relationship with yourself, your anxious mind and body, and your world. This is how you will attain real relief from anxiety and fear and genuine happiness and satisfaction with your life!

THE TAKE-HOME MESSAGE

We took a risk in evaluating this workbook, and it paid off. In truth, we would have been fine if the results didn't turn out as they did. But, across the board, the results show that the workbook works well and works in many ways.

But it only works for those who actually work with it. Readers in our study spent an average of four hours per week working with the exercises and material in the workbook, and most reported that it significantly changed their lives.

What this means is that to benefit, you need to be willing to take time with the material and allow yourself a chance to learn new skills. This is a point we stress throughout the workbook and another reason we keep coming back to old themes and concepts throughout. All the skills you learn must be nurtured and carried into your life from this point forward. They are not to be tried and then forgotten. They must be lived and become your guiding light from here on out. It's all up to you.

This is actually one of two studies we did to evaluate *The Mindfulness and Acceptance Workbook*. To keep things focused, we don't spend a lot of time discussing our second study, which compared the workbook to a more traditional cognitive-behavioral workbook for anxiety (Russo, Forsyth, Sheppard, & Promutico, 2009). Nor do we cover another large study by Eifert and colleagues looking at the benefits of the ACT approach for highly anxious people receiving more traditional face-to-face therapy (Arch et al., 2012). But these studies support everything we've shared with you here.

Many other researchers are also exploring ACT for anxiety concerns, with positive outcomes. We know there's more work to do, but you can be confident in knowing that you're not walking into a blind alley without reason. There is hope for you to find genuine happiness and to get your life moving in ways that matter to you. Now it's time to commit to doing that important work yourself.

We hope that the updates, new exercises, and materials we've included in this, the second edition of *The Mindfulness and Acceptance Workbook*, will set the stage for you to break free from anxiety and fear so that you can embrace and live your life to the fullest.

Introduction

There are two primary choices in life:
to accept conditions as they exist,
or accept the responsibility for changing them.

—Denis Waitley

We'd like to start off with a simple "yes" or "no" question. Read it slowly, but don't read into it. Listen to your gut. This isn't about labeling yourself with a diagnosis. We're not asking you to judge yourself either. Just answer honestly "yes" or "no." That's it. Now, here's the question:

Is anxiety and fear a major problem in your life?

If you answered "yes," you're not alone. If you answered "no," you're in good company too. But a "yes" is different than a "no." If you answered "yes," then you're probably suffering in some way. It's not that you just have anxiety. You have a *problem* with anxiety.

You may be suffering from anxiety, fears, panic, unsettling thoughts, painful memories, and worry. More deeply you may know, with absolute certainty, that anxiety has brought ruin to you and your life. You may feel frustrated and exhausted. You may feel broken, damaged, and at your wit's end. You may think something is wrong with you. And you are looking for a way out. We can tell you this much: you're not alone.

All of us experience worry, anxiety, and fear. You, too, can learn to experience anxiety and fear without it being a problem for you. We'll show you how in this book.

FREEDOM FROM ANXIETY MANAGEMENT

There's no way to escape the simple fact that anxiety is *part* of life. The emphasis here is on the word "part." Many people do live well, even with significant anxiety and often with the same anxieties and fears you may be experiencing. You may wonder how they do that and what little secret they have that you somehow lack. There's really nothing remarkable about what they do.

At a very simple level, they've learned to put anxiety and other unpleasant feelings and thoughts in their proper place—where they are just a part of life, but not the whole of life. At a deeper level, they've learned to free themselves from the pull of constant struggle with anxiety. In short, they don't let anxiety, fear, worry, panic, painful memories, and the like stand in the way of doing what they care deeply about.

The book you have in your hands will help you do this too. Anxiety need not continue to cause you to suffer by putting a choke hold on you and your life. There's another way—a set of skills that we'll help you learn so that you can devote more of your energies to aspects of your life that matter to you. This new approach, supported by solid research, will help you tip the scales back to where anxiety and fear become just a part of living well.

To get there you'll first need to face up to the fact that just about everything you've tried up to now hasn't really worked to keep anxiety and fear at bay. If you're like most people, then you know how difficult it is to get a handle on anxiety. And you've probably done many different things already to manage or reduce your panic, fears, worries, and tension. The activity below will help you get a better sense of this.

Here you'll find a list of some common things people do when they struggle with anxiety and fear. Look it over. Place a check mark (√) in the box next to the strategies that you've tried.

☐ Running away from situations that make me feel scared, anxious, or nervous

☐ Avoiding activities or situations that may bring on anxious thoughts, feelings, and memories (e.g., going outside, driving, working, being in a crowd, experiencing a new situation, eating certain foods, exercising)

☐ Suppressing or pushing out disturbing thoughts and feelings

☐ Distracting myself from anxiety, fear, and worrisome thoughts

☐ Changing how I think—replacing the "bad" thoughts with "good" thoughts

☐ Talking myself out of anxiety, panic, fear, or worry

☐ Sticking close to "safe" people (e.g., friend, family member)

☐ Carrying objects or performing rituals (e.g., phoning, checking, counting, cleaning, washing)

☐ Talking or venting with a friend or family member about my anxiety

☐ Joining online support groups for people with anxiety problems

☐ Educating myself by reading books written by experts on anxiety disorders

☐ Turning to self-help books offering "better" ways to control worry, anxiety, and fear

☐ Using antianxiety medications, herbal supplements, or alcohol to dull the pain

☐ Going to psychotherapy

Here, we'll venture a guess that you checked at least one box, but probably more than one. That's fine. Now we'd like you to consider the following question: how have these anxiety management techniques worked for you? These strategies may have bought you some short-term relief. But how have your solutions worked in the long run? Look deeply here. Have these strategies delivered the goods? Or, have they cost you in some way?

Before going on, see if you can connect with at least one of the costs. What have you missed out on in an effort to solve your anxiety problem—that is, to avoid feeling anxious or afraid? Think about something you really care about, however small or big. Perhaps it's work, finances, or family. Maybe it's travel, exercise, a hobby, or your health. Or it may involve relationships, intimacy, your freedom, peace of mind, or spirituality. Take a moment and write that one important thing below. We'll come back to that later on.

Because of my anxious thoughts and feelings, strong fear and panic, worry, or disturbing memories, I

have missed out on or am unable to _____

_____.

Anxiety and fear are intense and action-oriented emotions that are hard to control and cope with. Your experience up to this point tells you as much, and it's right on. The truth is that anxiety may never go away entirely. You may never be able to reduce, let alone get rid of, the intense feelings of panic, the painful thoughts, or the bad memories. In fact, if someone, however well intentioned, tells you that you can, please don't buy in to it. There is no magical solution that will remove anxiety and fear from your life. Why?

Because we are historical creatures. Modern neuroscience tells us as much. Our nervous systems are additive, not subtractive. This means that what goes in, stays in. Right now, you probably have a history that creates a good deal of anxiety and fear—and has taught you how to deal with it. It's all in the mix. The good news is that you can change the mix. That's how you'll get new outcomes—you create new history.

To change the trajectory, you'll need to learn how to take control over your life and not let anxiety take over and get the in the way of the things you want to do, the things you care about doing. You can end your suffering. You can get out from under anxiety and fear without having to get rid of anxiety and fear. You can get your life back! We'll teach you how.

A NEW WAY OUT OF YOUR WORRIES, ANXIETIES, AND FEARS

This book will take you on a journey of sorts. We can't tell you for certain where you'll ultimately end up, but we can say this much: the journey will be quite unlike anything you've tried before. This is good.

We aren't about to take you down the same old path. We won't offer you strategies that keep fanning the flames of fear and anxiety and don't work in the long run. You won't find anything in this book about teaching you "more, better, different" anxiety management and control strategies. This book is much bigger than that. It's about your life!

We're going to take you down a path that will challenge you in many ways. We'll show you how to change your relationship with yourself and the history you've had up to this point, including all the thoughts, memories, and images that trigger anxiety, the uncomfortable and scary feelings themselves, and your natural inclination to do something to make it stop, or to avoid it all together.

Inside the "anxiety is a problem" mind-set is often a relationship with anxiety that's hostile and unkind. This simply feeds and strengthens anxiety. And, as anxiety grows, you'll tend to struggle with it and resist it more—and on and on it goes in an endless cycle.

The most powerful antidote to this never-ending cycle is to learn how to bring acceptance, kindness, and compassion to your anxious thoughts and feelings. Developing acceptance and compassion for the more painful parts of your inner emotional life will weaken the power of anxiety to keep you stuck and suffering. And, it will do something else too—something that is larger and far more important than anxiety itself. It will allow you to create space to discover, or perhaps rediscover, what you want to be about in this life and where you want to go. As that space grows, you'll learn to refocus your energies on the people and experiences that matter most to you. In short, you'll get your life back. We wrote this book to help you do just that. Period.

Nobody wants to be about anxiety now and forevermore. Yet this is what you can become so long as anxiety is met with negative energy. That negative energy is packaged in the form of active resistance, denial, struggle, suppression, avoidance, and escape. As you read the book and do the exercises, you'll learn why this is so. And as you learn how to meet your anxiety with a kinder and gentler response, you'll find that the things you spend your time doing will change. New possibilities will emerge. You'll learn how to live out your dreams. You can have that without first having to win the war with your anxiety monsters.

These ideas are not fluff. They're backed by a growing research base showing that anxiety management and control feeds anxiety and fear, shrinks lives, and promotes the suffering you know about firsthand (Eifert & Heffner, 2003; Eifert, McKay, & Forsyth, 2005; Hayes, 2004; Hayes, Follette, & Linehan, 2004; Hayes, Luoma, Bond, Masuda, & Lillis, 2006; Hayes, Strosahl, & Wilson, 2012; Salters-Pedneault, Tull, & Roemer, 2004; Yadavaia, Hayes, & Vilardaga, 2014). This is why, instead of teaching you new ways to control anxiety, we'll go to the root of the problem in a way that will increase your vitality and your ability to create the kind of life you want to live—a full life, free of the pain of ongoing struggle with anxiety.

And, as strange as it may sound now, you'll learn how to engage in your life more fully and deeply with whatever your mind and body may dish out from time to time. When you do more of that, you can expect to think and feel better too. Acting to control your worries, anxieties, and fears is no way to live. Are you curious or suspicious? Good—read on.

HOW TO USE THIS BOOK

Many chapters include exercises that provide you with new experiences, skills, and ways to approach anxiety and your life. In fact, the exercises are the most important parts of this book. They bring to life in a personal way what you've learned and need to learn to break free from a place where anxiety and fear control you and your life. They'll also help you make contact with what works and what doesn't work. Some exercises show you how you can experience all of your worries, anxieties, and fears without acting on them. Understanding this is certainly helpful, but only experiencing it for yourself will make a difference in your life. The approach we'll teach you in this book is not some intellectual exercise where you'll suddenly achieve some great insight and all will be just fine. You need to *do* something with the material. This book will help you and work for you—but only if you work *with* it. How can you do that?

Put Taking Care of Yourself on Your To-Do List

To benefit from this workbook, you'll need to make an intention to work with it. You'll need to consider whether you and your life are as important as the mundane tasks that you and everyone else place on to-do lists each day. We think you're important enough to be at the top of such a list. So put taking care of yourself on your to-do list every day. We know that this may sound silly, but when people do it, they get results.

Make Reading a Priority

Make reading a priority in your schedule. Commit to it! Set aside a reasonable amount of time each week to read this book and practice the exercises. Be flexible. If you planned on reading in the morning and missed that reading time for whatever reason, allow yourself time to do it later on. The most important thing is that you do it.

Be Patient and Pace Yourself

Change takes time. You haven't arrived at this place overnight. We understand that you might feel the urgency to fix things quickly, but getting a different outcome in your life can't be done overnight. We strongly recommend resisting the temptation to read several chapters at once because you may end up feeling overwhelmed, and it will be hard to practice applying the new concepts and skills in your life. You need time to think about and work with the material—let it seep in. Be patient with yourself.

We suggest that you pace your reading at a rate of one chapter per week and do the exercises every day. This is a great way to take care of yourself. Chapters in part 1 can be read more quickly, but when you get into parts 2 and 3, *slow things down!* We've structured the chapters to be read this way.

It takes time to learn any new skill. And it takes time to counter the old habits that have kept you stuck and miserable. Ultimately, you should take as much time as you need with the material in each chapter. This isn't a horse race. Don't move on too quickly; instead, trust your experience. When you're able to apply new skills in your life, then you're ready to move on. Let that be your benchmark for progress.

Some Concepts and Themes Will Be Repeated for a Reason

Some themes will come up again and again. This repetition is deliberate. Repetition is your clue that a concept or skill is important. And when you see something show up again in later chapters, we're simply helping you learn how to apply that skill in new ways. Concepts are not to be read, forgotten, or left behind. But that's exactly what all of us tend to do with self-improvement books. We forget. We fail to see the bigger picture. We miss how skills apply to new challenges unless we're taught to make the connection.

We've also built in some repetition because this is exactly what would happen if you were working with a good therapist or life coach. And, we understand that you may be going this alone, without the benefit of a therapist to guide you. This can be hard. But the good news is that we know this workbook works when people use it on their own (see the prologue). So you can certainly benefit from this workbook without a therapist.

We understand that you may not like being reminded of this or that. In fact, your mind may resist it. But this is exactly the problem. Your mind may get hooked on judging this very workbook you're using in an effort to change your life. We can almost guarantee that your mind will jump in now and again with judgment and evaluation, calling exercises "stupid," "silly," "hard," or "too repetitive." Your mind may even tell you to put the book down. Whenever that happens, you'll need to take the reins.

Don't buy in to your mind's efforts to keep you stuck in the old and familiar—the very places that led you to pick up this book in the first place. You have a choice here—to move forward in new ways, or not at all.

If we could be with you in person as you use this workbook, then we would also return to earlier themes and concepts over time. Core themes are just as important in the later sections of this book as they are in the beginning. So think *familiar-sounding themes are important themes*. The work is to make them a habit in your life. That takes time, repetition, commitment, and practice.

Use the Worksheets, Audio Files, and Other Resources from the Workbook's Companion Website

Worksheets for some of the exercises are included in the workbook and can also be downloaded freely by visiting New Harbinger's workbook companion website at http://www.newharbinger.com/33346. Use the website to print out as many clean copies of a worksheet as needed for your personal use. These worksheets are clearly marked in the right-hand margins of this book with the computer icon shown here.

A few exercises are best listened to with your eyes closed, as we know from our own experience with the exercises and from people just like you. Being able to listen can pull you more quickly into the spirit of the exercises and guide you in learning the skills. You'll see what we mean soon enough. For these and other reasons, audio versions of some key exercises are freely available for download by visiting the workbook companion website at http://www.newharbinger.com/33346. These audio exercises are clearly marked in the right-hand margins of this book with the musical-note icon shown here.

Lastly, the workbook website also includes a listing of other print and online resources that we think you'll find helpful on your path of continued learning and growth.

Use the Workbook on Your Own or as Part of Your Therapy

This book was written as a stand-alone workbook to help anyone who may be struggling with anxiety problems, in whatever forms they may take. You need not have been told that you suffer from an anxiety disorder, which you'll learn more about in chapter 2, to benefit from this workbook.

If you happen to be working with a therapist for anxiety problems, you might also find this book helpful to complement the therapy. Therapists with experience and training in newer cognitive behavioral therapies, such as acceptance and commitment therapy (ACT), will know the approach in this workbook inside and out. If you're currently seeing an ACT therapist, you may find that the chapters roughly correspond to the material your therapist covers with you each week. If you are looking for an ACT therapist, you can find one at http://www.contextualscience.org/act_for_the_public.

OUR JOURNEY: WHY WE WROTE THIS BOOK

We wrote this book because we know that what it contains can be of enormous benefit. And we wrote it out of our sincere desire to help. Many paths led us to these goals. Here, we'd like to share with you a bit about us and our journey.

We were trained as clinical psychologists and researchers, with most of that training in what's commonly known as cognitive behavioral therapy (CBT). We've devoted a good part of our work to understanding the causes and treatment of anxiety and anxiety disorders. More broadly, we are united in our goal to find better ways to alleviate human suffering by cultivating psychological health and wellness.

We used to teach anxiety sufferers state-of-the-art CBT techniques. We focused on helping people gain mastery and control over their unpleasant thoughts and feelings using numerous techniques, many of which offered "new, different, better" ways to change thoughts and feelings. You probably know about this approach. Maybe you've learned how to identify catastrophic negative thoughts, to see that they are unrealistic, and then to replace those thoughts with more realistic thoughts. If so, you have a taste of what CBT is about.

Another major part of all effective treatments for anxiety involves having anxious people expose themselves to the things they most dread. Usually these are cues and triggers for anxiety and fear. Some triggers can be found in your mind and body, and many more lurk in the world around you. With exposure, and more exposure, people gradually learn to face their fears. And, with time, many get relief from anxiety. These and many other related techniques have strong research support. They work for some people, some of the time. But they are far from being curative.

In our own research and clinical work, we've seen time and time again people getting better—meaning less anxious—then returning later for more help. They come back because their anxiety and fears have returned. In trying to make sense of this, we began to wonder whether some of the techniques used to manage anxiety had lost their punch. This observation is not unique to us. Partial or full return of anxiety following traditional CBT is more common than many of us would like to believe.

Many people seeking help with anxiety problems have been through the mill of sensible strategies, often with limited results. Something there didn't seem right to us. And, as we stepped back, we began to question whether CBT was sending the wrong message. That message is this: anxious thoughts and feelings are *the* problem and are what keep you from creating a better, richer, and more meaningful life. From this perceptive, the only way into a better life is to alleviate the problem. Often this means learning ways to control and change what you think, feel, and remember.

Inherent in this approach is the idea that it's not okay to be you. Or, put another way, it's not okay to have the history that you've already had up to this point in your life. And along with that comes the idea that it's not okay to think what you think and feel what you feel. Many people who seek therapy think this way too, at least early on. And many therapies for anxiety problems promote this message. They focus on changing how you think and feel. And when and if you're successful doing that, you'll be happy and thrive. But the message that it's not okay to be you still lives inside this approach. And that message itself is hurtful. There's just no healthy way to go forward while holding on to the idea that something is fundamentally wrong with you.

The very idea that living well follows from thinking and feeling better (meaning less anxious and afraid) didn't sit well with us. And neither did the CBT solution to anxiety, with its focus on teaching better anxiety management. But the CBT message is part of a much larger cultural theme about solutions to anxiety and other forms of emotional pain. You've no doubt heard it—fix your pain and you'll be happy and live well. But the fundamental question is this: must we fix the pain first to live well?

It might be tempting to think that because we know a thing or two about anxiety, somehow we've escaped its darker side. In truth, both of us have gotten stuck now and then trying to get a handle on our mental and emotional hurts, only to find that our trusted bag of CBT strategies didn't seem to work well in the long run. Yes, even the two of us—the anxiety experts—can't get rid of our anxiety. And you know something? That's okay. Our collective personal and professional experience tells us that getting anxiety under control is no guarantee of a vital life. Thinking and feeling well does not automatically translate into living well, nor is it a path to genuine happiness.

As CBT expanded, new ideas began to emerge. These ideas seemed to challenge just about everything we'd been taught and were trying to apply in our own lives. This newer work was suggesting that perhaps thoughts and feelings aren't the enemy. Perhaps they need not be managed to live a vital life. This new wave of CBT was even going so far as to suggest that the *struggle* with our minds and bodies is the root source of human suffering.

In place of anxiety management, this work pointed to something radical, fresh, new, and, yes, even counterintuitive. That idea was this: Perhaps the struggle is unnecessary and even part of the problem with anxiety. And if that's true, then we ought to be teaching people how to develop comfort in their own skins. And we ought to help people redirect their energies to managing things that they can control and ought to manage—their actions in the service of doing what they care about.

That new approach involved a very simple idea and a powerful set of research-supported strategies and skills to help people bring acceptance, compassion, and gentleness to their unpleasant thoughts, feelings, memories, and even their sense of self. A shift in perspective was underway. Struggling to think and feel better was no longer part of the anxiety solution. The solution now focused on helping people change their relationship with their inner emotional life while also learning how to live better with whatever they might be feeling or thinking. A radical idea? You bet!

This work was building on several lines of research like those we outlined early on, showing that when you add management and struggle to normal human pain you often get more pain. In fact, you get suffering. You get pulled out of doing what most people consider important in life.

ACT is part of this new approach and forms the fabric of the ideas we'll be sharing with you in this book. We've spent a good part of our careers expanding ACT to help people just like you. We've also been using it in our daily lives—at work, with our kids, in our relationships, with our health, in our communities, and while doing things that we enjoy.

Here's what's different. When the inevitable pain of life rears its ugly head, we no longer resist and struggle with it. We are now meeting that pain with kindness, gentleness, mindful awareness, and a heavy dose of compassion. In a way, both of us are practicing drawing a line in the sand by letting go of needless struggle and making meaningful life choices. We're simply unwilling to let our emotional pain stand between us and where we want to go. This has given us more time and energy to focus on doing what really matters—living our lives in ways that resonate with our cores. And as we do more of that, we've noticed that we tend to think and feel better too.

We're not saying any of this is easy. It takes practice and commitment. But the payoff can be profoundly life altering. Our lives have been enriched in so many ways simply because we've learned how to put our energies to good use. We're less caught up in our painful heads and hearts and more engaged in doing what we care about. And we've seen this work with those who have sought our help, including thousands of people who have used our book.

Our intention is for you to make the most of your one precious life too. Everything that we know, we've crammed into this workbook to help you on the way. Now it's your turn. We hope that you make the most of it and see what this book can offer you. If you give it a real chance, we think you'll be pleasantly surprised. Your life will be better for it too.

BEGIN YOUR JOURNEY

This book is designed to help you get something different by doing something different. Reading this book—and internalizing what you learn—is part of this process. But there's no book on the planet, no pill, no person that can make you live your life in a certain way. It'll be up to you to put what you learn into action. You are the only person who can make the changes you need to make. In the end, you control the direction you want your life to take—that's your choice.

There is a Buddhist saying that the journey of a thousand miles begins with one step. Getting your hands on this book is a step in a new direction. Reading this book, even up to this point, is yet another step on your journey out of your anxiety and into a new life. Congratulations on getting this far! Now comes the hard part: keeping yourself moving forward.

A life lived well is the end product of a number of small moments. It takes a lifetime to create a life. Living according to your values is something we will help you do more of, one step at a time. On your journey, you'll learn, progress, and see life in a way that you may never have experienced before. The important thing is that you are taking steps, for even tiny steps will eventually take you up a mountain.

We invite you to make this book your travel guide. Use the information here to help you decide where you want to go. As you commit to putting your values into action, the quality of your life, and of those around you, will begin to improve.

PART 1

PREPARING THE WAY FOR SOMETHING NEW

We can't be afraid of change.
You may feel very secure in the pond that you are in,
but if you never venture out of it,
you will never know that there is such a thing as an ocean, a sea.
Holding onto something that is good for you now,
may be the very reason why you don't have something better.

—C. JoyBell C.

CHAPTER 1

Choose a New Approach to Get a Different Outcome

Your life is a sacred journey. And it is about change, growth, discovery, movement, transformation, continuously expanding your vision of what is possible, stretching your soul, learning to see clearly and deeply, listening to your intuition, taking courageous challenges at every step along the way. You are on the path ... exactly where you are meant to be right now ... And from here, you can only go forward, shaping your life story into a magnificent tale of triumph, of healing, of courage, of beauty, of wisdom, of power, of dignity, and of love.

—Caroline Adams

This chapter is about preparing the way for something new in your life. As much as we hate to admit it, we know that to get a different outcome we need to change what we're doing *now*. We've put this simple idea in the form of a mantra to help you remember it. The mantra is this:

If I continue to do what I've always done, then I'm going to get what I've always got.

Write it down and keep it with you as you work with the material in this book.

YOU HAVE CHOICES

You have the power to make choices, but having anxiety is not one of them. Anxiety just happens. It's not a choice. Nobody chooses to be anxious or afraid. But you certainly can choose a new approach to your anxiety to get a different outcome in your life. This new approach is what you'll find in this workbook.

You'll see that the material in this book will help you act differently on your anxiety and your life by putting you in control of what you can control. Put simply, you *can* control and change how you *respond* to your anxiety-related feelings, thoughts, and worries:

- You can stop trying to cope with worries, anxieties, and fears (if coping and other management strategies have not worked in a lasting way).

- You can learn to leave worries, anxieties, and fears alone and simply experience them as thoughts, sensations, feelings, or painful memories.

- You don't have to act on your anxiety, and it doesn't need to drive what you do. As much as you feel like running from intense anxiety, you can learn to act differently. You can learn to watch anxious feelings and worrisome thoughts and *not* do what they tell you to do.

- You can learn to nurture a kinder and friendlier relationship with yourself and your emotional life instead of reacting to anxiety as an enemy or unwelcome guest.

- You can learn to move with your anxious discomfort and do something that's potentially vital in your life.

We know from research and clinical experience that the solution to anxiety, worry, and fear isn't more struggle. It's not about trying to get rid of them. It's also not about replacing negative with positive thoughts like you might do when swapping out a worn-out spark plug in your car. None of this really works with anxiety and fear. And yet, many people do struggle. You probably do too.

You know this battle firsthand, and so do we. You may think that you must win it—perhaps by trying harder, struggling more, learning better strategies, reading about anxiety problems, finding a new medication, venting, and so on.

But here's the hard truth. Nobody can win this kind of battle. We get that this may sound depressing, and you may even feel a bit hopeless. But there's good news lurking inside this hard truth: you don't need to win this battle in order to begin living the life you want to lead. As you work with this book, we'll show you why.

For now, we ask that you entertain the possibility that the solution to your anxiety problems is not to fight "better or harder." The solution is to change your relationship with, and your response to, your anxious thoughts and feelings. You can choose to stop fighting. To get there, you'll need to learn how to acknowledge anxious thoughts and feelings without "becoming" them, acting on them, and doing what they say.

Our sincere goal is to help you spend your precious time on this earth doing what you care deeply about rather than spending your time and energy trying to control anxiety. Keep this in mind as you work with the material in the book. The prize we're after is a life lived well—your life lived to its fullest!

LEARNING TO BE RIGHT WHERE YOU ARE

Before moving on, we'd like to invite you to settle in for a moment to practice a simple centering exercise. You could also think of it as a grounding exercise, or as a skillful way to train yourself to be present wherever you are. This exercise, and other ones like it that you'll see in this book, have a purpose.

Anxiety and fear will make you contract and will pull you into dark places that are far from where you are in the moment. So, to counter that natural tendency, you'll need to learn how to come back to where you are.

The centering practice will teach you skills that will help you be right where you are *and* become more consciously aware of what matters to you. This practice will also help you come back to the present in your daily life when anxiety or other painful experiences try hard to pull you out of the moment.

Be mindful that there is no right or wrong way to do this practice. Just follow along as best you can. All you need to do is get in a comfortable position where you won't be disturbed for five minutes. Download the audio file from the book companion website (http://www.newharbinger.com/33346), and then just close your eyes and listen along. You may also use the script below, though we've found that it is better to listen and follow along with this exercise.

If you'd rather keep your eyes open, you can do that too, but it's best to focus on a spot, say on the floor just in front of you, so you don't get too distracted. We'll end the exercise with a small chime and tell you when to open your eyes and move on.

EXERCISE: SIMPLE CENTERING

Go ahead and get in a comfortable position in your chair. Sit upright with your feet flat on the floor, your arms and legs uncrossed, and your hands resting in your lap. Allow your eyes to close gently. Take a couple of gentle breaths—in … and out … in … and out. Notice the sound and feel of your own breath as you breathe in … and out …

Now turn your attention to being just where you are. Notice any sounds that you may hear close to you and then farther away. Notice how you're sitting in your chair and feel the place where your body touches the chair. What are the sensations there? How does it feel to sit where you sit?

Next, notice the places where your body touches itself, and bring your awareness to the spot where your hands touch your lap or legs. And now, imagine your awareness pouring down over your hips to where your feet touch the floor. How do your feet feel in the position that they are in? Notice too that your feet are firmly grounded to the floor and earth beneath you.

Now gently expand your awareness and just notice sensations in the rest of your body. If you feel any sensations in your body, just notice them and acknowledge their presence. Also notice how they may, by themselves, change or shift from moment to moment. Do not try to change them.

Now let yourself come back to being just where you are, here with this workbook. See if you can feel the investment of yourself here, right now. What are you here for? If you're thinking this sounds strange, just notice that and come back to the sense of integrity here. Be aware of the value that you are serving by being here.

And, see if you can allow yourself to be present with what you are afraid of. Notice any doubts, reservations, fears, and worries. See if you can just notice them, acknowledge their presence, make some space for them, and allow them to be there. You don't need to make them go away or work on them. With each breath, imagine that you are creating more and more space for them, more space for you to be you, right here where you are. Now see if for just a moment you can be present with your values and commitments. Why are you here, working with this workbook? Where do you want to go? What do you want to do with your life?

Then, when you're ready, let go of those thoughts and gradually widen your attention to take in the sounds around you, and slowly open your eyes with the intention to bring this awareness to the present moment and the rest of the day.

Let's take a moment to reflect on your experience with the Simple Centering exercise. What's important here is that you begin to notice your experience and what it teaches you. This will give you a sense of where you are as you begin your journey. So, let's start there.

What showed up for you as you considered your intentions and why you are here, working with this workbook now to make changes in your life?

_____

_____

What sensations, if any, were you able to notice in your body?

_____

_____

List any thoughts that showed up that seemed to pull you out of the exercise (e.g., _I can't concentrate; this is boring, I'm not doing this right_). Be specific.

_____

_____

Were you attached to any particular result by doing the practice—like feeling more relaxed, calm, or at peace? If so, note this below.

_____

_____

We encourage you to practice this Simple Centering exercise daily. Find a time and place that's right for you. It will help you create the space you need to show up to your life and do what you care about.

WHAT IS ACT?

This workbook offers you a way out of your anxiety and fears and into your life, based on a revolutionary approach called *acceptance and commitment therapy* (ACT, pronounced like the word "act"). This pronunciation is important because it summarizes what ACT ultimately stands for: committed ACT*ion*.

Accept—Choose—Take Action

The easiest way to get the gist of ACT is to focus on the three steps that the letters represent: Accept—Choose—Take action. Put another way, ACT is about letting go, showing up to life, and getting yourself moving in directions you want to go. Don't worry if this strikes you as too general or idealistic. We'll get more specific as you move on and practice the exercises. For now, we'll unpack the ACT acronym just a bit to give you a sense of what's to come.

Accept

This is the first step in ACT and a step that we'll help you nurture again and again in this workbook and, we hope, throughout your life. It involves active skills that'll help you to respond differently—with kindness, compassion, gentleness, and less engagement—when anxieties, fears, worries, panic, and other sources of emotional and psychological pain show up. The idea is to accept what you're already experiencing. This skill disarms the struggle you're having with unwanted thoughts and feelings. As you learn to let go, the need to eliminate or change those thoughts and feelings washes away, and so does the suffering.

After you drop the rope in your tug-of-war with your anxiety monsters, you'll notice that your hands, feet, mind, and mouth will be freed up to be put to use for the things in your life you truly care about. In the process, your life will grow and develop in ways that may have seemed impossible until now. Acceptance will help you make anxiety just a part of your larger life.

Choose

The second step is about choosing a direction for your life. It involves identifying what you value in life and what you want your life to stand for. Here, you'll get a chance to discover what is truly important to you—what you value—and then make a choice. What kind of child, sister or brother, student, or friend do you want to be? What types of activities are meaningful to you? Answering these kinds of questions is about choice—choosing to go forward in directions that are uniquely yours *and* accepting what is inside you and what accompanies you along the way. It's a step you'll take time and time again.

Here your life is asking you an important question: are you willing to contact and stay in touch with what your mind and body are doing anyway, fully and without avoiding or trying to escape from it? If the answer is no, you'll get smaller and your anxiety will grow larger. If the answer is yes, you'll get bigger and your life will get bigger too. Living well will become your focus, not living to feel and think well.

Take Action

The third step involves taking steps toward realizing your valued life goals. It's about making a commitment to action and changing what you can change. This means learning to behave in ways that move you forward in the direction of your chosen values. As you work with the material, you'll begin to see that there's a difference between you as a person, your actions, and the thoughts and feelings you have about yourself. And you won't find us asking you to simply face your fears in the hope of a better life. Our goal is to foster your willingness to take your inner emotional discomfort along with you in the service of your life goals and dreams.

You may feel intimidated by these three big bold steps. In fact, you may be quite scared. You may say, "This is too big—I can't do this." If you do feel this way, that's perfectly okay. This is what minds do. All we ask is that you hold your thoughts lightly. Just keep the book in your hands. Use your eye muscles to keep on reading. Let the thoughts be what they are and let them do what they do. Like other thoughts and feelings, it's okay if they come, it's okay if they stay, and it's okay if they go.

WHY ACT?

What we share with you in this workbook is supported by research showing that anxiety management and control efforts are unnecessary and costly. They can even be counterproductive. Paradoxically, these strategies tend to increase the very suffering you've been trying to reduce, and they also greatly restrict your life.

Recall the list of anxiety management and control strategies we covered in the introduction. They may look different from one another, but they're all about one thing—reducing painful thoughts and feelings. They're about struggle. Here's a brief synopsis of what the research tells us about struggle with emotional and psychological pain:

- **Increases activity of the sympathetic branch of your nervous system.** This system is the engine that ignites when you feel anxious, angry, or when your life is in danger. It makes you feel ramped up and more uncomfortable.

- **Worsens memory for important life events.** This is because reducing or getting rid of unpleasant thoughts and emotions demands your attention. Focusing attention on your anxiety and hurt is pulling attention away from other more vital life areas.

- **Is effortful.** Another way to think about this is that it's hard work to push against unpleasant thoughts, feelings, and memories. Think of it as trying to use the palm of your hand to hold back a stream of water gushing out of a garden hose. It doesn't work and you just end up getting soaked.

- **Works just well enough in the short term.** This is why people keep doing it—pushing against thoughts and feelings often will buy you some temporary relief. In the long run, though, it doesn't work. People continue to suffer and pay a price for short-term relief.

- **Doesn't change the quality of negative thoughts and feelings.** In fact, people tend to feel as bad or worse during and after fighting unpleasant thoughts and feelings. And, on top of that, it's exhausting.

- **Pulls you out of your life.** This is the most important finding. People who fight their thoughts and feelings on a regular basis report poorer quality of life, feel less authentic, have fewer close relationships, and generally feel limited in what they do. They feel stuck.

These and other findings point to one conclusion: trying to change anxious thoughts and feelings doesn't work. ACT capitalizes on this research by offering a way out of anxious suffering without more management, struggle, and control. That way out begins with doing something that goes against the grain of what you've been doing up until now. You do the opposite of anxiety management. You change your relationship with your anxious discomfort—especially how you act in the presence of it—by no longer fighting it.

Changes like this will open doors. They'll give you wiggle room and energy to get into your life more fully. This is what we mean when we say that ACT is all about allowing yourself to feel what hurts while doing what works and is important to you. In a nutshell, it is about acceptance *and* change at the same time. If you're 100 percent willing to give this a shot, then you'll learn to accept and live with your uncontrollable, anxiety-related thoughts and feelings *and* take charge of what you can control: your behavior, or what you do.

WHY ACCEPTANCE AND ACTION ARE VITAL

Like most people, you probably gauge whether you're successful or not by what you spend your time doing, not by what you think or how you feel about it. This is another way of saying that your actions in life, however large or small, add up to what your life is about. It's only with your actions—what you do—that you move your life in the directions you want it to go.

When you act in ways contrary to your aspirations, you become emotionally and psychologically stuck. This is why we won't offer any cheap or quick fixes like the ones you hear every day from the media and our culture in general. You know the message—get rid of your pain and suffering, and then you'll be happy and have the life you want.

Being pain free is no guarantee of a vital life. Quite a few people seem to have no pain and hardly any worries, and yet they're unhappy with the life they lead. We also know that many people live with enormous pain and hardship and still manage to find meaning and dignity in their lives. They go about living each day as if it were their last. You can do this too. When you live each day as if it were your last, things that had seemed very important suddenly seem much less important—several exercises build on this idea in the chapters to come.

Learning to watch your thoughts with gentle, dispassionate interest and without entanglement will also help you learn how to stop letting anxiety continue to be a monster seemingly controlling your life. It'll position you to break loose from anxiety by making space for it. As you do that, you'll be free to put your attention and energy into living a life that you care deeply about. As that happens, anxiety and fear will become just a part of your life, not the very fabric of your being.

You've probably heard the basic message of ACT in another form—the well-known serenity creed: *Accept with serenity what you cannot change, have the courage to change what you can, and develop the wisdom to know the difference.* Most people find that it is much easier to agree with the serenity creed than to do what it says. That's because many people simply don't know what they *can* and *cannot* change. Many more don't know how to accept and live with thoughts and feelings that hurt. Even then, few know how to apply this profound statement to their daily lives. We'll show you how to put the serenity creed into action.

When you read this book and do the exercises, you'll learn how to make the important distinction between what you can and cannot change. When you practice the mindfulness and acceptance exercises, you'll learn how to make space for all of your experiences—the good, bad, and ugly ones. And with acceptance and compassion, you'll learn how to refocus your precious time and energy on doing what matters to you. This will start you on a new path out of your worries, anxieties, and fears and into your life.

ACT CAN HELP YOU WITH YOUR ANXIETY AND IMPROVE YOUR LIFE

Anxiety and fear come in many shapes and guises. Many people with anxiety problems experience the powerful rush of panic: intense bodily changes (e.g., racing heart) together with thoughts that something terrible is about to happen, feelings of terror, and a sense of gloom and doom. For some, panic attacks seem to come out of the blue. Others find that panic-laced thoughts and feelings show up in specific situations (e.g., in social situations, in front of a group, on an airplane, at certain heights).

Some people with anxiety are haunted by memories of traumatic experiences they once endured. Still others are consumed with intrusive, obsessive, recurrent thoughts, impulses, or images that bring on overwhelming anxiety. To reduce their distress, some people engage in ritualistic acts like checking, counting, or hand washing. These acts buy them a short-term honeymoon from anxiety. And then there is the large group of anxious people who worry day in and day out about all sorts of things (their past, future, daily hassles) without being able to resolve any of them.

In the next chapter, we'll do our best to explain what we know about all these worries, anxieties, and fears and how they're not as different from each other as they appear to be. If you have any of these experiences and are fed up with the toll they've been taking on your life, the ACT approach we describe in this book can help you get unstuck. Yet words are only words unless you get out there and put the words into action.

If you have any doubts about the importance of action, think about how you learn to ride a bike. You learn not by reading about bike riding or by watching a bicycle race. The only way to learn how to ride a bike is to get on one and start riding. You also need to be willing to fall once in a while, because you will. There's no other way to learn. It takes practice, commitment to learning how to do it, willingness to experience pain and falls, and recommitment to getting back on the bike after a fall. You just have to do it, and do it again and again.

In a similar way, learning about anxiety and fears with just your head, without taking steps to put your learning into action, is a dead end. You probably know this already from your own experience. Studies have shown that people learn best when they practice what they learn. In short, the best learning is active learning. So the challenge is to apply what you learn from this book in your daily life. This will take hard work on your part.

HOPE AND CHANGE: THE ACT WITH ANXIETY WAY

Before wrapping up this chapter, we'd like to pull together some key elements of this workbook to help you see what you are getting into and what you can expect. We'll do this with some cartoons and a few text prompts. Just imagine that you are the person illustrated in the cartoon.

This image is about what most people want. Notice that you're moving toward the very things that you care most deeply about in this life. You are free, engaging life to its fullest.

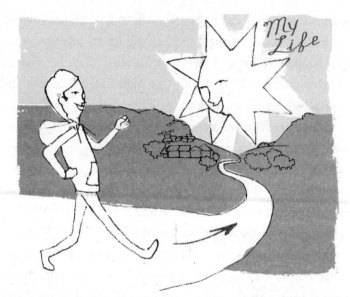

And then as you do that, all kinds of things show up—sometimes unpleasant things.

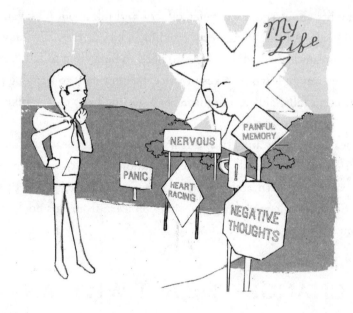

And so you stop.

You think.

You fret, wallow, and stew.

And you do what seems to be the most sensible thing to do. You try to get the "bad" stuff out of the way because it seems to stand between you and your life.

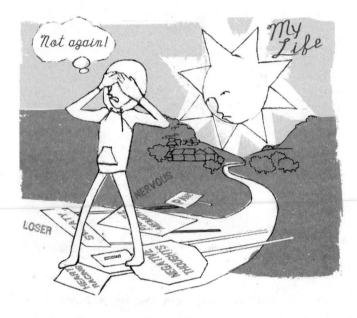

As you're trying to get a handle on your discomfort, you turn around—turning your back on your life and where you wanted to go. And your life notices this too: "Huh … what about me?"

Your life waits as you pour your energies into getting a grip. You try many different ways of coping, but nothing seems to work.

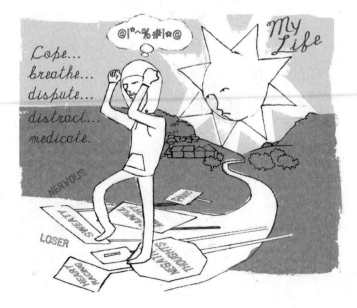

On and on it goes—a scene that has played out countless times. All the while, time is ticking by … ticktock … ticktock. There you are struggling, and your life is waiting, just waiting. And your life becomes sad too, because it knows the outcome. And here it is: you pull out of life. Now look at your life—living is not getting done.

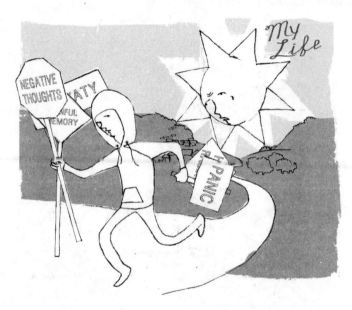

When you pull out, you never truly get away from your hurts. Notice that when you run, you take all those hurts with you too.

You're left feeling exhausted, frustrated, at your wit's end, head hung low.

And your mind is still at work—feeding you more negative news. *Why can't I be normal? Why can't I get a handle on my anxiety and fears?*

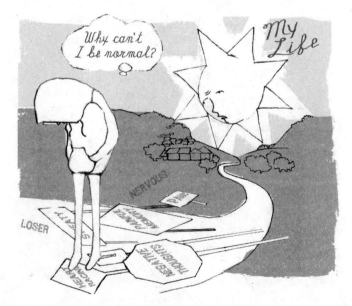

So there you are, stuck, wallowing in this "out of my life" place with pain on top of pain. You feel bad, broken, like a loser, and without hope. You may even feel sad that you've once again missed out on important things in your life. You might feel cheated, even mad at yourself too. Notice that your life is sadder than before and is still waiting for you.

But then something changes.

Something profound and beautiful happens.

You see what's really going on.

You take stock.

You say enough is enough.

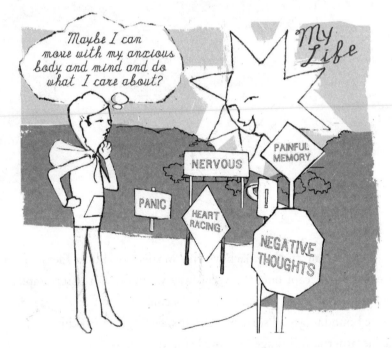

You open up to other possibilities.

Maybe, just maybe, your thoughts and feelings are not barriers at all. Maybe they're just part of you. Perhaps you can bring them along with you as you do what you care about.

Your life seems to like this idea.

So you take a step—a bold and courageous step forward in directions you want to go. You bring compassion and kindness to whatever shows up inside your mind and body. You're moving. You're headed back into your life and doing what matters to you.

Your life notices right away. Others notice right away. You notice right away.

You commit to doing what you care about with whatever your mind or old history dishes out.

You run toward life. And as you do more of that, your life improves. Your life enjoys spending time with you!

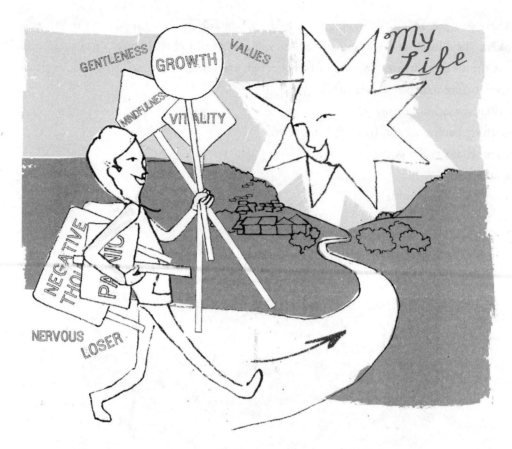

This last illustration sums up the approach we take in this workbook. Elements in all the preceding scenes will be addressed too, except one: there's no way we know of to stop unpleasant thoughts and feelings from showing up from time to time (see the second cartoon in this section). When you run toward your life, you're bound to get all sorts of thoughts, feelings, and bodily sensations. You can't have one (a life) without the other (a full range of thoughts and feelings).

But we can teach you how to keep your anxious mind and body from standing between you and your life. You'll learn to stop turning your back on your life in the service of anxiety management. You'll learn how to stop struggling with your emotional and psychological hurts. You'll develop skills to be kinder to yourself so that you don't wallow or beat yourself up with more negative judgments and blame. Most importantly, we'll show you how to win the war with your anxiety, not by defeating it, but by welcoming it as you engage in your life one step at a time.

Living well is how you'll defeat anxiety. It starts by acting on your anxiety differently than you have done before. This is the way to create the conditions for your genuine happiness!

YOUR COMMITMENT TO CHANGE

Commitment is a central component of any effort to change your life. Are you ready for that commitment and willing to learn another way to approach your worry, anxiety, and fear—and your life?

Answering "yes" means that you're one step closer to taking control over your actions and committing to move yourself in life directions you truly value. If you answered that way, great!

If you answered "no," then stop. Ask yourself, *What is getting in my way?* Look inside yourself first, and then look for barriers in the world around you. Write the barriers down in the space below and be as specific as possible.

_____

_____

_____

_____

_____

_____

Look at them. Take some time with them if you need to do that. We're not asking you to overcome any barriers. We're only asking if you're willing to learn a different way of relating with your anxieties, fears, and the like. Only you can decide whether to allow the barriers to continue to stand between you and getting something different out of your life. When you're 100 percent willing to make this commitment, do it, and do it again and again with each new chapter.

Commitment doesn't mean you have to get everything right and that you'll never go back to your old ways. We know there will definitely be times when you'll go back to old patterns. Commitment only means that you're committed to do your very best at what you set out to do.

And if you end up breaking a commitment, it doesn't mean you've failed or, worse, that *you* are a failure. Give yourself a break. This is just your mind talking. Beating yourself up for being human is never helpful. In fact, it's a surefire way to feel worse.

Breaking a commitment simply means you've fallen off the bike, as we all do from time to time, particularly in the beginning when we're still learning to ride. When you realize you've "done it again," you can choose to recommit, mean it, and do what needs to be done the next time.

Here's why we think commitment is so important: Without commitment to action—if you don't complete the exercises—nothing much is going to change in your life. We've touched on this theme already in this chapter, but it's worth repeating the mantra: *If I continue to do what I've always done, then I'm going to get what I've always got.*

Many people attribute this quote to Anthony Robbins and before him Albert Einstein, Henry Ford, Mark Twain, and even Steven Hayes and the developers of ACT. Regardless of the origin, what matters is the same point that all these smart people have made over the years: if you want to change the end result, you need to change the way you do things. This means that to get a different outcome, you need to do something quite different than you've done before. Just *reading* this book without *doing* anything new is a guaranteed way to continue to get what you've always got.

Let's pause for a moment and sink into what that might mean. When you commit to doing something new, what possibilities lie ahead for you? Do you even know? Have you stopped to consider what your life could become? The next brief exercise will help you get in touch with that.

EXERCISE: YOUR LIFE BOOK OF POSSIBILITIES

It's impossible to go forward in new ways while always looking back, focused on what's wrong with you and your life, repeating the same old patterns that led you to this place. And, it's next to impossible to commit to anything unless you can see it clearly. So, let's shift the perspective and get some clarity.

Take a few moments to pause and allow your eyes to close gently. Bring your awareness to your breath and where you are, right now, at this moment in your life. Simply settle into the now and give yourself permission to just be here. And when you're ready, slowly open your eyes and continue reading.

Go ahead and hold out your hands in front of you, palms facing up, and imagine that you're holding a book called *Your Life*. This is a book that you know all too well. As you look at this book, you'll notice that several of its pages are already written. They cover the familiar events and experiences you've lived through from the moment you were born up until now. You see large and small moments, joys, and perhaps enormous hardship and pain. This book also includes your struggles with anxiety and fear. You know the story.

But, as you flip through this book, you may also notice that the story ends abruptly. There's nothing written on the opening page of the new chapter called "Tomorrow." In fact, each and every page from this moment forward is blank. All you see are pages upon pages of plain white paper.

You may think, *That's strange … maybe I bought a defective book.* But what you're noticing isn't strange at all. In fact, what you don't see is exactly the way it is. Your life story from here on out has yet to be written. It's full of possibilities, experiences, and new journeys. Allow yourself to pause again and sink into that truth for a moment. And when you're ready, continue reading.

Now ask yourself this: *What do I want the next page to say about me and my life?* Will the chapter called "Tomorrow" be just a repeat of yesterday and the days, weeks, and months that came before? If you could put anything down on the next blank page of the book called *Your Life*, what would it be? What do you really want to be about from this moment forward?

This is the place where your commitment comes in. It needs to be specific and you need to become consciously aware of it. In the space below, take a moment to jot down what you would like the next page of your life book to say. Be specific. Think in terms of possibilities. Think in terms of what you (and only you) can do. Just write down a few words or sentences that capture the essence of what you'd like to be about and what you'd like to become. What you say here could be as simple as "I'm going to spend fifteen minutes reading and working with the material in this workbook to change the course of my life." Or, "I'm going to start my day with the Simple Centering exercise I learned about in the Introduction."

_____

_____

_____

LIFE ENHANCEMENT EXERCISES

For this week and the weeks to come, we will recommend several activities that you can do right now to get something new in your life. We call them Life Enhancement exercises because that's what they are about—enhancing the depth and quality of the life you wish to lead. We invite you to review them and commit to what you can reasonably do.

For now, we recommend the following activities:

- Commit to doing the Simple Centering exercise.

- Get a sense of your commitment to this workbook and why this is important to you now.

- Make reading and working with this workbook a priority in your life.

THE TAKE-HOME MESSAGE

Change can be scary and liberating at the same time. It involves some risk. Yet the risk of doing more of the same ought to be more frightening. To get something new, all of us need to do something new. It's that simple. And it starts with you making a choice and a commitment to do that. When you start ACTing on your anxiety differently, you have much to gain and really nothing to lose.

Preparing Myself for Something New in My Life

Point to Ponder: To get something new, I must do something new.

Questions to Consider: Am I ready to choose a new approach with my anxieties, fears, and worries? If not, then what is getting in the way?

31

CHAPTER 2

You Are Not Alone: Understanding Anxiety and Its Disorders

The truth is that our finest moments are most likely to occur when we are feeling deeply uncomfortable, unhappy, or unfulfilled. For it is only in such moments, propelled by our discomfort, that we are likely to step out of our ruts and start searching for different ways or truer answers.

—M. Scott Peck

YOU'RE NOT ALONE

Many people suffering with anxiety feel utterly alone. You may feel that way too. You may think that your anxiety is so intense and that nobody could possibly understand what it's like to feel the way you feel. In a sense, you're right; nobody knows your experience better than you. But that doesn't mean that you're alone in this either.

As you read this chapter and discover some facts about anxiety, you'll see that there are countless people all over the world who share your fears, your struggles, and your behavioral tendencies. You'll also see that your anxiety problem is well recognized and understood. In fact, anxiety and fear are the best understood of all emotional challenges. As you learn more, we hope you'll discover that there is hope *and* you're not alone!

People with anxiety disorders are everywhere. They live in every town, state, and country. Anxiety disorders affect the rich and the poor alike. In fact, anxiety disorders are among the most common of all psychological disorders, affecting up to 30 percent of the population at some point in their life-times (Kessler et al., 2005). That's about forty million people in the United States alone. To bring the numbers home, imagine that one day everyone with an anxiety disorder decided to wear a red hat. If that were so, then you'd be hard pressed to go about your day without seeing someone wearing one.

Anxiety disorders also tend to be chronic, costly, and debilitating. This means that without some changes on your part, the problems tend to stick around and may even get worse over time. With so many lives affected by them, it's not surprising that anxiety disorders are associated with enormous personal, social, and economic costs. In fact, the total estimated annual cost of anxiety disorders in the United States is approximately $45 billion, with only 25 percent of that pertaining to the costs of treatment (Barlow, 2004). This figure, which amounts to the budget of a small country, doesn't even address the many hidden costs of anxiety disorders. You know these hidden costs and so do we. They can be summarized in four words—reduced quality of life.

PAUSE AND GET CENTERED

Before we get into the meat of this chapter, we'd like to slow things down a bit and invite you to allow yourself five minutes to do another centering exercise. This one is a bit different from the exercise we shared with you in chapter 1, but the practice is basically the same.

As before, be mindful that there's no right or wrong way to do this exercise. Just follow along as best you can. All you need to do is get in a comfortable position where you won't be disturbed, and then just close your eyes and listen along. If you'd rather keep your eyes open, it's best to focus on a spot, say on the floor just in front of you, so you don't get too distracted. We'll end the exercise with a small chime and tell you when to open your eyes and move on.

EXERCISE: CENTERING INTO YOUR HEART

Go ahead and get in a comfortable position in your chair. Sit upright with your feet flat on the floor, your arms and legs uncrossed, and your hands resting in your lap. Allow your eyes to close gently. Take a couple of gentle breaths—in … and out … in … and out. As you're doing so, notice the sound and feel of your own breath.

Now turn your attention to being just where you are. Notice any sounds that you may hear close to you and then farther away. Notice how you are sitting in your chair. What are the sensations there?

Next, notice the places where your body touches itself, and bring your awareness to the spot where your hands touch your lap or legs. And now, imagine your awareness pouring down over your hips to where your feet touch the floor. How do your feet feel in the position that they are in? Notice too that your feet are firmly grounded to the floor and earth beneath you.

Now gently expand your awareness and just notice sensations in the rest of your body. If you feel any sensations in your body, just notice them and acknowledge their presence. Also notice how they may, by themselves, change or shift from moment to moment. Don't try to change them.

When you're ready, go ahead and allow your awareness to drift back, ever so slowly and gently, to your breath and just be here, right where you are. Notice that your breath is still with you, and along with it, the rising and falling of your chest and belly as you breathe in … and out. Imagine that with each breath in, you are creating more and more space inside of you to just be here. Let each breath expand your heart, creating more space within you as you breathe in … and then slowly out. Notice the space within you growing even just a little bit with each inhale you take, and then softening with each exhale.

Now, bring your awareness to that space within you just about in your center in the middle of your chest. Imagine settling your awareness in that special space close to your heart, however large or small it may be. Let your awareness settle and rest easily there, breathe gently and sense your breath going into that space around your heart.

And as your awareness settles in that heart space, we'd like to invite you to get in touch with your intentions. Why are you here? What do you want to be about? What do you want to become? And breathe. Soften to what shows up for you.

As we conclude this practice, we'd like to invite you to hold your intentions lightly, as you might hold a small butterfly or a tiny baby in your arms. Don't let go, just see if you can bring lightness, care, and gentleness to yourself and the intentions you hold dear.

And then, when you're ready, go ahead and take two deep cleansing breaths by filling your lungs fully, and then slowly releasing the air. Repeat that once again, and then slowly open your eyes while gently holding your intentions close to your heart as you go about your day.

WHAT IS THE NATURE OF ANXIETY AND FEAR?

All humans are born with the capacity to experience anxiety and fear. If you're reading this book, then you certainly have this capacity—or, more likely, think you have "too much of it." And you've probably educated yourself a bit about the nature of anxiety and fear too.

Here, our intention is to add a bit to what you may know already. And we'd like to offer you a slightly different perspective on what you may have read before. This fresh perspective involves getting a sense of the difference between "normal" and "abnormal" anxiety and fear.

Before you read on, take a moment to jot down what you think best describes three critical differences between normal and abnormal anxiety and fear. For instance, you might think that normal anxiety is *less extreme* compared with abnormal anxiety.

1. Normal anxiety/fear is _____ compared with abnormal anxiety/fear.

2. Normal anxiety/fear is _____ compared with abnormal anxiety/fear.

3.   Normal anxiety/fear is _____ compared with abnormal anxiety/fear.

Hold your ideas lightly as you read on, starting with the most basic and primitive of all emotions—fear.

Fear—The Present-Oriented Basic Emotion

Fear is an intensely felt alarm response. It arises in a flash and often in response to real or perceived threats in the world around you. But you may also be afraid of physical sensations, thoughts, and images that show up inside your skin.

You need fear to survive because it helps you take protective action when your safety or health is threatened. When you experience this emotion, your body will do a number of things to help you to get moving to take care of yourself. For instance, you may experience rapid heartbeat, breathlessness, smothering sensations, or increased blood pressure; you may feel hot, sick to your stomach, or dizzy; or you may break out in a sweat. You may even feel as though you're about to pass out.

Your body and brain are also kicking into overdrive. A number of other bodily systems are activated. All of this activity may leave you with a feeling of heightened energy—the adrenaline rush. These bodily changes are necessary to help you take decisive action. They represent a powerful tendency to fight or flee from signs of threat or danger.

Fear also tends to heighten awareness of your surroundings so that you may quickly detect sources of danger. This heightened awareness helps you stay focused on whatever triggers the fear (Barlow, 2004) and helps you to take quick action to protect yourself.

Anxiety—The Future-Oriented Emotion

Anxiety, by contrast, is a future-oriented mood state. This means you're anxious about something that has yet to happen. Perhaps it's a trip, or a health checkup. Maybe it's an exam, or a job evaluation. Anything in your future is a potential target for anxiety.

When you're experiencing it, you may notice apprehension or a sense of foreboding, worry, and muscle tension. You may feel keyed up and on edge. You may detect that the bodily changes associated with anxiety are much less pronounced and dramatic than with fear. Yet anxiety and worry can last much longer than fear, often ebbing and flowing for days, weeks, months, or even years. This is possible, in part, because anxiety tends to be fueled more by what your mind does than by real sources of danger or threat.

And as hard as it may be to experience anxiety, it's important to be mindful that you still need the capacity to experience anxiety. Why? Because it can help motivate you to get things done and can keep you out of harm's way.

EXERCISE: CAN YOU TELL THE DIFFERENCE BETWEEN ANXIETY AND FEAR?

Below is a list of circumstances that may help you get a sense of the difference between anxiety and fear. Read each item and then circle (A) if you think the event would mostly likely cause anxiety or (F) if you think the event would bring on fear.

• Seeing a bear in the woods A F	• Possibility of seeing a bear in the woods A F
• Being mugged in the city A F	• Chance of being mugged in the future A F
• A car almost hitting you A F	• Chance of getting hit by a car A F
• Suffering a serious injury A F	• Possibility of being seriously injured A F
• Being in a house fire A F	• Chance of your house burning down A F

What you should notice is that all the situations in the left column are present oriented, whereas those in the right column are future oriented. So you should end up with all Fs in the left column and all As in the right column.

The point of this activity is to help you get a sense of one critical difference between fear and anxiety: the present versus future quality. People are typically anxious about something that may happen in the future, whereas fear is a reaction to what is or could be happening in the moment. As an example, you might experience anxiety about the possibility of living through an earthquake and its aftermath, but fear would be your experience when the earth is actually shaking.

Behaviors most closely linked with anxiety have to do with what you think and say to yourself (e.g., worrying, ruminating over something, even making plans), whereas behaviors most closely associated with fear involve overt actions (e.g., running, fighting, taking cover, freezing). If it helps, you can think of the differences this way: fear requires little thought; anxiety needs big thought.

Normal Fear and Anxiety Keep Us Out of Trouble

Experiencing fear and anxiety is healthy and adaptive. Both emotions serve the purpose of keeping you and everyone else out of trouble and alive.

For instance, fear is necessary when you find yourself faced with real danger or threat. In these circumstances, fear will mobilize all of your resources and motivate you to take defensive action—get away or, if necessary, fight to defend yourself. Everything going on in your body and mind during fear is for one purpose: to help keep you safe, period.

Some of these actions are so automatic and hardwired that you don't need to learn them. You just react without having to think. As an example, do you remember a time when someone jumped out from behind a door, scaring the living daylights out of you? Your reaction was likely to startle, along with feeling like your heart was pounding out of your chest.

That's what we mean by an automatic reaction. It just happens. But you can also *learn* to respond with fear, often with the help of language. In fact, our capacity to use language makes it possible to run in fear in response to someone yelling "Get out—the building is on fire!"

Anxiety and worry often can be useful and adaptive. In fact, it would be maladaptive not to worry about future events that could truly threaten your health and welfare. We know that a bout of anxiety and worry can help motivate people to take appropriate steps to plan for the future. So you might put together an action plan to prepare yourself for potential threats to your health, employment, safety, or the welfare of your family. A good example would be a family coming up with an action plan in the event of a house fire. The plan may be simple or elaborate, but the goal is the same: to help you take effective action when faced with actual threat.

What About My Fear and Anxiety?

You may be wondering how your situation fits into this picture. For the following exercise, think of a recent example where you experienced intense fear that was very useful. By "useful" we mean a situation where you were suddenly faced with real danger—perhaps a car on the road that you didn't see or a person or animal that threatened to harm you. You can pick a recent example or one that happened a while ago that was a "big deal"—where experiencing fear and doing something to save yourself (or someone else) made a real difference, perhaps even saved your or someone else's life.

This activity may be difficult because you probably see your anxiety and fear as unwelcome intruders. You're not in a place yet where you can see your anxieties and fears as assets, or even as "friends or allies." That's fine and totally expected from the vantage point of where you are now.

Still, we'd like you to see if you can dig deep here and give yourself some time to do this exercise. See if you can put the "worrying, anxiety, and fear are bad" idea to the side for a moment as you think about at least one example from your life where fear and anxiety were helpful for you. Doing this little exercise will also be useful later when we'll help you figure out when acting on fear and anxiety is helpful and when it is not useful and can make matters worse. So, let's get started by focusing on a situation where you felt strong fear, after which we'll move on to have a look at anxiety.

EXERCISE: HAS RESPONDING WITH FEAR AND WORRY BEEN USEFUL TO ME?

On the lines below, briefly describe the threatening/dangerous event, your response, and how your response was useful. The point is to look at how fear mobilized you to do something for your own safety and welfare (and that of others too).

What was the threatening/dangerous event?

_____

What was your response (thoughts, feelings, actions)?

_____

How was your response useful?

_____

Now think of a situation or event where being anxious and worrying about a possible negative event or outcome helped you make a plan and where having a plan and acting on it was somehow useful to you. On the lines below, briefly describe the event, your response, and how your response was useful.

What was the potential problem you were anxious or worried about?

_____

What was your response (thoughts, feelings, actions)?

_____

How was your response useful?

_____

The reason this exercise is so important is that it ought to help you see that fear and worrying have served you well in the past and that you'll likely need to draw on your capacity to experience both in the future. Do not forget this fact as you go through this book. Write this down if it helps: *I need the capacity to experience worry, anxiety, and fear just like I need air to breathe, water to drink, and food to eat.*

This doesn't mean that you ought to be anxious 24/7. We understand that you probably feel like anxiety is with you all the time. And it probably seems that more often than not, your worry, anxiety, and fear are more hurtful than helpful. They happen too often or too intensely. They show up when you're at no risk of being harmed. Your worries may seem like they stretch to infinity. Your thoughts are too disturbing and almost impossible to turn off.

All of this and more has certainly interfered with you living your life the way you want to live it. In fact, interference with life is probably one of the chief reasons you picked up this book in the first place. It turns out that life interference is actually one of the key litmus tests that professionals, such as medical doctors and psychologists, use to determine when fear or anxiety move away from being adaptive and shift into the realm of an anxiety *disorder*.

Let's have a closer look at how this applies to you.

IDENTIFYING YOUR TYPE OF ANXIETY PROBLEM

Self-help books written for people with anxiety disorders typically focus too much on describing the various types of anxiety problems and helping people diagnose themselves. We don't want to lead you down this path because we don't think it'll be of much use to you.

Labeling yourself with a diagnosis or two will not make your life more livable or help you in other ways. In fact, the label can even become a self-fulfilling prophecy—something you become. It's hard to shake labels once they're applied. What you need to learn is how to accept what needs to be accepted and change what can be changed.

Your most important task here is this: to identify the root of what turns *your* fear, anxiety, worry, trauma, or obsession into the life-shattering problem or disorder. To get there, you need to be absolutely clear about what it is that you've been struggling with for so long. This kind of clarity has another purpose too. We've found that people do better with treatment when they focus their efforts on their most vexing concerns. We've also noticed that as they do that, other related or less pressing concerns tend to improve as well.

In the following sections you'll find a description of each of the major anxiety disorders. Be mindful that we do not agree with the recent decision by the psychiatric community to move obsessive-compulsive disorder and post-traumatic stress disorder into their own unique categories. In our view, the root of the problems with obsessions, compulsive behaviors, and a traumatic past are the same. You'll see why in a moment.

You'll also get a chance to read about real people who have struggled with anxiety problems. We've kept their stories brief and have gone to great lengths to protect their identities. You may see some of yourself in the stories we share. As you read on, you'll notice that all the real-life examples are different from each other in many ways. But we'd like to invite you to look for the commonalities among the different stories. See if you can find those. What is the golden thread that binds all anxiety problems together?

Panic Attacks

A *panic attack* is a sudden rush of fear. It's accompanied by intense physical sensations, a strong urge to escape or get away from the situation or place where those sensations occur, and a sense of impending doom—the feeling that something really bad is about to happen.

Below is a list of experiences that the American Psychiatric Association (2013) uses to define a panic attack. Check (√) all items that you experience when you have a panic attack:

☐ Pounding or racing heart

☐ Chest pain or discomfort

☐ Shortness of breath or smothering sensations

☐ Trembling or shaking

☐ Feeling of choking

☐ Sweating

☐ Dizziness, unsteady feeling, or faintness

☐ Nausea or abdominal distress

☐ Feeling you or your surroundings are strange or unreal

☐ Numbness or tingling in face, hands, or legs

☐ Hot flashes or chills

☐ Fear of dying (e.g., fear of having a heart attack)

☐ Fear of going crazy

☐ Fear of doing something uncontrolled

Panic attacks often occur quite unexpectedly—"out of the blue"—without obvious sources of real danger or threat. They're also called "false alarms" for this reason. This makes the experience even more frightening because the panic attack makes no sense and doesn't seem to serve any purpose.

We know from large research studies that panic attacks are common; about ten to thirty-three people out of one hundred experience at least one panic attack in a given year (Barlow, 2004). Having much stress in your life can certainly make panic attacks more likely, but panic attacks can happen during periods of calm too. They can even show up when you're asleep in bed at night.

Take the case of Jeff, a thirty-four-year-old web developer. His panic attack happened as he was about to go out on a date.

■ *Jeff's Story*

I was getting ready to go out on a date with Claire. She and I met online and had become good friends. I hadn't dated anyone in a very long time, and I remember that I was so excited to finally meet Claire in person. But that never happened. As I was getting ready in my apartment, I broke out in a cold sweat. It came on all of a sudden. My dress shirt was completely soaked. And as I scrambled to find another shirt, my heart felt like it was pounding out of my chest. I wasn't able to stand up or focus. I was really lightheaded and couldn't catch my breath. I tried sitting down, but that didn't help. I started freaking out and thought that maybe this is it, and that I'm having a heart attack and am going to die here. There was no way I could go out like this. I called 911 and ended up in an ambulance and spent the evening in the emergency room. No heart attack. No date. The next day I texted Claire and made up a lame excuse about why I stood her up. I couldn't tell her what really happened. I was too afraid of what she might think of me if I did.

How Panic Attacks May Turn Into Panic Disorder

Having many unexpected panic attacks without an obvious trigger or cause is *one* of the official standards used by mental health professionals when diagnosing panic disorder. Yet this isn't the whole story. Even if you've had many panic attacks and continue to have them as often as once a month, several times a week, or every day, it doesn't mean that you have *panic disorder*.

A diagnosis of panic disorder requires that you also worry about when the next attack will strike and the possible consequences of an attack. For instance, you might worry that you'll die, lose control, faint, go crazy, vomit, or have diarrhea. You may even think that you'll humiliate yourself, lose your job, or end up in the loony bin. All of these thoughts can certainly make things worse, but they are not the most important feature of panic disorder.

To get a sense of what we mean here, go ahead and tell yourself this: *I'm going nuts.* This thought likely had little effect on you at the moment you just had it. During a panic attack though, this thought and the strong urges that go along with it can lead you to do things that make you withdraw from your life; this withdrawal, or pulling out, is key.

In fact, the critical feature that makes panic a problem is this: a change in your behavior in order to cope with the attacks or prevent them from happening again. We've summarized some of the more common behavioral changes for you below (Antony & McCabe, 2004). As you'll see, the behaviors look different from one another, but underneath, they are really quite similar—they all serve to make people feel safe (or at least safer) from panic. As before, check (√) all behaviors in the list that you engage in to manage your panic:

☐ Sitting near exits at the movies or in a restaurant

☐ Checking where the closest exit is when visiting a shopping mall

☐ Carrying medication, money, cell phone, pager, water, or other safety items

☐ Avoiding activities (e.g., exercise, sex, thriller movies) that might trigger physical arousal

☐ Drinking alcohol to combat feelings of panic

☐ Avoiding caffeine, alcohol, or other substances (e.g., MSG, spicy foods)

☐ Frequently checking your pulse or blood pressure

☐ Distracting yourself from the panic experience (for instance, reading a book, watching TV)

☐ Insisting on being accompanied when leaving the house

☐ Always needing to know the whereabouts of your spouse, partner, or other "safe" person

Some people with panic disorder don't avoid situations where panic attacks may occur. With courage and determination they refuse to let panic attacks dictate where they go and don't go or what they do or don't do. Most people with panic disorder, however, develop some degree of *agoraphobia* over time. This simply means they avoid places or events where panic attacks might happen. These are often places from which a quick escape is difficult and where they might feel confined or trapped.

Some of the most common situations people avoid are listed below. Again, check (√) all situations in the list that you avoid so you won't have a panic attack:

☐ Crowded public places (e.g., supermarkets, theaters, malls, sports events)

☐ Enclosed and confined places (e.g., tunnels, bridges, small rooms, elevators, airplanes, subways, buses, hair salons, and long lines)

☐ Driving (especially on highways and bridges, in bad traffic, and over long distances)

☐ Being away from home (Some people have a safe distance around their home beyond which they find it difficult to travel; in rare cases, leaving the home may seem completely impossible.)

☐ Being alone (at home or in any of the situations listed above)

Let's look at how some of this played out with Donna, a thirty-year-old stay-at-home mom. Her frequent experiences of panic attacks have morphed into panic disorder: she's worried about future attacks. And she's changed her behavior to avoid having them. Like many people with panic disorder, over time she's developed some *agoraphobic avoidance*: she avoids places where panic may attack.

■ Donna's Story

I've had many panic attacks, but the worst one happened while I was driving to meet up with my entire family at a lake house we had rented for the summer. I was driving with my newborn daughter in the back seat. My husband had left earlier, and we had planned to meet him at the lake house later that day. During that drive, I started feeling a sharp pain in my chest. And then I began thinking about how my uncle had a heart attack while driving. He ended up dying because his car slammed into a utility pole. My mind was consumed with thoughts about him and about me. Maybe I'll have a heart attack and end up swerving off the road, and then my daughter will be dead and so will I. As these thoughts swirled around in my head, my breathing became shallower and I started feeling woozy. I then felt the tingling in my arms and in my lips. That was it. I found a safe place to pull over and called my husband. I told him that I wasn't feeling well enough to make the trip, and once I calmed down, I made my way back home with my daughter. Since then, I've stopped driving and have a hard time leaving the house alone. My husband understands my struggle with panic, but when I'm with anyone else, I just make up excuses about why I can't do this or that. I often feel like I must be nuts or something. If I don't feel completely safe, I just take a pass on doing things. I'm really sick of having panic attacks and am tired of feeling like I'm losing it or going crazy all the time. I also worry about what my daughter will think of me—the crazy mom who can't do anything because she's too afraid of having another panic attack. This is no way to live.

Specific Phobias

Just about everyone has something that they're afraid of. You probably do too. But specific phobias are more than just extreme fear of something. You also need avoidance. Those who struggle with a specific phobia experience a strong urge to get away from the feared object or situation. Many are quite successful at doing just that, but for others the avoidance can be quite costly.

Large surveys teach us that about 10 percent of the population will struggle with a specific phobia during their lifetime (Kessler et al., 2005). The most common specific phobias (in descending order) are fear of animals, heights, closed spaces, blood and injuries, storms and lightning, and flying.

We also know quite a bit about the fear in people struggling with specific phobias. In fact, many people experience an alarm reaction that is virtually identical to a panic attack. Even though specific phobias and panic disorder share the experience of a panic attack, they differ in one important way: the presence or absence of an obvious cue or trigger for fear. The alarm response in specific phobias is almost always triggered by a feared object or situation, whereas in panic disorder, the alarm response happens unexpectedly without a clear trigger.

People with specific phobias also recognize that their fear is excessive or unreasonable. But this awareness has no impact on the fear itself or the urge to run from and avoid feared objects. And it does little to help them control or minimize the unpleasant emotional discomfort that's triggered by feared objects or situations.

Take a look at the list below and check (√) all items that give you an intense panic-like response when you encounter them:

☐ Situations (e.g., heights, closed spaces, dentists, elevators, airplanes or flying)

☐ Animals (e.g., snakes, rats, spiders, dogs)

☐ Natural environment (e.g., heights, storms, lightning, water)

☐ Illness or bodily harm (e.g., diseases, injuries)

☐ Sight of blood or needles

☐ Other (e.g., choking, eating certain foods, vomiting)

Most people with specific phobias never seek treatment. They simply avoid the feared object. This is fairly easy to do because the object of fear is clearly known. In other cases, contact with the feared object is so unlikely that it never gets in the way of what they need to do. So if you have a shark phobia and you live in Idaho, it's highly unlikely that you'll have much difficulty with this phobia. There's no chance of running into a shark in Idaho (other than in movies or on TV).

At other times, "successful" avoidance may come at a high personal cost. For instance, we once worked with an Australian family who used to spend weekends visiting a beautiful island just three miles offshore. The island was a popular weekend getaway destination for the family and many people in the area. The family stopped going because the mother had a shark phobia. She couldn't stand the thought of sharks swimming underneath the ferryboat during the crossing.

The critical question this woman faced was this: what's more important—my family or my fear? The answer was obvious to her—family. Coming to terms with that choice made a real difference in her life. But getting there wasn't easy. Life was asking her to make a choice between two options. She could choose to spend time with her family in a beautiful setting *and* allow herself to feel the fear while getting there. Or, she could stay at home without fear *and* miss out on fun time with her family.

Evelyn is a thirty-four-year-old mother of two children who has a phobia of crickets. She was also facing some tough choices.

■ *Evelyn's Story*

I know it's totally unreasonable, but I'm terrified of crickets. My anxiety skyrockets when I'm outside because I feel like they're everywhere. Sometimes I can hear them at night through my window. To blot out the noise I turn the TV on and crank up the volume. I end up staying awake all night because of the noise. Just thinking about them gets my pulse racing. I can even feel my breathing become very shallow and strained. When I hear them, or even worse, see them, I hyperventilate to the point where I'm sure I'll pass out. It's gotten so bad. I can't even go to the park with my kids for fear that I'll see one. The kids don't understand what it's like for me, and I feel terrible that I can't overcome my fear for their sake.

Social Anxiety Disorder

Many people will, at times, feel anxious, self-conscious, or awkward in social situations, but social anxiety disorder is more than that. It's more than shyness too. Inside social anxiety is an intense fear of embarrassment or humiliation. Usually, this fear shows up when you're exposed to the scrutiny of others or you must perform while being watched. You may fear that you'll say or do something that will lead others to judge you as incompetent, weak, or stupid. You may also worry that others might detect your social discomfort.

Social anxiety disorder is also more than extreme anxiety in social situations or fearing embarrassment, judgment by others, or humiliation. People who are truly suffering with social anxiety end up doing things to avoid having anxiety in social situations. As you might imagine, trying to avoid interactions with other human beings is extremely hard to do without significant costs.

Social anxiety is more common than you might think. In fact, it ranks number one of all the anxiety disorders, with about 3 to 13 percent of the population suffering from it at some point during their lives. Let's take a closer look.

Below is a list of social fears that people often experience, leading them to try to avoid these situations. You'll see that fear of public speaking tops the list. It's the most common trigger for social anxiety and a concern shared by many. As before, check (√) all social fears that apply to you:

- [ ] Fear of public speaking

- [ ] Fear of blushing in public

- [ ] Fear of choking on or spilling food while eating in public

- [ ] Fear of writing or signing documents when others are present (e.g., at grocery checkout)

- [ ] Fear of being watched (e.g., at work, working out, shopping, dining out)

- [ ] Fear of crowds

- [ ] Fear of using public toilets

Some people with social anxiety also experience panic attacks. Mostly, these panic attacks are related to a specific type of social situation or being embarrassed and humiliated rather than being confined or trapped.

To minimize or reduce their discomfort, people with social anxiety typically avoid social situations (such as speaking in public, meeting or talking with people of the opposite sex, attending group meetings or social gatherings, speaking on the telephone, and using public restrooms or public transportation) as much as they can. More than 90 percent of all people diagnosed with social anxiety fear and avoid more than one social activity (Barlow, 2004).

But some do not avoid social situations, even while experiencing intense anxiety around people. In fact, performers (such as stage actors) and people whose jobs require them to make presentations will do their work day after day *and* take their anxiety along with them. How do they do that? We'll return to that question in chapter 5.

For now, let's take a look at Steve, a twenty-eight-year-old teacher struggling with social anxiety. As you read through Steve's story, see if you can detect how he's not only distressed in social situations—he also does whatever he can to avoid and get rid of that distress.

■ *Steve's Story*

I've been suffering from social anxiety for as long as I can remember, at least as far back as first grade. Then, I remember getting on the bus for the first day of school only to be harassed by the older kids—they taunted and teased me about my hair, my glasses, my weight, the way I looked, and my backpack. The teasing and bullying just continued at school, mostly on the playground, where my head was the prized target in games of dodgeball. I remember becoming very self-conscious back then and was extremely apprehensive about meeting new kids. It wasn't that I was shy or anything like that. I just believed they were judging me or that I would do something to make a fool of myself and then bear the brunt of that. I still feel this way now, some twenty years later. I fear that people are judging me constantly. Even when I'm not with people, I believe that they're judging me. I think that every time I say something or do something (or don't do something) they could suddenly not like me anymore. I feel very uncomfortable around people and am convinced they can see that in me. It doesn't matter if it's people I know or complete strangers, I still think they're looking at me in a harsh way. I stopped running in the mornings too—too many drivers who will judge me—and have gained about twenty pounds. I know I'm extremely negative and critical of myself, but I can't see a way out. It's so damn frustrating. I work so hard to get through the day. I start student teaching in a little over a week. I'm terrified about that, but I'm trying not to be—trying to tell myself that I'll be fine. Life has become a burden and I don't know what to do anymore.

Obsessive-Compulsive Disorder

Being neat, tidy, orderly, organized, and following rules can be a blessing in many situations in life. But when these behaviors are carried to the extreme, they can become disruptive and take over a person's life. When they do, it's called *obsessive-compulsive disorder* (OCD).

Obsessions are recurring and persistent thoughts, impulses, or images that bring on intense anxiety. Examples include images or thoughts of hurting or harming someone, being contaminated with dirt or germs, or fearing you left your lights or stove on or your door unlocked. People typically experience these thoughts or images as intrusive (that is, happening despite efforts to resist them), unreasonable, and distressing. Obsessions can become so intense, so consuming, that some people spiral into full-blown panic attacks. This reaction is similar to that seen in panic disorder except that the feared objects in OCD are thoughts or images rather than bodily sensations or fear of panic itself.

Here's a list of some common obsessions. As before, check (√) all items that apply to you:

☐ Thoughts that you might harm yourself or others

☐ Violent or horrific images

☐ Fear of blurting out obscenities or insults

☐ Fear of acting on unwanted impulses (e.g., to stab a friend)

☐ Fear of stealing things

☐ Fear of being responsible for something terrible happening (e.g., fire, burglary)

☐ Sexual thoughts, images, or urges

☐ Fear of acting on "forbidden" impulses (incest, homosexuality, aggressive sexual acts)

☐ Concern with sacrilege and blasphemy, right and wrong, or morality

☐ Concern that someone will have an accident unless things are in the right place

☐ Fear of saying certain things because they might come true

☐ Fear of losing things

☐ Intrusive nonviolent images, nonsense sounds, words, or music

☐ Concerns about dirt, germs, or bodily waste or secretions (e.g., urine, feces, saliva)

☐ Concern about getting ill from possible contaminants

☐ Concern about environmental contaminants (e.g., asbestos, radiation, toxic waste)

☐ Excessive concern with household items (e.g., cleansers, solvents)

☐ Excessive concern about animals (e.g., insects)

Compulsions are repeated ritualistic behaviors (for example, checking, hand washing) or mental acts (such as counting, praying). The purpose of performing rituals is to reduce anxiety and suppress or neutralize the disturbing intrusive thoughts or images. Attending to obsessions and ritualizing is enormously time consuming. And it puts so many constraints on life that people literally run out of time to do what they need to do. This cycle interferes with daily routines and social functioning. In extreme cases, hospitalization may be needed to break the cycle.

Here's a partial list of common compulsions. As before, check (√) all behaviors that seem to apply to you:

☐ Excessive or ritualized cleaning (e.g., hand washing, bathing, tooth brushing, grooming, toilet routine)

☐ Excessive cleaning of household items or other inanimate objects

☐ Checking locks, stove, appliances, and so on

☐ Checking that you did not/will not harm others or yourself

☐ Checking that nothing terrible did/will happen

☐ Checking that you didn't make a mistake

☐ Needing to repeat routine activities (e.g., jogging, going in or out door or up or down from chair, brushing your teeth, rereading, rewriting)

☐ Compulsively collecting or not being able to get rid of useless objects (e.g., junk mail, old newspapers, garbage, and other objects such as ear swabs, wrappers)

☐ Performing mental rituals (other than checking or counting, such as repeating a mantra or prayer)

☐ Excessive list making

☐ Needing to tell, ask, or confess, or touch, tap, or rub

☐ Ritualized eating behaviors

☐ Engaging in superstitious behaviors (e.g., carrying something for good luck)

☐ Compulsive hair pulling (top of head, eyelashes, eyebrows)

With OCD, you may or may not realize that your obsessions and compulsions are excessive and unreasonable. You may even have tried to ignore or stop them. But that only increases your distress and anxiety. So, you feel driven to perform compulsive acts, chasing a sense of relief that comes about by struggling to neutralize unwanted thoughts and associated anxiety.

The problem is that rituals typically only reduce anxiety for a short while, and then anxiety and tension come right back. The same is true of the thoughts that trigger the anxiety in the first place. In fact, there's solid evidence showing that attempts to ignore or suppress unwanted thoughts and images can actually backfire. Instead of lasting relief, you get more of the very thoughts and images that you don't want to have in the first place (Hayes, Wilson, Gifford, Follette, & Strosahl, 1996; Wegner, 1994). This process keeps the vicious cycle going with OCD, as Ray knew all too well.

Ray is a forty-year-old office clerk who feels completely controlled by the endless cycle of recurring obsessions, anxiety, and compulsive washing.

■ Ray's Story

For as long as I can remember I've been terrified of germs and the prospect of getting diseases. When I go to stores, I can't even open the door myself. I have to stand outside and wait for someone to go in or come out and then I try to catch the door with my elbow. I can't stand to even think about touching public property and wouldn't ever leave the house without antibacterial hand gel. I can't eat off plates or silverware at restaurants, so I never eat out with my friends. Even in my own house I eat off paper plates and use plastic silverware. My hands bleed because I wash them so much. I must wash ten times, repeating "Ten times fine because it takes care of the grime." I can't sleep if I feel like I might have germs on me, and so I have to shower ten times before falling asleep. My mantra in the shower goes like this: "Ten showers gives the germs no power." As much as I want to enjoy normal activities like everyone else, I can't make the anxiety go away. My washing rituals take hours out of my day and are the only thing that seems to help. But the anxiety always comes right back again and again. Will it ever end?

Post-traumatic Stress Disorder

In your lifetime, it is likely that you'll be exposed to a traumatic event. In fact, estimates suggest that about 60 percent of men and about 50 percent of women will witness or experience a trauma at some point in their lifetime (Friedman, Keane, & Resick, 2014). Although there's still some debate about what qualifies as a trauma, these events are generally thought to be experiences that would produce intense fear, terror, and feelings of helplessness in just about anyone. These include being the victim of a violent crime (such as rape, assault, or abuse as an adult or child), combat situations (for instance, wounding of self and others, committing or witnessing atrocities), natural disasters (such as earthquakes, tornadoes, floods), and accidents (such as car or plane crashes, fires).

Going through a trauma can be enormously challenging, but it doesn't mean you'll automatically develop *post-traumatic stress disorder* (PTSD). In fact, estimates suggest that only about seven or eight out of every one hundred people with a trauma history (still a large number of people) will go on to struggle with PTSD at some point in their lives. Even experiencing a horrific event such as the bombing of the World Trade Center doesn't mean that you or anyone else is destined to develop PTSD. In fact, research with survivors shows that "only" about 25 percent of those who were caught in the buildings after the 9/11 attack developed PTSD.

People suffering from PTSD may notice a number of changes a month or more after the traumatic event. Some changes affect how they experience their world, perhaps seeing the world as a dangerous place, feeling emotionally numb, or feeling a sense of detachment from one's self or surroundings—like an out-of-body experience. Other changes are more behavioral and may include being startled easily, scanning the environment for threats, having frequent nightmares, and attempting avoidance or escape. These changes tend to creep up on people over a period of several months after the traumatic event.

As you read through the items in the list below, check (√) all items that apply to you:

☐ Repetitive, distressing thoughts about a traumatic event

☐ Nightmares related to the event

☐ Intense and vivid flashbacks, leaving you feeling or acting as if the trauma was happening again

☐ Attempts to avoid thoughts or feelings associated with the trauma

☐ Attempts to avoid activities or external situations associated with the trauma—such as driving after you have been in a car accident

☐ Emotional numbness—being out of touch with feelings

☐ Feelings of detachment or disconnection from others (e.g., loved ones, friends)

☐ Losing interest in activities that used to give you pleasure

☐ Always feeling on edge—difficulty falling or staying asleep, difficulty concentrating, startling easily, scanning the environment for signs of danger or threat, and irritability and outbursts of anger

☐ Elevated bodily arousal that can spiral up into a full-blown panic attack

Many people with PTSD are anxious and depressed. The trauma seems to be there as "background noise" all the time. Regardless of the type of trauma, people suffering from PTSD often go to great lengths to avoid thinking about the traumatic event. They also avoid any cues or situations that may remind them of the event. Here, you may think that avoidance wouldn't be a bad thing. After all, who wants to think about some terribly awful, frightening memory from the past, and along with it, all the images and painful feelings? And yes, you would be right about that, at least to a point.

The main purpose of avoidance within PTSD is to prevent reexperiencing the emotions and psychological pain associated with the trauma. The problem here is that it's next to impossible to keep painful memories from popping into our awareness now and then, so avoidance tends not to work as a lasting solution. But many continue to do it because of the short-term relief it offers. Over time, avoidance tends to grow to infect many areas of life that may have little to do with the original trauma. So, in the end, avoidance ends up greatly restricting life functioning.

Mary, a thirty-eight-year-old secretary, is a good example of someone who's exhausted by her unsuccessful struggle with PTSD. Her story shows how PTSD can interfere with just about all aspects of a person's life.

■ Mary's Story

Less than two years ago I was attacked and mugged outside my car one night after work. Since then I've been in a constant state of extreme anxiety and panic whenever I walk alone, day or night. I can't sleep without having intense nightmares of the attack, and often I wake up soaked in sweat with my heart pounding out of my chest. Even during the daytime my mind will often wander off and I'll have vivid flashbacks of the event: I can't seem to stop my mind from replaying the event over and over again. Lately, I've been trying to get my mind off this memory by taking up new activities so that I'm constantly busy. But nothing keeps my interest for long, and it doesn't seem to make a difference anyway. No matter what I do, I can't control the flashbacks, the awful feelings, and the dread when they come. Simple tasks like going to the grocery store are unbelievably difficult. Harder things like work have become nearly impossible. All of my limited energy goes into trying to make the memories stop, but they keep coming. I'm completely exhausted.

Generalized Anxiety Disorder

Just about everyone worries now and then about things such as family problems, health, or money, but people with *generalized anxiety disorder* (GAD) find themselves extremely worried about these sorts of things, as well as many other issues, even when there may be little or no reason to worry.

In a nutshell, people with GAD worry excessively about a number of events and activities. They commonly report feeling stressed and overwhelmed by everyday life experiences, or "daily hassles."

Worrying typically occurs more days than not and causes significant distress or impairs functioning either at work, at home, or both.

Approximately 5 percent of the population will suffer from GAD at some point in their lives (Barlow, 2004). GAD typically develops slowly over time, often beginning at an earlier age than other anxiety disorders. Because of this, many GAD sufferers think that they "have always been a worrier" and "an anxious person." Worry and anxiety tend to be intense during periods of high stress and to decrease during periods of low stress.

As you read through the items in the list below, check (√) all that apply to you:

- ☐ Inability to stop worrying even if it doesn't seem to solve anything and is unproductive

- ☐ Worrying as an attempt to reduce anxiety (see explanation below)

- ☐ Restlessness—feeling keyed up

- ☐ Muscle tension

- ☐ Being easily fatigued

- ☐ Difficulty concentrating

- ☐ Irritability or edginess

- ☐ Difficulties with sleep

People with GAD often have a pervasive feeling that they can do little to predict and control stressful events in their lives, so they end up worrying about them. There's now convincing evidence that people engage in worry as a way to avoid this unpleasant imagery and the physical tension associated with anxiety (Bandelow et al., 2013; Borkovec, Alcaine, & Behar, 2004).

This avoidance works in the short run—it buys the person some relief. Yet in the long run it doesn't work. People get caught in a loop. They tend to experience even more intense anxiety followed by efforts to reduce anxiety by engaging in more worrying. All the while, they are unable to work through their problems and arrive at active solutions. This is what we mean by the worrying being unproductive. Marianne's case highlights this vicious cycle.

Marianne is a forty-year-old accountant working for an investment firm—a job that feeds right into her anxiety problem. She cannot remember a time without GAD, and she feels her mind has gone on "worry autopilot" in recent years.

■ Marianne's Story

I've always been a chronic worrier, fretting over things I have little to no control over. I'd even worry about the things I did have control over, always thinking about the way in which they'd go wrong. At work, I constantly second guess myself, and my accounting reports are usually late because I re-run the figures again and again looking for errors—I never find them, but I can't stop thinking they might be there. And I often worry about things that are so unlikely and unimportant. I shouldn't be thinking about them at all. Just yesterday I couldn't go on a ski trip with friends because I couldn't shake the fear that I might break my leg, or worse, kill myself in a skiing accident. And, to top it off, what if the ski lift got stuck, or the cable broke? What if one of my friends hurt themselves on the slopes? I also worry constantly about death and getting some serious illness or disease. Logically, I know I'm in good health, but that doesn't keep me from spending hours on WebMD looking up any new symptom I may be experiencing. For a time, I even thought my shoulder pain was a sign of a tumor. Now I know it's part of my anxiety. So yeah, I worry about everything—what I'll wear for work, what to eat, about my health, about whether I'll keep my friends, about my safety, about the planet even. My sleep is terrible too, and often I lie in bed for hours because I can't shut my mind off. I just wish I could get a handle on this so I can be happy and enjoy life.

ANXIETY DISORDERS HAVE MUCH IN COMMON

Each of the anxiety disorders we've covered may seem quite different from one another. And that's true up to a point, but don't let the apparent differences fool you. Now more than ever, we're coming to terms with the fact that anxiety disorders are more similar than we've made them out to be. And it turns out that the similarities are much more important than the minor variations when it comes to helping people like you. Have a look at the list of similarities below to get a sense of what we mean.

- **Anxiety and fear are triggered by something.** There are an infinite number of possible triggers for anxiety and fear, including stress. The triggers can spring forth from within you (thoughts, images, memories, or bodily sensations), from the world around you, or from some combination of both. For some types of anxiety disorders we can pinpoint what actually brings on fear and anxiety. And when the source of fear and anxiety is known, you can anticipate it reasonably well. Examples of anxiety problems with obvious triggers include specific phobias, social anxiety disorder, and PTSD. With panic disorder, OCD, and even GAD, the triggers tend to be subtler and more difficult to spot. Yet not knowing what your triggers are doesn't mean that your anxiety and fear isn't triggered by something. The triggers are there and simply need to be revealed.

- **Duration and intensity of anxiety and fear ebb and flow.** Our bodies cannot sustain anxiety and fear 24/7. In panic disorder, specific phobias, and social anxiety disorder, the fear and accompanying physical changes people experience are intense but relatively short-lived—typically no more than half an hour and rarely beyond one hour. People who experience such difficulties may report the feelings lasting longer, but this has more to do with our minds than our bodies. Our bodies cannot keep up panic or extreme anxiety for long periods of time. In GAD, the anxiety and related physical reactions are less intense, and they persist over much longer periods of time than fear. In OCD and PTSD, anxiety and tension may vary greatly in intensity and duration over time. None of it lasts forever.

- **Fear is fear, and anxiety is anxiety.** It turns out that the experience of fear and anxiety doesn't differ in form or substance across the anxiety disorders. Fear is fear. Anxiety is anxiety. Both emotions characterize all anxiety disorders. And, at a basic level, the nature of fear and anxiety that people with anxiety disorders talk about is identical to fear and anxiety experienced from time to time by people without anxiety disorders.

- **Similar treatments work well for all anxiety problems.** If anxiety problems were truly different in kind and substance, then you'd expect that we'd have special treatments matched to each unique anxiety problem. This turns out not to be the case. Research shows that similar treatment strategies work for all anxiety disorders. In fact, most effective treatments for anxiety problems share a small set of common exercises and skill-building tools. We've wrapped those effective elements into this book. This is good news for you.

This list highlights what we've learned from research over the last decade or so. It shows that anxiety disorders have some striking commonalities. Yet the most important commonality of all is not on that list. We left it out. It's time to state it boldly: *people with anxiety disorders struggle with, avoid, and run away from their fear and anxiety.*

This tendency defines the actions of just about every person with an anxiety disorder. And struggle turns out to be *the* most toxic element that constricts lives and transforms anxiety from being a normal human experience into a life-shattering problem. You got a glimpse of where avoidance can take you with the cartoons in chapter 1. We'll focus more on this critical issue in the next chapter.

OTHER PROBLEMS WITH ANXIETY DISORDERS

Studies in the United States and elsewhere around the world (Craske, 2003) show that more than half of the people struggling with an anxiety disorder also have other significant emotional and behavioral problems such as depression and drug abuse. Quite a few are also taking some form of medication for anxiety or depression. We cover these concerns below because there's a good chance that they might apply to you.

Depression

Depression is a persistent mood state where people feel very sad, "down and empty," worthless, and hopeless about the future. Some people say that depression feels like a black curtain of despair has come down over their lives. And just about everything they do is cast in darkness by this curtain. Many question whether their life situation will ever improve.

Lack of energy and fatigue are common complaints, and many report difficulties concentrating, remembering, and making decisions. Many also have sleep difficulties. Others feel irritable and restless all the time for no apparent reason. They often lose interest in hobbies and activities that they once enjoyed, including sex.

Depression is by far the most common co-occurring emotional problem experienced by people with anxiety disorders. In fact, about half of all people with an anxiety disorder will also experience significant depression at some point (Barlow, 2004). At times depression may develop before an anxiety disorder, but it's more common for depression to creep up on people after they've been suffering from an anxiety disorder for a while.

Given the way anxiety and fear can get in the way of meaningful life activities, it's not surprising that people start to think and feel that life is no longer enjoyable or worth living. The good news is that this workbook can help lift the veil depression may have on you. Our own research, which we discussed in the prologue, looked at people with severe anxiety and severe depression. What we found is that many showed significant declines in their depression when they practiced what we'll teach you in this book.

Alcohol Abuse

Virtually all people with anxiety problems engage in similar strategies to cope with their anxiety—strategies that have not worked very well and have caused more problems in the long run. For instance, men in particular have been found to "self-medicate" their anxiety problem with alcohol to make their life situation more bearable (Barlow, 2004). But women also turn to alcohol as a way to cope. This self-defeating strategy is chosen by at least one in every four people with an anxiety disorder.

As with avoidance, this tactic blunts the emotional and psychological pain for a short while, but over time the pain comes right back (often worse than before), and now the person has two problems—a more entrenched anxiety disorder and budding alcoholism.

If you think that your drinking is in the service of managing your anxiety, fear, and even stress, we strongly encourage you to take stock and seek additional help if necessary. As you work on learning the skills in this book, you may find that drinking to take the edge off no longer has a purpose. You may also find that you are unable to stop drinking alcohol to excess, even after using this workbook, because you have developed a dependence on alcohol. Take this as another sign to get the support and help you need.

Medical Conditions

Many medical conditions can mimic signs and sensations associated with anxiety and fear. This makes it hard to distinguish a medical problem from an anxiety disorder on your own. This determination is best left for a trained professional.

For this reason, it's important to rule out any medical conditions or possible drug-related factors that may be contributing to your anxiety and related difficulties. Examples of medical disorders that can trigger symptoms of panic or anxiety include thyroid problems, balance disorders (e.g., inner-ear disturbances), seizure disorders, asthma, and other respiratory or heart conditions. Use of stimulant substances (like cocaine, caffeine, diet pills, and certain other medications), withdrawal from alcohol, and use of other drugs (like marijuana) can also trigger panic-like feelings.

So before assuming that you have an anxiety disorder, it's important to talk with your doctor and have a full medical workup to help determine whether there's a physical cause for your problems. You can also think of this as a good way to take care of yourself. Once physical causes are ruled out, you can be much more confident when using the strategies described in this book.

Medications for Anxiety and Depression

Many people with anxiety disorders are prescribed medication. You may be one of them. In fact, we know from our own research that about 40 percent of readers were taking some form of prescription medication for their anxiety and/or depression while they were using this workbook. So if this applies to you, you're in good company.

We also know from our research and that of others that medications alone are no real cure. This is because medications tend to offer some short-term symptom relief, but in the long run, studies show that people actually tend to do worse when on medications alone or in combination with gold-standard treatments like CBT. In fact, the best long-term outcomes are found in people who are working to make significant changes on their own, with or without the help of a therapist, using proven strategies.

Our intention here is not to cover all the medications that are available for anxiety problems—that is best left to your primary care physician or a psychiatrist. This is also not the time for you to stop taking your medication as prescribed. You should first consult with your doctor before making *any* changes to your medications. The good news is that you can benefit from this workbook even if you are taking medications for anxiety, depression, or both.

As you work with this workbook, you may want to reflect on why you are taking antianxiety or antidepressant medication. Look at your intentions here. Are you taking medication to get rid of or control your anxiety? Look also at how the medication is working. Are you anxiety- and depression-free while taking your medication?

Many people struggling with anxiety and depression do not wish to be taking medications their entire lives. You may feel that way too. Some of the skills in this workbook will help you learn to be with your anxiety and depression just as they are. This new way of relating with your emotional life may then lead you to have a conversation with your doctor about reducing or discontinuing your medication entirely.

TAKING STOCK: A LOOK AT YOUR ANXIETY PROBLEMS

At this point, it might be helpful to go back over some of the checklists and anxiety disorder summaries in this chapter. You may find that you fit neatly into one particular anxiety subtype. Although that's possible, it tends to be somewhat rare. Research studies and our own experience have taught us that most people do not fit neatly into one category. In fact, about half of those struggling with one anxiety disorder also suffer from another anxiety disorder (Barlow, 2004). All this means is that most people simply have a mix of anxiety problems.

You may notice that some of the problems described in the depression section apply to you too—perhaps not all, but some of them—even if just to a mild degree. You also may have started to engage in behaviors to give yourself relief from anxiety (for instance, excessive use of alcohol or other drugs).

As you read on, you'll see that much of what feeds and perpetuates your suffering with anxiety and fear has to do with buying into what your "critical mind" says about your anxiety and also buying into what you have learned from our culture about what can and should be done about anxiety.

THE SHINING LIGHT AT THE END OF THE TUNNEL

The good news is that it doesn't really matter whether your experience fits neatly into the features of one or more anxiety disorders, if you have a unique mix, or if you have anxiety with or without some depression. It doesn't really matter if someone has told you that you have an anxiety disorder either. What really matters is your answer to the question we posed in the introduction to this workbook: *Is anxiety and fear a major problem in your life?*

To get unstuck from your current situation, you don't need to figure out what your "correct" anxiety disorder diagnosis is. It is much more important that you do this: identify what is feeding your anxiety and keeping you stuck.

The key is to start with the most problematic aspects of your anxiety. That may be panic, or fears of an object or social encounters. It could be PTSD, and struggles with memories of a painful past trauma. It could be obsessions and compulsions.

It is important to ask yourself this question: *What are the most disturbing and interfering aspects of my problem with anxiety?* Find your answer to this question by going over the checklists we covered, and then write down what stands out to you in the space below. Think about problems that lead you to pull out of your life in a flash, where you'll try like crazy to avoid the anxiety and fear. You can also go back and review the case examples to help you choose events, situations, and behaviors to work with later on in the exercises.

_____

_____

_____

_____

_____

_____

_____

_____

LIFE ENHANCEMENT EXERCISES

For this week, we invite you to do the following:

- Do one of the centering exercises daily—simply choose the one you like best.

- Spend time with the material in this chapter.

- Before moving on, be clear about what anxiety problem is most challenging for you!

THE TAKE-HOME MESSAGE

Fear and anxiety are two unpleasant emotions that can be healthy and adaptive. Both emotions propel us into action and serve the purpose of keeping us alive and out of trouble. Labeling yourself with a diagnosis for your anxiety problem will not help you or make your life more livable. Diagnostic labels are just that, words, and these words can often be self-limiting. So, instead of playing the label game, we're going to help you identify the root of the most problematic aspects of your anxiety problem: What is it that turns *your* fear, anxiety, worry, or obsession into the life-restricting problem it has become? What is it that *you* have been struggling with? Facing these questions squarely is the key to making changes that will move you in directions that are truly important to you.

Discovering the Differences Between Normal and "Disordered" Anxiety

Points to Ponder: Finding the "correct" professional diagnosis won't help me get my life back. What I need to do is look into how the drama of managing and avoiding anxiety plays out in my life so that I can start taking steps to do something about that.

Questions to Consider: What exactly are my problems with anxiety? What are the most disturbing and interfering aspects of my problem with anxiety?

CHAPTER 3

Confronting the Core Problem: Living to Avoid Fear and Anxiety Is No Way to Live

If you are facing a new challenge or being asked to do something that you have never done before don't be afraid to step out. You have more capability than you think you do but you will never see it unless you place a demand on yourself for more.

—Joyce Meyer

Thoughts and feelings of panic and anxiety are unpleasant, intense, overwhelming at times, and even terrifying. But they're not the real enemy. The real enemy is rigid avoidance of fear and anxiety.

In fact, as we touched on earlier, the weight of research shows that excessive avoidance is the most toxic element responsible for turning worries, anxieties, and fears into potentially life-shattering problems and psychiatric disorders. Remember the image in chapter 1 of the person turning away from life and struggling with discomfort. That's the problem as far as your life is concerned.

As you saw from the case examples in the last chapter, toxic avoidance takes many forms, such as avoiding people, places, activities, and situations that might lead to anxious and fearful feelings; using substances to minimize the occurrence of such feelings; and running away from situations where you experience unpleasant emotional states.

A life lived in the service of not having anxiety and fear is quite limiting and may have come to define how you live your life—an issue that we'll explore more in chapter 6 and throughout this book. For now, though, the key thing to remember is that avoidance, particularly when rigidly and inflexibly applied, gets in the way of the things you want to do and the directions you want to go. There's no way to embrace a vital life while avoiding emotional and psychological pain.

STAYING WITH YOUR BREATH INSTEAD OF RUNNING AWAY

Before moving on, we'd like to invite you to settle in for a moment with another centering exercise. It builds upon the skills you have already started to practice. In this exercise, we learn how to come back to the breath, again and again, and notice that it is always with us wherever we are. This "coming back again and again" is an enormously useful skill. It will help you when anxiety, fear, or any life circumstances threaten to take over.

All you need to do is get in a comfortable position where you won't be disturbed for five minutes. Locate the audio file on the book website (http://www.newharbinger.com/33346), and then just close your eyes and listen. You may also use the script below, though we've found that it is better to listen and follow along with this exercise.

If you'd rather keep your eyes open, you can do that too, but it's best to focus on a spot, say on the floor just in front of you, so you don't get too distracted. We'll end the exercise with a small chime and tell you when to open your eyes and move on.

EXERCISE: LET'S GET PRESENT BY COMING BACK TO YOUR BREATH

Go ahead and get in a comfortable position in your chair. Sit upright with your feet flat on the floor. Place one hand on your chest, just above your rib cage. Then place your other hand on your belly, just over your belly button. Allow your eyes to close gently. Take a couple of gentle breaths: in … and out … in … and out. Notice the sound and feel of your own breath as you breathe in … and out.

Now turn your attention to the movement of your hands as you simply breathe in … and out … in … and out. Allow your breathing to be natural here as you simply notice the movement of your hands as they rise and fall with each breath. There's nothing else to do, no state to be achieved. Simply notice and watch.

As you settle in, you may notice that your attention gets pulled elsewhere. Maybe you notice thoughts … thoughts about you … thoughts about this exercise. That's okay. When you notice your attention being pulled into your mind, simply acknowledge that, and then bring your awareness back to the movement of your hands as they rise and fall with each breath.

You may also notice that your attention is drawn to sounds around you, maybe sounds in the room, or outside nearby. That's okay to notice too. Simply acknowledge those sounds, and then gently bring your attention back to your hands as they move with each breath in … and out … in … and out. Remind yourself too that your breath is always with you even if your attention goes someplace else.

There may be moments when your attention gets pulled into physical sensations in your body, or even strong emotions. Dull ones are fine too. Maybe you're tired, or bored, or feel a grumbling in your stomach. The practice here is still the same. Gently acknowledge where your attention led you, and then kindly bring your awareness back to your hands and to the breath. Notice again that the breath is always with you.

As this time for practice comes to a close, let go of any thoughts and slowly widen your attention to take in the sounds around you. As you do, take two or three cleansing breaths in and out. With each cleansing breath, fill your lungs as much as you can with each inhale, pause for a moment, and then slowly exhale. Repeat that one or two times, and then slowly open your eyes with the intention to practice bringing your attention back to your breath—your safe refuge.

AVOIDING ANXIOUS DISCOMFORT IS THE PROBLEM

Discomfort avoidance is the common thread that binds all anxiety problems together. How people avoid anxiety and fear may differ from person to person and across anxiety disorders, but avoidance is avoidance no matter how it's done.

For instance, people with panic disorder, specific phobia, and social anxiety avoid the situations, objects, and events that could bring on fear—particularly situations where they have experienced intense anxiety in the past. People with PTSD avoid painful memories and people and places that may remind them of past trauma. People with OCD may avoid contact with objects or dirt so as not to experience the unpleasant feelings that may arise by touching things that have germs on them.

So you might avoid people or situations where there's a chance of thinking and feeling anxious or afraid. You may avoid things like sex, exercise, certain movies, unfamiliar or new activities, or foods that activate your internal triggers. And when you find yourself in a hot-button situation, you may do many things to cope as a way to keep anxiety and fear in check.

Now, if and when all of this fails, you can cut and run too—pulling out of situations after anxiety and fear kick in and threaten to overwhelm you. And in the aftermath of the storm, you'll likely say and do things to regain a foothold—repeating positive things to yourself, lying down, taking medications, breathing, thinking pleasant thoughts, and on and on.

Let's take a closer look at how this plays out with the people we talked about in chapter 2.

Panic Disorder

Donna's experience gives us an important insight into what people with panic disorder fear most: they are afraid of fear itself. If you asked Donna, she'd tell you that she wasn't all that afraid of cars or driving itself. Instead, her number one fear was of having another panic attack. Donna also needed to feel "safe" before doing this or that, which meant having her husband close by just in case she panicked. At the core, each and every safety behavior has one purpose: to help avoid experiencing a panic attack, minimize its impact, or make it go away as quickly as possible. Period. Safety behaviors are just another form of avoidance.

Specific Phobias

As you saw, Evelyn's cricket phobia changed her behavior and restricted her life. Recall that she couldn't go to the park and was deeply concerned about how her fear was impacting her kids and her ability to be a good mom. At first glance, it seems like the purpose of not going to the park was to avoid a cricket encounter. But deep down Evelyn knew that the crickets weren't her real problem. What she really dreaded most was the panic and terror she experienced—the discomfort when encountering a cricket or when just thinking about one. She didn't want to experience the panic she knew would come if and when she saw a cricket. This was the deeper and more critical issue. By avoiding crickets, what Evelyn was really avoiding was the possibility of fear itself—just like someone with panic disorder.

Social Anxiety Disorder

Steve's story shows that the problems with social anxiety go well beyond a fear of specific social situations or public events. The central issue is being afraid of experiencing fear and anxious discomfort in those contexts or of somehow failing in front of others. But the main problem again is avoidance. Steve's avoidance was of the discomfort—the anxiety and unease of being humiliated, vulnerable to scrutiny, or embarrassed in social situations.

Obsessive-Compulsive Disorder

Here again, the most problematic features of OCD—the compulsions—are actions designed to reduce or minimize anxiety, tension, and other discomfort related to unwanted thoughts and images. Compulsions are avoidance. As you saw with Ray, compulsions pull people out of their lives in a flash—consuming enormous amounts of time, energy, and resources. Absent the compulsions, you're left with emotional discomfort and unpleasant thoughts. And without engaging in the compulsions, you'd be free to engage in other potentially more vital behavioral options too.

Post-traumatic Stress Disorder

The trauma is past, but the pain remains, often resurging at times when it's most unwelcome. It's what people do about the memories of the trauma—and the current painful reminders they encounter along with unpleasant physical sensations—that accounts for much of the suffering with PTSD. Mary's story tells us as much. As painful as these memories and flashbacks undoubtedly are, they're not the real problem. The real problem with PTSD is the avoidance of emotional and psychological pain related to memories of past traumatic events.

Generalized Anxiety Disorder

Marianne's life was consumed with never-ending worry about many areas of her life. She had tried to control it, but nothing worked. This struggle left her exhausted and keyed up most of the time. What was hardest for Marianne to face was the reality that her worry was, in fact, her mind's clever way of keeping her at arm's length from contacting deep feelings of fear and the uncertainties in life. Things do sometimes go terribly, horribly wrong, and no amount of worry will change that. But avoiding that truth by worrying needlessly was incredibly costly to her.

THERE IS HOPE—YOUR LIFE CAN BE DIFFERENT!

In chapter 6 we'll help you figure out what solutions to your specific anxiety problem haven't worked for you and why. This is the first step toward making room for a completely new approach—one that is radically different from anything you've done before.

There's an impressive and growing research base that points to one conclusion: avoidance is costly and can even make things worse (see Hayes et al., 2006). This hard conclusion covers a broad swath of strategies where you might try to reduce, control, or somehow "manage" your anxiety and fear. It doesn't matter how creative or sophisticated your avoidance efforts might be. This is not about effort or willpower either. The hard truth is that avoidance doesn't work.

We understand that you might be frightened reading this. You might even think, *If that's really the case, then there's no hope my life will ever get any better.* But the conclusion that avoidance doesn't work can be liberating too, for it points to a more hopeful solution. The next metaphor hints at that.

Poison Ivy and the Anxiety Itch

Poison ivy is a plant that produces a strong skin irritant. Most people avoid touching the plant because they know what they'll get: a nasty, red, blistering rash that itches like hell. Maybe you've had a poison ivy rash before and know what it's like. It leaves you with a strong urge to scratch. And when you do that, you make matters worse. You end up with open sores on your skin. And if you haven't washed the plant oils from your hands and exposed areas, you may spread the allergic reaction to other parts of your body. No amount of scratching will cure the inflammation; you need to stop the scratching and allow your body to heal itself.

The anxiety itch is like this too. The discomfort rages through your head and body, and you have a strong urge to get relief. So you avoid. You struggle. The problem is that you can't avoid exposure to anxiety in the same way you can avoid a poison ivy plant. Anxiety can show up anytime or anywhere. When you scratch your anxiety itch with avoidance or struggle, it makes the anxiety worse—the anxiety grows and spreads to infect most of your life. And all that avoidance scratching pulls you out of your life too.

How Do You Scratch Your Anxiety Itch?

This reflection points to hope and liberation too. Nobody asks for poison ivy. No amount of blame and struggle will make it go away. The same can be said for anxiety and fear. So take heart. You aren't to blame for your anxiety troubles. The moral isn't that if you'd only tried harder, then you could've overcome your anxiety by now. The message is that you've done what you thought was best. Now you need to stop scratching.

Before moving on, give yourself a few moments to reflect on how you scratch your anxiety. What do you do when anxiety and fear shows up? How do you scratch it? Use the space below to jot down what comes to mind.

_____

_____

Become Mindful When Your Mind Beats You Up

People struggling with anxiety problems are some of the strongest people we know. They're survivors. But they can also be very harsh with themselves. We've seen this again and again in working with people just like you. In fact, many constantly beat up on themselves. They feel that they're not good enough; they're too weak; they're not trying hard enough; they just haven't got what it takes to lead a more fulfilled life. It all amounts to this: they're somehow broken. No book talks about self-loathing as a feature of an anxiety disorder—and yet it's there.

This judgmental virus of the human mind is active all the time. It can poison many aspects of your life if you let it. But there is an antidote, a way out of this toxic mind virus. It starts with catching the self-loathing before it consumes you. We'll get into this more deeply as we move along, but for now, take a moment or two and consider this: What does your mind tell you about you and your anxiety problem? How does your mind beat you up? Jot down a few thoughts that come to mind in the space below.

_____

_____

Catching the ways your mind beats you up is something you can start doing now. Later on, we're going to blend this with exercises and skills for cultivating your capacity for self-kindness and compassion—one of the most powerful antidotes to cut off the mind virus at its source. As we teach you to do that, you'll slowly discover that your life can be different. Your life need not be determined by how much or little anxiety you have. You don't have to be one of those people who continue down the dark path of more anxiety management and control when they know it doesn't really work. You can learn how to ACT on your anxiety differently! This is the kind of hope and liberation we're after in this book.

Don't Believe Us or Your Mind—Trust Your Experience

So if managing anxiety doesn't work, what else can you do? As we suggested in chapter 1, the way to get back into your life is to go into your anxiety and let it be—no more running. Instead, you choose to experience anxiety for what it is and start doing what you care about doing. The skills we'll teach you in this book will help you observe anxiety and relate to it in kinder, gentler, less engaged ways. This will position you to make more vital life choices. We know this may sound strange. And yes, some of what you read in this book is going to sound odd at first, even silly and bizarre.

You don't need to believe what we say. And you don't need to understand it all right away either. We guarantee that your mind will throw many arguments at you as to why this or that sounds impossible, is too difficult, or doesn't make any sense—*This book is rubbish; just put it down* or *You can't do it; this is all far too difficult.* When such thoughts show up, thank your mind for each of them. Then move on.

You need not argue with your mind. Don't get stuck trying to convince yourself of anything. The only thing we ask is that you stay open as you learn new ways of relating to your anxieties and worries, that you do the exercises and check out whether, over time, they start working for you.

You have little to lose and much to gain by approaching your problems with anxiety in a radically different way. We'll show you the way. Just keep on reading and doing the exercises—and then trust that experience and let your mind do its thing.

LIFE ENHANCEMENT EXERCISES

For this week, we once again invite you to work with the material in this workbook by spending time with the following:

- Do one of the centering exercises daily or as often as you can.

- Take stock of how avoidance plays out in your life.

- Continue reading and working with this book, but don't rush it!

THE TAKE-HOME MESSAGE

The most critical element that separates normal from problematic anxiety and fear is this: avoidance, avoidance, and more avoidance. It's the common tie that binds all anxiety disorders together. Avoidance of fear and anxiety feeds fear and anxiety, and it shrinks lives. It's toxic for this reason. This is why we're going to help you cut it out with actions that are kinder, gentler, and more compassionate. These powerful skills are the salve that will cut avoidance off at its root and allow your life to grow.

Discovering the Toxic Root of "Disordered" Anxiety

Points to Ponder: Avoidance can turn normal anxiety and fear into a life-shattering problem. Attempting to control and run from my anxious discomfort may be the real problem I need to face and do something about.

Questions to Consider: How do I avoid my emotional and psychological pain? Am I willing to meet my anxious discomfort with actions that are kinder, gentler, and more compassionate so I can lead a better life?

CHAPTER 4

Myths About Anxiety and Its Disorders

Think about any attachments that are depleting your emotional reserves. Consider letting them go.

—Oprah Winfrey

A good deal of what you read earlier in chapter 2 ought to have resonated with you. There's comfort in being able to put a label to your suffering. Yet do you really want to be known and defined by your anxiety problem now and for the rest of your life?

Think about it—Bill "the social phobic," Anita "a panicker," John "a worrier," Lisa "the lady with PTSD," Scott "the agoraphobic," or Tom "an obsessive-compulsive." You might even do this yourself—my name is _____, "the _____ [insert your anxiety problem]."

Labeling is seductive. It implies that knowing more about your problems will lead to discovering a solution or way out. You might pause here to ask if this is true of your experience. Has knowing more about anxiety and its disorders really helped you move forward in vital and lasting ways? Has learning about how others cope with anxiety or staying on top of the latest research, self-help techniques, and so on really helped? These activities may make you feel good temporarily and will, over time, make you more of an anxiety expert. Yet that expertise and fleeting sense of comfort won't get your life back on track.

Once you buy into the label of "your disorder," you can quite literally become it—thinking and behaving like someone with an anxiety disorder. This kind of information is useless as far as your life is concerned. Anxiety disorders are not things that people really *have*. Labels are a ruse, strings of words that were created by members of the psychiatric community to summarize experiences people share, and more importantly, what people do. That's it really. You certainly do not need to buy into the story that you *are* your disorder.

Simply ask yourself if the label has been useful to you. Has it brought a greater sense of peace, freedom, dignity, vitality, and freedom to your life? Or, has it limited your options and kept you stuck and wallowing in worry, anxiety, and fear? You're enough of an expert about your anxiety and your life already. Maybe what needs to happen is for you to do something radically different than you've done before.

David Allen (2002), in his book *Getting Things Done*, teaches us that useful knowledge helps you achieve practical results and points you toward actions that make a difference in your life. And it's by your actions—what you spend your time doing—that you create your life, one step at a time. This is what others will see about you too. This is the kind of change we are about in this book. So let's start by focusing on actions that are potentially vital and different from what you've done before.

> If I continue to do what I've always done, then I'm going to get what I've always got.

You can start by allowing yourself to let go of the label. You are much more than an anxiety disorder—the label isn't you. This chapter will start you down a new road, beginning by dispelling some common myths about anxiety and fear.

COMMON MYTHS ABOUT ANXIETY AND FEAR

It seems like every day we're learning something new about anxiety and its disorders. This entire workbook stands on the shoulders of hundreds, if not thousands, of research studies. Each has explored what turns anxiety and fear into life-shattering problems and, most importantly, what you can do about it.

You probably also know quite a bit about anxiety and its disorders already. Some of this you know from your own experience. You may have picked up other pearls of wisdom from newspaper and magazine articles, books on the topic, TV, the Internet, conversations with family members and others, or from what your doctor has told you. You may have heard that anxiety disorders are a disease, just like diabetes or cancer, or that some people inherit anxiety disorders. You may have heard that anxiety disorders can be treated with herbal remedies or by changing your diet. Others have told you that anxiety disorders are caused by your brain's neurochemicals run amok, so you need medications to repair chemical imbalances within your faulty brain.

In fact, you may feel overwhelmed by all the new research and sound bytes about the causes and potential cures for anxiety. Scientists and the media are just as guilty of promoting messages that are not necessarily helpful. As an example, we recently learned of a new study claiming that injections of a natural hormone known as cortisol can block intense fear reactions, and that medications for high blood pressure can weaken how your brain forms and stores emotional memories following exposure to traumatic events. Inside this work, of course, is the message that it's not okay to feel fear, and that remembering a painful past is bad too.

Still others are promoting untested practices, often preying on the desperation and suffering of people just like you. They get away with it because they exaggerate their claims, and exaggeration sells. Sadly, there's just no evidence that magnets, aromatherapy, Bach flower therapy, biofeedback gadgets, brain wave synchronizers, thought field therapy, hypnosis, homeopathy, passion-flower tea, or special diets cure anxiety and panic. In fact, even our best available scientifically supported treatments do not cure anxiety in the sense of making it go away and for good. So, when you see a claim of a new cure, please be mindful of your wallet.

The message behind many of these claims is that it's abnormal to experience intense fear and anxiety. You may even think so too. And you might think that this means you are weak, broken, or on the verge of losing it and going crazy. Perhaps you've heard that learning better ways to manage and control your thoughts and feelings is a way out of your anxiety—another pervasive message promoted by our culture.

These are all common experiences and beliefs about anxiety, and even some mental health professionals accept them. Yet none of them are true. Each is a myth or, at best, a partial truth. They are unhelpful because they keep you and others like you stuck in old patterns that don't work. They leave you wanting, waiting, and struggling to get a foothold. They feed patterns of thinking that you are unlike most people who seemingly glide through life happy and carefree. This isn't so.

So let's take a look at the myths and reveal them for what they are.

Myth #1: Anxiety Problems Are Biological and Hereditary

Too often we hear people say, "Anxiety runs in my family, so that's why I'm anxious." Or, "My doctor said my anxiety disorder is caused by my family's genes, so the best I can do is take medication to manage it." You may even think this way yourself. Both of these statements are widely supported by the medical establishment and popular media. Fortunately, both also turn out to be false.

Yes, it is true that anxiety often runs in families, but that's because of learned behavior, not because of genes. You may also inherit some predisposition to be anxious or afraid, just like you inherit predispositions to be outgoing, introverted, intelligent, muscular, or athletic. But inheriting a *predisposition* to be anxious is not the same thing as inheriting an anxiety *disorder*.

In fact, there's no compelling evidence that you or anyone else is born with any anxiety disorder. At best, genes contribute about 30 to 40 percent to your anxiety problems (Leonardo & Hen, 2006). What this also means is that about 60 to 70 percent of your difficulties have little to do with your biology or genes. And newer work with epigenetics is showing that genetics are not as fixed as we once thought.

Many genes seem to operate like light switches, turning on and off in response to the environment and what we do. What this means for you is this—genetics is not destiny. Whatever your genetic make up, there is room to grow and change.

The bulk of what makes anxiety a psychiatric problem has nothing to do with your biology or genetics. That other 60 to 70 percent has to do with how you relate with your anxiety and fear—what you do about your anxious thoughts and feelings. This is the more important part because it's something you can control and change. You cannot change your genes, nor can you change your biology in any permanent sense, by resorting to medications. But you can change your life (and even your biology) by changing what you do. This is why we'll focus on helping you work on what you can control and change—your actions, or what you do when you have anxious feelings.

> *People don't inherit anxiety disorders.*

Myth #2: Intense Anxiety Is Abnormal

One of the main reasons people seek help for anxiety is this: they do not like how they think or feel. The anxiety and fear seems overwhelming, the painful memories too much to bear, the thoughts and worries paralyzing or next to impossible to turn off. In a word, anxiety is too intense.

It's certainly true that intense anxiety tends to go hand in hand with all anxiety disorders. It's also true that intense anxiety doesn't constitute an anxiety disorder. We need the capacity to feel intense emotions like anxiety and fear. Even newborn babies have this experience. Most children and adults report strongly felt anxiety at some point in any given year, often more than once, and even in situations where there's no risk of being harmed. All humans are wired to experience a range of emotions at varying levels of intensity. It would be abnormal for this not to be so.

As you saw in chapter 2, intense fear and anxiety has one purpose—to ready you for action when faced with real danger or risk of harm. Life-threatening events such as combat, sexual assault, abuse, accidents, and natural disasters fall into this category. In these situations, most people will experience intense anxiety and fear. And without the capacity to feel such emotions intensely, we wouldn't have survived as a species. These reactions are 100 percent normal.

Your mind might be saying, *Yes, but I experience anxiety and fear in situations where I'm not at risk of being harmed … Surely that's a problem.* And when that happens, you likely do what most people would do when at risk of being harmed or even killed: you freeze, drop what you were doing, and then attempt to run away. Here you ought to notice where your intense anxiety and fear go when you do that. They go with you, right? You can't run away from them. They're a part of you. You can't run from you.

Take stock of what else happens when you act in ways to avoid or run from anxiety. You likely feel better temporarily, but in the meantime, you're not doing the things that you care about. Over time, your life space shrinks and you get stuck. Intense anxiety may seem like a barrier that stands between you and your life. And it will remain a barrier as long as you continue to buy into the myth that strongly felt anxiety is a problem.

The short of it is this: intense anxiety doesn't make anxiety a problem. Many people experience intense anxiety, even panic attacks, in their daily lives *and* continue to do what's important to them. Intensely felt emotions need not be a barrier to the life you want to lead. They can be welcomed in as a vital *part* of you. This is why we are going to help you to learn new ways of relating with your anxious thoughts and feelings and then how to take them with you. If you're willing, this approach will get you unstuck and back on track toward the life you want.

Myth #3: Anxiety Is a Sign of Weakness

Anxiety isn't a sign of weakness, personality defect, poor character, laziness, or lack of motivation. Anyone can get stuck and off track because of emotional or psychological pain. All human beings have pain. Having pain is built into the human condition.

You may buy into the idea that anxiety is a sign of weakness because other people in your life seem so well put together. You see others making it, doing things that you'd like to do, seemingly without the shadow of anxiety hanging over their heads. This great illusion is fueled by two sources. The first one is the tendency for our minds to make inferences based on very limited information. When you see and interact with others, you may not see them as anxious or actively suffering. You may think, *Why can't I be that way?* And next, *something must be wrong with me.*

What is needed here is some perspective. Imagine that you're able to shadow one person who you think has it all together. You can watch this person's every move 24/7, and know what he or she is thinking and feeling at any time. If you were able to do this, you'd have a hard time ignoring this simple fact—that person is not so different from you.

As you open up to this person's humanity, you'd see someone who experiences a whole range of thoughts and feelings just like you—pleasant, unpleasant, and everything in between. Someone who needs to eat, drink, sleep, and use the bathroom, just like you. Someone who, like you, will at times feel frustrated, be worried about this or that, or experience sadness, loneliness, regret, and anger. And someone who, at times, will also be anxious or afraid.

Anxiety isn't a sign of weakness.

The second source that fuels the weakness myth is social comparison. When you narrowly view your life as full of anxiety and emotional pain and see others as dancing through the lily fields of life, happy and carefree, you'll naturally feel that something is wrong with you. You'll think that you're missing something they have.

The truth is that you have everything you need. You aren't broken. The capacity for change lies within you. You and only you are responsible for what you do with your precious time and energy. This is why we'll be nurturing your capacity for responsibility. With that, you'll create change in your life by refocusing time, energy, and resources in those areas that you can control and change—the things you do with your hands, feet, and mouth.

Myth #4: Anxiety Can and Must Be Managed to Live a Vital Life

Of all the myths, this one is the most damaging. It's fueled by social rules and expectations, or what we call the *culture of feel-goodism*. These rules set up emotional and physical pain as barriers to a life lived well. The message is this: *In order to live better, I must first think and feel better. And once I start thinking and feeling better, my life will improve for the better.* This is a trap.

The bait for the trap is the emotional and psychological pain you experience with anxiety, panic, worries, unwanted thoughts, or memories. In your mind, this pain isn't just pain. It's *bad* pain. Your mind has judged it as unacceptable and has linked it with not being able to do what you care about. When anxiety pain shows up, you go after it to weaken it or drive it away. You also do this or that to prevent that *bad* pain from showing up in the future, and on and on it goes.

EXERCISE: DON'T THINK ABOUT A PINK ELEPHANT OR WORSE

This brief exercise will help you see what trying to suppress and control unwanted thoughts gets you. Go ahead and get in a comfortable position. Now, when you're ready, we'd like you to close your eyes and try this: Don't think about a PINK ELEPHANT! Try hard. Give yourself a few minutes to really work at it. After you've given it a go, open your eyes and read on.

If you're like most people, you'll find this task difficult or practically impossible. The reason is that you cannot do what the instruction says without thinking of the thing you aren't supposed to think about. Put another way, the thought *Don't think about a PINK ELEPHANT* is itself a thought about pink elephants. So there you are, stuck with the very thing you don't want.

Your mind may have come up with other clever tactics to accomplish the goal of not thinking about a pink elephant. You might have tried thinking about something else. This seems reasonable. Yet how did your mind do that? How did you know that the other thought was not a pink elephant? In order to think of something that is clearly not a pink elephant you need to compare it to a pink elephant. So there you are, back with the thought of a pink elephant again.

Your mental programming has lots of links that surface automatically, just as the thoughts of pink elephants did, because you've learned them. Here are a few. Go ahead and complete the blanks without giving them much thought.

Twinkle, twinkle, little _____   Practice makes _____

Don't spill the _____   Actions speak louder than _____

Look before you _____   The early bird gets the _____

Now, we'd like you to pick one of these statements and read it slowly, but don't think about the word that completes the phrase. For instance, read "Twinkle, twinkle, little" but don't think _____ ("star"). What happened? Could you do it? Let's take this a step further.

Imagine that "star" is one of those really distressing thoughts, bodily sensations, feelings, or memories that you struggle with and wish not to have. You're now in a situation where your automatic programming kicks in. Here it comes—"Twinkle, twinkle, little _____"—but you can't have what comes next. What do you suppose will happen here? You end up with more of the thing you don't want to experience. And you'll probably do this or that to avoid it in the future.

When you take the bait, look at what happens to the pain and your life. You're devoting enormous time, energy, and resources to keeping the anxiety and panic at bay. You keep doing this because it has often bought you some temporary relief. You also do it because this is what you've been taught to do in our culture, whether or not it actually works for you over the long haul.

If you suffer from panic disorder, then you may know what this is like. Having a panic attack at the grocery store or elsewhere is a highly unpleasant experience. And it may lead you to do things to prevent it from happening again: stop shopping, shop with a "safe" person but not alone, only go to the store late in the evening when few people are around in case you panic again, and so on. All the while, you may be concentrating on relaxing as you also watch for signs of a possible panic attack.

If your difficulties are with social anxiety, you may take many steps to minimize or avoid having anxiety in social encounters. This is hard to do in a highly social world like ours and so can be quite crippling. Imagine going about your day without interacting with people for fear that you might panic or humiliate or embarrass yourself. Now imagine how that might feel knowing the truth that none of us can control how other people respond to us.

> *Anxiety management and avoidance leave you feeling safe and less anxious in the short term and greatly limit what you can do. This inaction is a problem.*

We could go on outlining the different strategies people use to control and manage their anxieties and fears. And, as we explored earlier in this workbook, you have probably tried many yourself, to little or no avail. In truth, only creativity and resources limit the possible universe of strategies that people can devise. Despite your best efforts, your anxiety comes back, perhaps even stronger the next time.

Worse, time spent trying to manage and control anxiety is time and energy away from doing things that you care deeply about. So anxiety management and control actually double your pain: on top of the pain of more anxiety, you also get the pain of loss or regret that comes from an unfulfilled life. This other pain will creep up on you over time when you take a pass on doing something that's important to you because of the fear and anxiety. Both forms of pain are a natural consequence of fighting a battle with your unpleasant thoughts and feelings.

But don't fault yourself for doing this. Everyone can get stuck in a loop of trying to make their pain go away. And many studies show that people get more of the very thing they don't want when they try to push it out of their mind. So, when you don't want anxious thoughts and feelings, you'll naturally get more of them. And the more you don't want them, the more you're stuck with them. We'll elaborate on how this works in a moment. For now, the important thing to remember is that these actions fuel your anxiety and slam the trapdoor shut on your life.

The exercises in this book are designed to help you recognize the anxiety management and control myth for what it is—a rigged, no-win game that has brought much unnecessary suffering to your life. You can avoid getting sucked into the anxiety trap by learning not to take the bait. You can learn to live better without first having to think and feel better. You can learn to bring comfort to the unpleasant experiences your mind and body are serving up and do what matters to you.

WHERE THE MYTHS WILL TAKE YOU IF YOU LET THEM

Each of the myths feed anxiety and can keep you stuck and cut off from the life you want to lead. The myths are, in a sense, like a sticky spider web. When you get caught up in the web, the natural reaction is to struggle to get out. And the more you struggle, the more tangled up you become. On and on it goes; eventually you become the anxiety management expert, searching, hoping, perhaps praying, for that magic cure or new solution.

The hard truth is you won't find a cure for anxiety in a pill, an online support group, or even in some solid psychotherapies known for offering "new, better, different" strategies for getting control over your anxious thoughts and feelings.

Whenever your mind tells you otherwise, look at your experience. Have these and other options worked in the long run? Does your experience tell you that they will work if you work harder, longer, or better at them? Do you want to be about dealing with anxiety for the rest of your life? Haven't you worked hard enough?

■ *Sharon's Story*

Sharon, one of our recent clients, shared a story with us that illustrates where the myths can take you if you let them. She came to us at the age of forty-five after twenty years of crippling struggle with anxiety, panic, and depression. She struggled with thoughts of meaninglessness in life. She believed that something was biologically wrong with her. She thought of herself as the kind of person who had been dealt a bad hand—a life filled with too much emotional pain and anguish. Her runaway mind was constantly feeding her doom and gloom, self-blame, and negativity. Sharon didn't think she had much of a chance for a bright future.

She feared having a nervous breakdown if she ever found herself stuck, away from home, and isolated from family and friends. She feared the dark, being out alone, and driving at night. She saw her life ticking by, and feared being put in a hospital, medicated, doped up, and cut off from her children and her life. When she wasn't seeing herself carted away to the hospital or waiting for hospice, she imagined being isolated and alone, unemployed, with her kids in an orphanage.

Sharon had been on and off antidepressant and antianxiety medication and in and out of cognitive behavioral therapy, often finding that such treatments left her with a renewed sense of hope, a honeymoon from the crippling panic, wrenching anxiety, agoraphobia, and disturbing thoughts. She bought a sun lamp to stave off the depression. She invested hundreds of dollars in professional and self-help books about anxiety disorders, belonged to many online support groups, and even attended seminars.

For about two years, Sharon was living better and seemed to feel better too. Armed with a solid set of tools to keep her anxiety and fear at bay, she was able to readily challenge her negative thoughts, relax away the tension, dismiss the worry, and breathe herself out of panic. And she had the sun lamp and the books to read when she found herself in a pinch. These strategies seemed to work, but she never fully escaped the lurking sense that someday, somewhere, the strategies wouldn't work—and then the shadow of anxiety and depression would return and take over. And that's exactly what happened and what ultimately led Sharon to us.

Sharon was at a tipping point and she knew it. For the first time in her life, she looked for new answers instead of old solutions. But it all began when she finally asked herself this question: Can I learn to live with feelings and thoughts that I don't like and not allow them to control me and what I do? You'll learn more about Sharon in the next chapter.

PAUSE AND COME BACK TO YOUR BREATH

Before wrapping up this chapter, we'd like to invite you once again to take a moment to pause and settle yourself just where you are. In this space, we strongly encourage you to go back and repeat the Centering into Your Heart exercise you learned about in chapter 2. This is a powerful exercise for many reasons. Anxiety can't grow in an environment that is spacious, open, and kind. It just can't. Anxiety needs negative energy and your active participation to grow. So, the skill here is to open up right where you are and connect with your heart—your safe refuge. Give yourself time to cultivate this important skill. And, if you wish, you may also go back and practice any of the other centering exercises. Each of them, in their own way, offers an antidote to your suffering with anxiety.

LIFE ENHANCEMENT EXERCISES

For this week, make a commitment to integrate the following activities into your daily life:

- Do one of the centering exercises daily—one that resonates with you.

- Practice coming back to your breath—your abiding refuge—during your day (e.g., while driving, walking, doing the dishes).

- If you are having difficulty doing any of the exercises we've covered so far, slow things down and look to see what's getting in your way. Then ask, is this stuff what has kept me stuck all along? Maybe it's time to do something that is truly new!

- Continue reading and working with this book, but go slowly.

THE TAKE-HOME MESSAGE

All of the myths about anxiety are set up and fed by Western notions of psychological health and wellness. The message is that happiness is normal. But what if happiness isn't normal? What if it is impossible for you or anyone to create a life free of significant psychological and emotional pain? When you look more closely at people's lives, you'll find that significant pain and struggle are companions that we all must take along on the road to a vital life.

Your anxiety problems may have something to do with you buying into the "happiness or bust" message. You might think that your worries, anxieties, and fears must go away first so you can start doing what matters to you. But perhaps the solution is to do something radically different than what you've been doing. Are you willing to take that step?

The Myths Feed Anxiety and Keep Me Stuck

Point to Ponder: All the myths of anxiety are limiting. They send the message that my anxiety and fear are unacceptable and a barrier between me and my life.

Questions to Consider: What myths of anxiety have I bought into? Have I let anxiety control my life? Am I willing to take responsibility for what I do about my worries, anxieties, and fears? Will I let go of the myths?

CHAPTER 5

Letting Go of Old Myths Opens Up New Opportunities

Bad things do happen; how I respond to them defines the quality of my life. I can choose to sit in perpetual sadness, immobilized by the gravity of my loss, or I can choose to rise from the pain and treasure the most precious gift I have—life itself.

—Walter Anderson

Dr. Seuss (1960/1990) wrote a wonderful children's story called *Oh, the Places You'll Go.* The story speaks volumes about what it takes to create a life that is meaningful. This is a story for the young and old, for it speaks to life, pain, and joy—and what it takes to live out the life you want to lead.

And as much as your mind might be telling you otherwise, you don't need to continue to do what you've always done. As Dr. Seuss teaches us, you don't need to be one of those people standing in line waiting, just waiting, because of _____ [insert one of your big anxieties and fears here], waiting for your life to begin.

THE PLACES YOU'LL GO WHEN YOU LET GO OF THE MYTHS

As Sharon worked with the material in this book, she began to let go of the myths. She stopped playing the waiting game. She stopped feeding her negative thoughts and instead learned to watch them, with kindness, curiosity, and at times with humor. She began to see what buying into the myths about anxiety had cost her. She stopped trying to manage and control her anxiety and depression and would no longer allow them to stand between her and her life.

Sharon learned that she could live better when she stopped trying to conquer her anxiety and depression. And when she started living better, she began to feel and think better too. For Sharon, this didn't mean being free from anxiety and fear, worries, or negative thoughts. It meant that when they showed up, she chose not to feed them. She was unwilling to dignify her anxieties, fears, and worries with more struggles. Instead, she met them with compassion and gentleness. She learned that she could start living her life without winning a war with her pain.

Some of the old habits remained. In fact, Sharon recently took a trip out of town with her husband and kids for a family vacation to the beach, something she'd never considered doing before. While packing for the trip, Sharon had stuffed a duffle bag full of her old safety myths: vitamins for her anxiety, her iPod loaded with ten gigabytes of relaxation tracks and self-help lectures, earplugs to blot out the noise of her kids screaming while they played in the hotel room, a sun lamp to ward off depression, and a dozen or so books on anxiety and its disorders. The weight of her baggage was enormous, literally and emotionally.

It turned out that all this antianxiety gear was unnecessary and next to useless. Over the weekend, Sharon didn't open her duffle bag once. With a chuckle, she said, "Sheesh … I had times over the weekend when I felt anxious and had anxious thoughts. And then I reminded myself that I didn't want to be about what was in the duffle bag."

For Sharon, being about the contents of her duffle bag meant being holed up in her hotel room, alone, popping vitamins, her iPod cranked up, reading the book *Anxiety and Its Disorders* in front of her sun lamp. Instead, she spent her time outside, playing with her husband and children on the beach, going for sunset walks, searching for seashells, and reading a fun book. She went out to dinner and took the kids to a Sunday matinee. She even had a chance to share quiet conversation with her husband over a nice glass of wine on the balcony of her hotel room after the kids went to bed. These are the things that Sharon cared deeply about.

At times she felt really good while doing all these things. And at other times she was quite anxious about the possibility of having a panic attack. She even worried whether the good feelings would last. And no matter what happened, she remained steadfast in one choice she'd made: she was unwilling to spend time struggling with her anxiety, panic, and the negative news that her mind fed her from time to time. She kept on going and gave herself some space to have all those experiences without attempting to resolve them. Her weekend at the beach left her feeling alive!

Sharon's story is typical in many ways. Your story may be different, but what may not be different is what has happened to your life. If you feel your life has shrunk to the size of a postage stamp, then you may be just as stuck as Sharon was.

So ask yourself: Has buying into the myths taken you out of your life and left you stuck and trapped in your anxiety? Is it possible that, just like Sharon, you don't need to think and feel better in order to live better?

Sharon found her answers not by blindly trusting what we said. In fact, she had serious doubts about what our treatment program could offer her. The ideas were new, sounded a bit strange, and cut against the grain of just about everything she believed could and ought to be done about her anxiety and her life.

We didn't ask Sharon to get rid of or resolve her doubts. And we won't ask you to do that either. All we ask is that you soften to the possibility that your old ideas about the solutions to your anxiety problems may not be serving you well and may be doing you more harm than good.

As Sharon began doing the exercises in this book, she learned to stop buying in to and feeding her judgmental mind, to trust her experience, and to act in ways that mattered to her. She began spending more of her time doing the things she cared about—sometimes with and sometimes without anxiety—and less time with her anxious thoughts and feelings and other sources of emotional pain that left her feeling hopeless and depressed. Sharon learned that things could be different when she approached her anxiety and her life in a new way. You have these options too.

WHAT FUELS THE MYTHS AND KEEPS THEM ALIVE?

There are four key factors that fuel the myths about anxiety, turn anxiety into a problem, and keep you stuck. Let's briefly have a look at each one.

The Mind Trap: Fusion with Your Thoughts, Images, and Memories

Like every human being, you have the capacity to become fused or tangled up with your thoughts. When you fuse with your thoughts, you'll tend to treat them "as if" they were the same thing as the experiences or events they describe.

For instance, the word "panic" may conjure up all sorts of associations. These may include images of having a heart attack, death, fainting, going crazy, losing it, or being carted off to the funny farm. Your mind will also throw evaluations into these associations, such as bad, dangerous, weak, stupid, humiliated, and so on. All of these judgmental labels have their own associations too, many of them quite negative.

What's important to see here is that the word "panic" is not a real panic attack, nor is it the same as the associations and evaluations linked with the word. The word "panic" is just a word. The evaluation "bad" is just a word. You could choose to treat them just as words. Or you could respond to the word, associations, and evaluations as if they are more than that.

When you go beyond seeing words as words, you're buying into the illusion your mind creates. The thoughts shift from being thoughts to being something dangerously serious. And when that happens, you'll often find yourself trapped in old behavior patterns that are neither helpful nor in your best interest. We call this a *mind trap*.

Consider this: what would happen if you responded to the word "panic" and its associations as if the word and its associations were the real thing? You might lie down, take a tranquilizer pill, listen to soothing music, call your doctor or a friend or relative, or go to the emergency room. In short, you'd respond to the word and its associations with behavior. This is what we mean by *fusion*: responding to words, images, memories, or evaluations with actions—with things you do—as though the products of your mind are the same thing as the actual life events they represent or are related to.

Fusion can be a hard concept to explain, let alone understand intellectually. This is why we're going to help you connect with it more experientially throughout the book. For now, all we ask is that you play with the idea that your anxious suffering is set into motion when you feed your unpleasant thoughts and feelings by getting tangled up and fused with them.

Your judgmental mind is at work here, and it's not your best friend at those times. When you allow your mind to take you down the fusion road unchecked, you'll naturally tend to react strongly to what your mind feeds you and to give thoughts more importance than they deserve. This can keep you stuck.

EXERCISE: GETTING TANGLED UP WITH ANXIETY

To get a sense of this process, take a moment to complete the following exercise. Select a thought, worry, emotional experience, or memory that's particularly upsetting for you. Once you have that in mind, jot down events or experiences that tend to go along with it. Here's an example of how Sally, who suffers from strong anxiety and panic attacks, did it.

My Experience	What Comes to Mind
Panic/strong anxiety	1. Jittery and shaky
	2. Can't think clearly
	3. Heart races, sweaty
	4. Can't be in a crowd, drive a car, go near heights
	5. Think I might be going crazy

Sally noticed a couple of things here. When she bought into her anxious thoughts and feelings and tried to eliminate them, she also bought herself everything else on her list and then some. She felt more anxious. (Remember the pink elephant.) Worse, she now became the very thing she wished not to be by fusing her sense of being with her anxiety, as in, "I'm anxious."

In fact, Sally told us, "I'm Ms. PAT (Panic-Anxiety-Terror)." Once she fed that thought, she became a person who was not only anxious, but also incapable of being in a crowd, driving a car, and going to work on the fifth story of her office building. And she didn't like herself very much anymore either. No surprise, given that she had fused with the very things she most disliked.

My Experience	What Comes to Mind
	1.
	2.
	3.
	4.
	5.
	1.
	2.
	3.
	4.
	5.
	1.
	2.
	3.
	4.
	5.

If you're like Sally, then you give a whole lot of importance to anxiety-provoking thoughts or feelings. That's because you've learned to buy in to what your mind tells you about your experience. The more you do that, the more you become fused with the label and evaluations and trapped by your mind.

You might be thinking, *Are they telling me that my fear and anxiety aren't real?* Absolutely not. The bodily sensations, the thoughts, and the images are all there and are real, in the sense of being parts of your experience.

What we're asking is for you to look closely at what you're responding to. Are you responding to the images as images, thoughts as thoughts, sensations as sensations, and memories as memories, *as they are*, unedited and untainted by negative evaluations? Or are your actions steered by judgments and evaluations of these experiences—the stuff your mind feeds you about them?

The critical question here is this: must you respond to experiences as though they are what your mind says they are ("The racing heart is a heart attack and not simply a fast heartbeat"), or can you just treat them as actual sensations, as thoughts consisting of words, or as fleeting memories or images of the past?

Perhaps you also feel like Ms. or Mr. PAT (or like Dr. Worry, the expert on worrying). And you may have had times when you've said to yourself, *I'm weak, I'm depressed, I'm a loser,* or *I'm going crazy.* Each of these statements may seem like they are who you are.

> *Your anxious thoughts and feelings are part of you—not you.*

Now think for a moment what would happen if all of a sudden you had the thought, *I am a banana.* To find out, close your eyes for ten seconds and keep thinking that thought: *I am a banana.* What happened? Perhaps you saw a yellow curved object in your mind. You may even have imagined the taste of a banana. Did having that thought turn you into a banana? Is that thought any more true or false than any other thought your mind might throw at you now and then?

Intuitively, you may already know that your thoughts are different than the events they describe. As we teach you how to step back and defuse or disentangle a bit, you'll see that the thoughts are simply thoughts, sensations are sensations, memories are memories, and feelings are feelings—nothing more, nothing less. We'll teach you skills so that you don't "become" them.

If you feel a bit confused, be patient and skeptical about what your mind may be telling you now, and keep on reading to discover for yourself what this might all mean and how it can help you.

Evaluating Your Experiences

Just about everything human beings experience and do is tagged with some sort of evaluation or judgment: good versus bad, right versus wrong, happy versus sad. Media and marketing are built around helping you experience a positive evaluation of products so that you go out and buy them.

Similarly, models of health and wellness are built around the idea that emotional and psychological pain is not simply pain, but "bad" pain. You can apply this habit of evaluation as readily to yourself and your private experiences as you can to most events in your world.

There's nothing wrong with evaluating your experience, provided that you recognize it for what it is: an evaluation of reality, not reality itself. To put it another way, you might call a duckling "ugly" or "cute," but that doesn't change the fact that the duckling is a duck. This is an important point that we'll revisit throughout this book.

Evaluations of your experience rarely add anything to the experience itself. When you buy into and feed your negative evaluations unnecessarily, you'll often fuel your suffering unnecessarily. It just plain hurts when we evaluate ourselves and our experiences negatively—as ugly, broken, screwed up, weak, worthless, stupid, crazy, foolish, and the like.

You may not be able to control the stream of evaluations, but you can choose to feed them or not. Here's a short story to give you a sense of what we mean by feeding your mind.

Feeding a Painful Wolf or a Compassionate Heart

A Native American grandfather was talking to his grandson about how he felt. He said, "I feel as if I have two wolves fighting in my heart. One wolf is the vengeful, angry, violent one. The other wolf is the loving, compassionate one." The grandson asked him, "Which wolf will win the fight in your heart?" The grandfather answered, "The one I feed."

In chapter 1 we talked about anxiety and fear as being a loose collection of bodily sensations, thoughts, and behavioral predispositions, all of which tend to hang together with other events and situations you've experienced. Go back and review what you wrote down about these areas as they apply to your experience with anxiety and fear.

With these thoughts, bodily sensations, feelings, and behaviors in mind, take a moment to write down words that best describe your evaluation of them. You may think of these as bad, unwanted, unpleasant, nasty, aversive, painful, screwed up, awful, annoying, or wrenching, or you may have other words that you routinely apply to them. Don't overthink this. Just write down any judgments that immediately show up.

_____, _____, _____, _____, _____, _____

Take a moment to pause and reflect. Look at what you tend to respond to more: your experiences just as they are—unedited—or your judgments and negative labels of those experiences? It will tend to be one or the other, not both. What is it for you?

When you buy in to the negative evaluations, you're left with only one sensible option—to do what you can to rid yourself of the bad and potentially damaging experience. You feed your anxious wolf.

Buying in to judgmental labels also leads to inevitable actions. Suppose one of your judgmental thoughts was *My panic attacks are so bad that they're eventually going to kill me*. If you completely believe this thought and only react to what it seems to say, then you are left with few options. The thought says that your life is in the balance so you *must* do something to alter that state of affairs—perhaps you won't leave the house or you'll take an antianxiety pill every few hours. The same principles are at work with obsessional thoughts that you might think will come true if you don't do something about them, like, *I might harm my children* or *I may have come in contact with germs*.

The bottom line is this: nothing else makes sense except acting on the thought. But here's the rub: as soon as you do that, you'll find yourself caught in the mind trap, feeding the hungry anxiety wolf one more time.

Avoiding Your Experiences

Avoiding or escaping from experiences that bring on the "bad" thoughts and feelings may leave you with a brief honeymoon from the pain and its source. In fact, this is exactly what keeps avoidance and escape behavior going. When you avoid or run from bad emotional experiences, you'll tend to buy yourself temporary relief. Countless studies have shown that this temporary relief makes it likely that you'll use the same strategy next time the "bad" anxiety or fear rears its "ugly" head (another evaluation).

Avoidance would be a sensible strategy, and something we might actually recommend, if the situations could harm or kill you. We might even suggest it if there was a healthy way for you to live your life wholeheartedly while avoiding unpleasant psychological and emotional experiences. But neither of these options applies here, and in fact, the second one is just flat out impossible. What may be difficult to see is that avoidance is unnecessary and is, in fact, enormously costly. We'll walk you through some of the costs in the next chapter.

For now, we'd like you to consider the possibility that the pain that lies beneath your "bad" anxiety and fear may not be so bad after all. It may actually serve a purpose and be a type of "growing pain." You may need it to get you moving toward the life that you so desperately want. What follows is a simple story that illustrates this point.

What Avoiding Pain Cost the Emperor Moth

One day, a man found a cocoon of an emperor moth. Being curious, he took it home, hoping that one day he could watch the moth come out of the cocoon. Then, on the fifth day, he noticed that a small opening appeared. The man dropped everything he was doing and sat and watched the moth for several hours, just watching as the moth struggled to force its body through that little hole. "This is it, the moment I've been waiting for," or so he thought. But it wasn't long before the moth stopped making any progress. It appeared to have gotten as far as it could. It just seemed stuck.

Then the man, in his kindness, decided to help the moth. So he took a pair of scissors and snipped off the remaining bit of the cocoon. The moth then emerged easily, but it had a swollen body and small shriveled wings. The man continued to watch. He expected that, at any moment, the wings would enlarge, fan out magnificently, and be able to support the body. None of this happened! The little moth spent the rest of its life crawling around with a swollen body and shriveled wings. Sadly, the moth was never able to fly.

What the man in his kindness and haste didn't understand was this: In order for the moth to fly, it needed to experience the restricting cocoon *and* the painful struggle as it emerged through the tiny opening. This was a necessary part of a process to force fluid from the body and into the wings so that the moth would be ready for flight once it found freedom from the cocoon. Freedom and flight would only come after allowing painful struggle. By depriving the moth of struggle, the man deprived the moth of health.

You may see a bit of yourself in this story. You wish to move on with your life without the pain of having anxiety and fear as a part of that movement. The story also hints at another possibility that may seem a bit wacky at first: Could it be that your worries, anxieties, and fears aren't your enemy? Is it possible that you need anxiety to "force fluid from your body into your wings" in order to have the kind of life that you so desperately want?

We're not suggesting that you just take off and fly into a happy life. All we're asking is that you open up to the possibility that your anxious thoughts, images, and feelings may serve an important purpose in your life. You may not see this purpose from where you are right now. That's okay. It's next to impossible to see any important purpose behind anxiety and fear when you're focused on getting yourself out of your anxiety cocoon.

This is why we're going to teach you skills that will help you learn to be with your anxiety, without being consumed by it. As you learn these skills, you'll learn how anxiety is necessary for you to take flight in life directions that are vital and meaningful for you.

Reason Giving for Your Behavior

Many people we've helped with anxiety have deeply rooted reasons for why they cannot do this or that. Here are a few examples:

"I can't fly in a plane because I might panic."

"I can't make new friends because I'll make a fool of myself."

"I can't be in crowds because it's too unsafe."

"I can't hug my wife because she's covered in garden dirt and germs."

"I can't date because I was abused as a child."

The content will differ across the reasons, but all have a familiar ring to them. Each includes an "I can't" and a "because." The part right after "I can't" points to an important life experience, and the part after "because" points to the problem that's getting in the way.

By now, you've probably come up with several plausible reasons why you *can't do* this or that *because* of your worries, anxieties, and fears (WAFs). These WAFs are barking at you much like a dog might do: WAF ... WAF ... WAF! And when others ask you why you can't do this or that, you may respond with lots of reasons that take this form—because of "WAF ... WAF ... WAF!"

With your WAFs in mind, we'd like you to go back and recall what you wrote down on page 3 when we asked you this:

Because of my anxious thoughts and feelings, strong fear and panic, worry, or disturbing memories, I

have missed out on or am unable to _____

_____.

We can turn this around in the form of a question and a response. We might ask you, "Why can't you do that one important thing in your life?" You might say, "because I might panic or get too anxious, faint, lose control, get hurt, humiliate myself, break down, or act on my disturbing thoughts" (WAF, WAF, WAF!).

In fact, it's common for people struggling with anxiety disorders to give themselves, or others, reasons that point to anxious thoughts and feelings. And many people will go along with what you say to be sympathetic, kind, and supportive. This only solidifies the link between your WAFs and your inability to take action.

The problem here is that you can start believing your "because of" reasons—your own stories: "I can't do _____ because of _____ [my WAFs]." Look at what happens. Like a big, fierce-looking dog, your WAFs have now turned into a barrier that stands in the way of going forward in your life. So, if you can't fly because you might have a panic attack, the only way you'll ever fly is if you can make sure you never panic—WAF!

Reasons that bind with anxiety and fear now become the causes of you being stuck. And when you buy into this story line, which is very easy to do in our culture, you'll be left thinking that the only way to go forward is to take care of the causes: *I must get rid of my WAFs.*

We've already given you a taste of what happens when you buy into thoughts like *Don't be anxious!* We are not about to snip off the opening of your life cocoon either. In the next chapter we'll help you get a better sense of what the struggle to control anxiety and fear has cost you and then help you develop skills to move with your anxiety and fear as a necessary part of a vital life.

LEARNING TO OBSERVE YOUR EXPERIENCE

One of the most courageous things you can do when your WAFs show up is to sit still with them and not do as they say. It's courageous because the impulse to cut and run is so strong and so automatic. Doing nothing about them is the more difficult path. It's important to learn this skill because the urge to act on and through your WAFs greatly diminishes your life. Practicing *mind watching* will teach you to become a true observer of your mind rather than taking and swallowing whatever nasty-looking stuff your mind dishes up for you.

Mind Watching

We know observing your mind filled with WAFs isn't easy. Your mind will be screaming at you to respond as you've done in the past. Through persistent practice, it'll get easier over time to observe and take note of thoughts, images, and urges rather than doing as they say. Here's how you get started.

EXERCISE: MIND WATCHING

Get in a comfortable place where you won't be disturbed for about five to ten minutes. Begin by closing your eyes and taking a series of slow, deep breaths. Keep this up throughout the entire exercise. Imagine your mind is a medium-sized, white room with two doors. Thoughts come in through the front door and leave out the back door. First, watch each thought as it enters. Keep on watching to see what it is doing next. Don't do anything with it. Your only task here is simply to watch the thought.

Simply watch the thought and don't analyze it. Don't engage or argue with it, and don't believe or disbelieve it. Just acknowledge having the thought—that's all; acknowledge it *and* do nothing with it. It can just be a fleeting moment in your mind, a brief visitor in the white room. Keep on watching the thought until it leaves. When it does seem to want to go, let it go and don't try to hold on to it.

If you find that you're judging yourself for having a particular thought, then just notice that. Don't argue with your mind's judgment. Just notice it for what it is and label it: *Thinking—there's thinking*. The key to this exercise is to notice judgmental and other unwanted thoughts rather than getting caught up in them. You'll know if you're getting caught up in them by your emotional reactions and by how long you keep each thought in the room.

Keep breathing … and keep watching. A thought is just a thought. A thought doesn't require you to react; it doesn't make you do anything; it doesn't mean you're less of a person for having it. Again, watch and notice your thoughts and treat them as if they were visitors passing in and out of the white room. Let them have their brief moment on the stage. They're fine the way they are—including the judging thoughts and any other uninvited visitors. The important thing is to let them leave when they're ready to go and then greet and label the next thought … and the next.

Continue this exercise until you sense a real emotional distance from your thoughts. Wait until even the judgments are just a moment in the room—no longer important, no longer requiring action. Practice this exercise at least once a day.

Take Your Mind and Body for a Walk

Another way to learn to be a skillful observer of your thoughts and feelings is to practice moving *with* them instead of *because of* them. To practice doing that, think of taking your mind and body for a walk. Start your practice by literally going outside for a walk, for fifteen minutes or longer, without listening to music.

EXERCISE: MINDFUL WALKING

As you walk, you'll notice that you don't need to think much about what your legs and body do while walking. They seem to go on autopilot. Here, we're going to learn to bring mindful awareness to the experience—probably something you've never done before.

As you begin this activity, focus on your breathing—deeply in and out—as you did with some of the centering exercises we've covered already. Walk naturally and bring your awareness to the rhythm of your steps and how your body feels as it moves. If your mind wanders to other things, just notice that. Then, gently bring your attention back to the experience of walking.

Notice the feel of your feet as they meet the ground with each step. Move your awareness to your hip area—experience how your hips move with each stride. What sensations are there? Then, move further up to your midsection, and allow yourself to feel all the movements there too. See how your body is in perfect rhythm and flow.

Notice how you're moving with your thoughts and feelings too—all of them going forward. Sense the vitality in this movement.

Silently reflect on this mantra as you walk: *I am whole, I am complete, I am in flow.*

Once you finish, allow yourself a few moments to reflect on your experience. What showed up for you as you walked? What was walking like as you became more consciously aware of the experience of walking?

As with any other skill, learning to be an observer takes practice. The more you practice, the easier it will be to catch yourself when you get caught in autopilot, reacting to life rather than being aware of it.

Stay and Ride Out the Storm

When anxiety and fear show up, they can drain away your strongest resolve. It can seem nearly impossible to be inside your own skin and stay where you are. We naturally want to get away from discomfort. The urge to do something can be uncomfortably strong, having the energy and explosive force of an intense storm. This can leave you feeling out of control and frightened.

Still, most storms begin small, way out on the horizon. Some will move in and over you, unleash their energy for a bit. Eventually, they all move on. You can learn to ride out the stormy weather of your urges to struggle and resist your WAFs by learning to ride along with the energy inside—the thunder of your impulses, the lightning of your fear, the relentless uncertainty of your anxiety, or the pounding wind and rain that drives your tendency to cut and run. You can practice just being with it, without letting it blow you away. This next exercise will give you more practice getting in touch with this energy without automatically doing what the urge commands. You'll need about five minutes and a quiet place where you can listen and follow along.

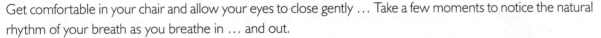

EXERCISE: RIDING THE STORM OUT

Get comfortable in your chair and allow your eyes to close gently … Take a few moments to notice the natural rhythm of your breath as you breathe in … and out.

As you settle, bring to mind a recent situation where you felt the strong urge to cut and run from your fear and anxiety. Take a few slow deep breaths and bring the situation alive in your mind as best you can … Where were you? … Who else was there? … What happened …? What did you experience then and what are you experiencing again right now?

As you bring the situation to mind, you may notice the storm of anxiety or fear rolling in. You can hear the thunder, or even feel the rumble of physical sensations. Notice any stormy physical changes in your body, including pain, pressure, or any other scary sensation that is kicking up and blowing around. There may be lightning strikes of thoughts, perhaps about your sensations and feelings. What's your mind telling you about them? … about the situation? … about you?

Next, bring your attention to the physical experience of the urge to act. Notice the wild energy there, as the pounding rain tries to wash away your resolve and all that you care about … Is there pressure, tightness, or tension? If so, where is it located? Does it have a shape? … a color?

Now, choose to ride the storm out … Imagine opening up, arms wide open, and staying with the wild energy below the surface of your experience. If you can, go ahead and open your arms as wide as you know how. This time you're not doing what you've always done. Look deeply into your experience without trying to fix it, fight it, or suppress it, and without acting on it. Find the pain and hurt driving the storm to new heights … Gently look at it, breathe with it, and bring kindness to it … ride it and let it be. Notice how the storm is trying to throw you off track and push you to act in unhelpful ways … Just stay there, your arms still wide open, bringing kindness and curiosity to the energy and pain, as you would do for a dear friend or loved one who is in pain and needs your help.

See if you can notice as the storm front within you starts to move on. Notice as things begin to quiet down and become still. And, as you rest in that stillness, notice what is new or different for you … See if you can connect with having done something good for yourself … your life … even if you were scared, feeling the strong urge to run or lash out.

As this time for practice comes to an end, acknowledge and honor the step you took with this exercise and commit to practice riding out your difficult urges in the service of your life. When you hear the bell, bring yourself back to the present and slowly open your eyes. Take a moment to reflect on what you've experienced and learned.

After a week or two of practicing mind watching, mindful walking, and riding out difficult urges, you'll be ready to apply the practice wherever you are in your daily life. So, look for ways to approach what you do in a more mindful way. Anything that requires movement could be done mindfully. You could even practice being more mindful as you do household chores like cooking, vacuuming, washing the dishes, cleaning, doing laundry, running errands, or with hobbies you enjoy. In truth, anything you do, including simply sitting and doing nothing at all as you ride out a WAF storm, is an opportunity to practice being mindful and present just as you are.

The point here is to practice being mindful of the experience of movement with your thoughts, feelings, and sensations. In fact, you can put a note in your pocket or purse or set an alarm to beep every hour as a reminder to simply notice your experience just as it is.

LIFE ENHANCEMENT EXERCISES

Many exercises covered so far aim to cut the fuel source feeding the destructive power of your anxieties and fears. These are skills that take practice. So, for this week, we invite you to do the following:

- Commit to making a centering exercise part of your daily routine.

- Practice mind watching, mindful walking, and riding the storm out.

- Remember that your breath is always with you—come back to it.

- If you haven't been doing this already, slow the pace down and work with the workbook so that it will work for you!

THE TAKE-HOME MESSAGE

Recognizing how mind traps keep you stuck is an important skill. It's a critical step out of the struggle-and-avoidance trap. You can get something different out of your life if you're willing to learn to relate with your mind, body, and feelings in a different way. This is a choice only you can make. We hope that you make it now and act on that intention as you continue working with the material in this book.

Mind Traps Keep Me Stuck

Point to Ponder: The mind traps that keep me stuck and feed my struggle with anxiety must be seen clearly and acknowledged. This is an important step out of the anxiety trap and into my life.

Questions to Consider: Can I learn to watch my mind rather than be jerked around by it? Am I willing to stop feeding my fear and anxiety wolves? Am I willing to face what buying in to my raucous and judgmental mind has cost me?

PART 2

STARTING A NEW JOURNEY

How strange that the nature of life is change,
yet the nature of human beings is to resist change.
And how ironic that the difficult times we fear might ruin us
are the very ones that can break us open
and help us blossom into who we were meant to be.

—Elizabeth Lesser

CHAPTER 6

Facing the Costs to Take Charge of Your Life

For a long time it had seemed to me that life was about to begin—real life. But there was always some obstacle in the way, something to be gotten through first, some unfinished business, time still to be served, a debt to be paid. Then life would begin. At last it dawned on me that these obstacles were my life.

—Alfred D'Souza

Life invites obstacles, problems, and pain. There is no escaping this simple truth. All human beings on this planet will confront this truth at some point in their lifetime, often many times over. The challenge is to find a way forward when pain and difficulty seem to block our path and drain our resolve. Moving forward requires us to pause and take stock, and look deeply at what our lives have become. Now is that time.

As Alfred D'Souza teaches us, we can literally squander our lives by living life in the service of dealing with obstacles. His awakening came only after he became willing to take a hard look at what he was doing and what he had become. Now it's your turn.

You have your anxiety obstacles. And, you have the real life you wish you could lead. It's time to wake up to what your struggle with anxiety has cost you before it's too late. Now—this very moment—

is your time to take stock and look clearly at where you've been, what you've become, and where you want to go. It's time to face the costs of waiting and struggling with your anxiety obstacles. It's time for your life to begin—finally.

This is an important moment. We all have a finite amount of time on this earth. And many of us plow through each day on autopilot, never stopping to take a good, hard look at what we're spending our time doing or asking: *Is this truly what I want to be about?*

Here we'll be asking you to face squarely the costs of your battles with anxiety. Some of this may be painful for you to do. Yet it's vitally important that you do it.

So long as you hold on to old ways of solving your anxiety problems, you'll end up exactly where you are now. And if you continue to treat your WAFs as obstacles standing between you and your life, you'll naturally spend your time and energy trying to figure out ways to conquer them. In short, you'll continue to get what you've always got—more suffering. WAF struggles will be your life!

As you fully, openly, and honestly engage in this process, you'll see how you're attaching importance to activities and experiences that don't serve you well and that keep you stuck. This may be painful, but there's a sober vitality—or a wakefulness—to this kind of pain that you may not have experienced before.

Roger von Oech (1998), in his wonderful little book called *A Whack on the Side of the Head*, likens the path of growth and creative change to a visit to a junkyard. As you know, a junkyard is a place where you'll find lots of stuff. But everything you'll find in that junkyard was once precious and valuable to someone. Looked at in this way, a visit to a junkyard can be a sobering experience, because it's there that we see the final destination of almost everything we once desired and were attached to.

You've certainly had precious things that have long since gone into the dumpster. You also have ideas about what needs to be done to get out from under your WAFs. And you've probably attached a great deal of importance to overcoming your WAFs so that your life can truly begin. These strategies are, in a way, precious and valuable to you. After all, your life seems to depend on finding a solution—and each new strategy seems to promise a solution. But you need to ask yourself if that's really so. Have the ways you've dealt with anxiety really worked? Are you free of anxiety? Are you living your life wholeheartedly? If not, maybe now is the time to let go of those WAF coping strategies and put them in the junkyard.

You've reached this moment—reading this book—because you want to be about more than your WAFs. More deeply, you are here because you're still struggling in some way with anxiety and fear. What needs to happen now is for you to wake up to what you and your life have become because of your battles with anxiety. Then you can take a stand and decide that you no longer want to be about that. This is a choice only you can make. We hope that when you reach the end of this chapter, you'll be willing to make that choice.

COSTS OF ANXIETY MANAGEMENT

Struggle with anxiety has cost you—in the coin of energy, time, deep and painful regret, missed opportunities, lost moments, financial burden, restricted freedom, relationships that might have been, and damaged or strained relationships with those with whom you have the closest bonds. Deep down you probably know that your best efforts at anxiety control haven't worked as intended. This failure at control has left a deep mark on you.

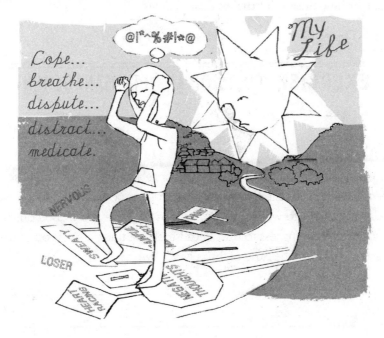

This is a good starting point. The difficult work is facing how you've struggled with anxiety and how that struggle has cost you in the various areas of your life. Remember the sobering process of wading through a junkyard.

Have you experienced broken and strained relationships, sickness and poor health, excessive stress, difficulties at school or work, poor concentration, or problems with alcohol or other substances? Or, in a more general way, have you lost any sense of freedom? Do you feel that you're unable to do what you care about because the WAFs seem to stand in the way? There may also be other less obvious costs or those you prefer not to think about.

The following Costs of Anxiety Management exercise can help you get a better sense of the costs linked with your WAF struggles. This will also give you a clear idea of what you've missed out on by responding to your WAFs with struggle and avoidance behavior.

You'll see that we're asking you to look at your personal experience with worry, anxiety, and fear across various life areas. Nobody is more of an expert about your experience than you. So as you wade through this exercise, gently remind yourself of this fact.

If your mind wanders, you can return to the spirit of the exercise by asking yourself this: *What does my experience tell me about the costs of WAF struggle?*

Are you willing to get started? If so, then use the lines below (or the downloadable version of this exercise, available at http://www.newharbinger.com/33346) to address some of the questions in each life area. An example of how Susan did the exercise follows.

EXERCISE: COSTS OF ANXIETY MANAGEMENT

1. Interpersonal costs

Summarize the effects of struggling with your WAFs on your relationships. Have friendships changed or been lost? Have family members been alienated? Do they avoid you, or do you avoid them? Have you lost a marriage or romantic relationship due to worry, anxiety, or fear? Or have you missed out on new social bonds because of fear, dread, or an unwillingness to trust because of past trauma? Are you unable to engage in your roles as a spouse, partner, or parent because of those pesky WAFs?

_____

_____

2. Career costs

Summarize the effects of struggling with anxiety on your career. Have you ever quit or been fired from a job because of attempts to get a handle on your anxiety and fear? This includes being late, being less productive, missing days of work, being unable to travel, avoiding tasks where WAFs might show up, skipping out on business and social interactions with colleagues and customers, or procrastination. Has a boss or have coworkers commented on your poor performance because of your anxiety management efforts? Have those efforts affected your school career (relationships with teachers, administrators)? Have they resulted in unemployment or being on disability or welfare?

_____

_____

3. Health costs

Describe the effects of managing your worry, anxiety, and fear on your health. Do you tend to get sick often? Do you have difficulties falling asleep and staying asleep? Do you sometimes ruminate and stew over anxiety and worry to the point of feeling sick or keyed up? Do you avoid taking care of your health because of your WAFs (e.g., avoid going to the doctor, having tests done, visiting a dentist)? Do you avoid exercise because it might bring on your WAFs? Have you spent quite a bit of time in the doctor's office or emergency room for your WAFs?

_____

_____

4. Energy costs

Outline how managing your anxiety has affected your energy. Do those efforts sometimes exhaust you? Have you put time and energy into disappointing efforts at WAF control? Are you often engaged in mental planning and fact finding in an effort to ward off or minimize your WAFs? Do you waste mental energy on worry, stress, fretting over distractions, checking, and negative thinking? Have you experienced difficulties with memory or concentration? Are you constantly reliving painful moments from your past, or feeling trapped in the doom and gloom your mind feeds you about the future? Do you spend needless time checking or performing rituals to feel more comfortable or to ward off catastrophe? Have your attempts to manage anxiety left you feeling discouraged, fatigued, frustrated, or worn out?

_____

_____

5. Emotional costs

What have efforts to get a handle on anxiety cost you emotionally? Do you feel sad or depressed about your WAFs? Have you tended to be on edge, perhaps exploding in anger in times of stress? Do you carry regrets and guilt because of what you have done or failed to do as a result of your WAFs? How do regrets about your WAF episodes affect you emotionally? Do you feel depressed or hopeless when your efforts to control anxiety aren't working? Do you feel as though life is passing you by?

_____

_____

6. Financial costs

How much money have you spent on managing your WAFs? Consider money you've spent on psychotherapy for your WAFs and related difficulties (e.g., depression, anger, alcoholism). How about the cost of medications, doctor's visits, anxiety books, audio or video recordings, or seminars? See if you can come up with a reasonable estimate of these monetary costs. You can include costs due to disability, lost wages, expenses related to missing important and enjoyable events (e.g., concerts, plane trips, dinners out), and missed work because of your WAFs too.

_____

_____

7. Costs to freedom

How have your efforts to control WAFs limited your ability to do what you enjoy and want to do? Can you drive near and far, with or without others? Can you shop, take a train or plane, or go for a walk in your neighborhood, the park, a mall, or a forest? Do the WAFs keep you from trying new foods, new activities, new forms of recreation, experiencing your dreams, and doing what you care about? Is your day arranged around avoiding feeling anxious, panicky, or afraid?

_____

_____

The Example of Susan

Here's how Susan, an office assistant, completed her Costs of Anxiety Management exercise:

1. Interpersonal costs

Few friends. Avoid making eye contact. I'd like to enjoy stimulating conversation but find myself too busy worrying about how awkward I am. I've avoided being intimate. I don't go to parties, large gatherings, and haven't been to the beach or a movie in some time. Always make up excuses about why I can't do something fun with people. I am a people pleaser ... always putting the needs of others before my own. I feel like I'm living in a shell. I'm turning into a real loner.

2. Career costs

Dropped out of college because I couldn't get my anxiety under control. Lost my previous job because I wouldn't drive long distances for business. My current work is only fifteen minutes from my house, but it takes me almost an hour to get there because I can't take the bridge. Just called in sick again because I'm having a shitty start to my day. Attending staff meetings is difficult, and I make up excuses for not going. Can't seem to get things done on time because I'm a perfectionist and worry that my work is not up to snuff. My boss has warned me about this.

3. Health costs

Constant tension. Getting sick a lot. I've been to several doctors and the emergency room, had EKGs, hormonal tests, chest X-rays, and saw a GI specialist. I've started to drink more booze to get my mind off my anxiety and panic, to the point of getting sick. Now my panic seems worse. I wonder if I have a drinking problem. The dentist is one of my big anxiety/panic buttons too—haven't been in for a checkup in ten years. I don't sleep well or digest food—upset stomach, feeling bloated. I've stopped exercising—the physical sensations are too much. Getting fatter too.

4. Energy costs

Getting a handle on anxiety is one big, constant challenge. I'm exhausted all the time—not just at night but also in the morning—must be all that tension. I try to stay busy to keep my mind from wondering when I'll have another panic attack. I can't concentrate and am easily forgetful because I'm always thinking about losing it, getting too anxious, or even having another panic attack. I can't seem to get a handle on my anxiety and I kick myself for being so out of control. I'm tired of not being able to enjoy life.

5. Emotional costs

Loneliness—my few friends have told me that I'm the biggest glass-half-empty person they know. Depression, disappointment, things aren't turning out, and all that shit. It feels like I have a noose around my neck, or I'm about to pop. Not going places because I feel "shaky," leaving food untouched in a restaurant because my stomach is upset from feeling shaky, lying to people about what's wrong because I'm afraid that the few people who love me will finally leave me and go find someone who isn't "broken." Feel like an angry nag—arguing more with my husband and yelling at my kids over little things. I really fear screwing up my kids and marriage.

6. Financial costs

I've been on a half-dozen anxiety medications (and still am on a few) … about a year of psychotherapy … and have bought a number of books. Bought several herbal remedies too. None of this has really worked. Counting all the tests and doctor and emergency room visits, I've probably spent close to $10,000 trying to kick this. This doesn't even include missed days at work, lost college tuition, and sick leave … Shit, if I add all that in, then the figure is more like $20,000. Sad really. I could think of so many other ways to spend that kind of money.

7. Costs to freedom

Basically anxiety is completely controlling me. I feel like I have no life—like I'm disabled. My buttle with anxiety and panic attacks has become a daily challenge. I can't go out to restaurants or to movies. Because I can't wait in lines at the grocery, I have to shop really early in the morning or late in the evening. I "rush" through the grocery store, and I REFUSE to go to the mall. I pretty much stay in my comfort zone, only going to the places I "know." I can't go to church or watch my children in their school plays. Missed my oldest daughter's graduation from college. I'd like to socialize at work but just can't do it. I'm just barely holding it together at my current job. I can't even take a family vacation beyond my backyard. Unfamiliar or new situations are out of the picture. Flying, buses, and trains are out too. I feel stuck—like I'm trapped in a time warp doing the same old things over and over. My kids are suffering too, and this really hurts me.

Completing your Costs of Anxiety Management exercise is a crucial first step in honestly facing how your WAFs have damaged your life and continue to do so. But it has a further purpose. It's important that you recognize and actually feel the effects of your WAFs despite all your efforts to change. When you do that, you position yourself to do something differently. So let's start there.

WHAT HAVE YOU BEEN DOING ABOUT YOUR WAFS?

In the previous exercise you faced the costs associated with managing your WAFs in some important areas of your life. We've hinted at what makes them costly for you. Now we'd like to come out and say it more boldly. The costs have little to do with your WAFs. The costs have everything to do with what you're doing *about* your WAFs.

Anxiety Manager at WAFs "R" Us

You may feel like you've been forced into a new job for WAFs "R" Us. You don't necessarily want this job, but there you are—promoted—the new anxiety manager. This job, of course, is a full-time position, meaning 24/7 with no breaks.

The position requires that you engage in your life fully while keeping your WAFs at bay. Sounds simple, right? You've got the tools at your disposal—your mind and your capacity to avoid. You're pretty good at figuring out when and where you might have the WAFs—your mind has this down—and so you plan, strategize, and the like to avoid these situations.

Sometimes you get caught off guard, but then you know that you can opt for other tools, perhaps distraction, being with safe others, breathing your way out of it, medications, disputing those unsettling thoughts, or the tried-and-true cut-and-run response—escape.

You're doing reasonably well at your job as far as the WAFs are concerned. True, they still show up and bite you now and then, but you're able to quell the storm enough so that you don't lose your job. The problem, though, is that you aren't fulfilling the other more critical aspect of your job description—engaging your life fully and moving toward your dreams.

You aren't able to do that because the other part of your job at WAFs "R" Us takes so much time and effort. Every time you try to do something you care about, you risk the old WAFs showing up. And your experience probably tells you that many things you do care about in life are linked with the WAFs. So when you stop doing what you care about to get a handle on the WAFs, you end up stuck in a funk.

Here's another way to look at your situation. Your employer at WAFs "R" Us is your mind, and it isn't serving you well here. It's given you a job description—just avoid your WAFs at all costs—that cannot be carried out without major costs in other areas of your life. In fact, there's no way to avoid your WAFs without also avoiding what you care about. So you get the pain of the WAFs now and then, and on top of that, your life is shrinking around you—and this shrinkage just adds more pain. You realize that this job may not be for you.

There's another option. This option involves a change in emphasis and a choice. Taking this route means that you choose to do what you care about, even if that guarantees you'll experience WAFs now and then. There will probably be some pain. Yet with that pain you'll get vitality that comes with being liberated from being a prisoner to your WAFs. You'll be living.

Right now, you don't need to decide whether any of this makes sense. In fact, we're pretty certain that your mind is dishing out all kinds of reasons why this stuff doesn't apply to you. Don't argue with your mind now, and instead ponder two questions:

1. Have your WAF management strategies made you less anxious *and* happier with life?

2. Has being an anxiety manager moved you in directions you want your life to take?

Below, we're going to help you make contact with what you've done about your WAFs and how well the struggle for control has worked for you. You need to feel this in your heart and not just understand it in your mind.

Why might this be? The simple and honest answer is that we don't want you to go about doing more of the same, especially when old WAF management strategies haven't worked for you. Successful anxiety transformation begins with facing—openly and honestly—each WAF management attempt, each past strategy, and then looking to see how it has worked and what it has cost you. This isn't easy, which is why we have designed an exercise to help you identify clearly what hasn't worked.

Taking Stock of Your Anxiety Management History

Right now, we'd like you to look back over the last month at your attempts to manage and control your WAFs. The following exercise will help you organize your memories across different situations and relationships.

EXERCISE: WHAT HAVE I GIVEN UP FOR ANXIETY IN THE LAST MONTH?

The purpose of completing this exercise is to let you examine how costly managing your anxiety is for you. Think about your life—all the things (big and small) you care about and want to do.

As you go through this exercise, ask yourself what you have given up in order to manage, reduce, and avoid your WAFs in the past month. What opportunities to do things that you like or that matter to you have you traded in to control and manage anxiety? Over the past month, what have you missed out on in the service of WAF management and control?

In the first column, record each situation or event that triggered your anxiety, panic, concerns, or worries. In the second column, write down your anxiety, bodily sensations, thoughts, concerns, or worries. In the third column, record what you did to manage your anxiety—your coping or management strategy. In the fourth column, record what effect your efforts to control or reduce your anxiety had on you. For instance, how did you feel afterward? In the fifth and final column, write down the consequences and costs associated with your efforts to manage your anxiety. What did you give up or miss out on?

Situation/Event	Anxiety/Concern	Anxiety Coping Behavior	Effect on You	Costs
Example 1: Was invited to go out with some friends.	Example 1: Fear of people judging me; was afraid of doing something stupid and embarrassing.	Example 1: Told my friend I was feeling sick; stayed at home and watched TV.	Example 1: Felt safer for a bit, but then lonely, sad, and angry with myself for being so weak.	Example 1: Lost out on good time with my friends; missed an opportunity to deepen friendships.
Example 2: Was about to get on a plane with my wife and kids for a business meeting and short vacation.	Example 2: Was afraid of freaking out on the plane, having a panic attack, going crazy, being hauled off the plane in a stretcher, making a fool of myself.	Example 2: Got on the plane, but then my heart started pounding and I felt claustrophobic. So, I got up and told the stewardess that we would be getting off the plane. We didn't take the trip.	Example 2: Relief once I told the stewardess we were leaving, but then felt terrible and sad; disappointed in myself; embarrassed in front of my family.	Example 2: Missed an important business trip; missed what would have been a fun time with family; shame at hearing my four-year-old son say, "Daddy ruined our trip"—he really wanted to fly in a plane; depression; loss of freedom.

Taking Stock of Your Coping Strategies

After completing this exercise, we'd like you to take stock of what you've learned. Have your efforts to control your WAFs worked? Have they increased your vitality and ability to engage in life to the fullest? Or have your WAFs simply returned again and again, crippling your life, and leaving you feeling stuck and hopeless?

If you're like a lot of people with anxiety problems, nothing you've done to control anxiety has really worked. You keep doing things you regret. You keep missing out on potentially vital life experiences. And you keep trading in more and more of your life flexibility in an effort to get a foothold. All the while, your life is slowly ticking by. What does your heart, your gut, tell you about your history with anxiety? What does your experience tell you about your response to your WAFs? Take a moment to take stock.

Anxiety and fear are powerful feelings that can sweep away your strongest resolve. Despite your best efforts to manage and control your WAFs, you still have the costs. You keep feeling bad about yourself. You keep doing things to avoid situations that trigger your anxiety. You want to change, but no amount of remorse or trying seems to stem the force of the WAFs when they show up.

You may wonder if you've got what it takes. You may think that you just have to try harder and apply more willpower. Check your experience and see if your mind is giving you good advice here. Haven't you gone down that road—perhaps even more than once? We suspect you have. And if this is true of your experience, then spending more of your time on Try-Harder Street, Effort Lane, or at the corner of Coping Avenue and More Willpower Boulevard isn't the solution.

How Have Your Coping Strategies Worked?

Each moment you spend struggling with your WAFs is a moment taken away from something you want in your life. What keeps this going and why doesn't it work? As we've said, it all boils down to avoidance of your WAFs. This avoidance, more than anything else, is what keeps you stuck, feeling that your life is shrinking around you. You probably keep doing it because avoidance buys you short-term emotional relief. But you suffer long-term costs to your life and freedom.

EXERCISE: ANXIETY MANAGEMENT COST-BENEFIT ANALYSIS

This brief exercise will help you connect with some of the short- and long-term benefits and costs of your WAF management efforts. To do this exercise, go back to the previous one and list each of your coping strategies. Note that some of them might also include less obvious ones, like therapy, use of alcohol, self-help, and anything you might think of that seems to be focused on avoiding, reducing, or getting away from your WAFs. Take your time with this.

As you do the exercise, watch for strategies that don't work in the long run and that tend to get in the way of you doing what matters to you in the short run. Don't be concerned about strategies that seem to work in a lasting way, or that don't interfere with your life.

Making the distinction between what works and what doesn't work can be tricky. Here's why: your mind may tell you the strategy works and doesn't interfere with your life. Yet, you ought to ask your mind, *What would I be doing with my mental and physical energy if I weren't spending it coping with my WAFs?* If you answer this question openly and honestly, then you'll likely come up with other activities that are new or potentially more important and interesting to you than successful WAF management.

Here's how Alice, a twenty-four-year-old college student, completed some of her cost-benefit analysis. We include her responses below as an example for you when doing the remaining parts.

WAF Coping Strategy	Costs		Benefits	
	Short-Term	Long-Term	Short-Term	Long-Term
Avoiding crowds	Can't go clothes shopping at the mall; feel bad about that	Keeps me out of many fun activities, like music, social events, movies; feel like a loser	I feel less anxious.	Nothing comes to mind.
Distraction	Can't focus on much else; tend to miss important details	Becoming more forgetful; others describe me as distant, like I'm in another world	Keeps my mind off my anxiety; anxiety tends to go down, but not always	Nothing

When Alice was finished, she noticed that most of the benefits she experienced had nothing to do with things she cared about in her life. They were all about buying herself some relief. And most of this relief was only fleeting.

She also spotted many costs and no long-term benefits to her anxiety management efforts. In fact, she suggested that we consider deleting the long-term benefits column. We haven't done so because we believe that you need to find out for yourself whether anxiety management and control buys you anything good in the long run. Go ahead and find out.

PAUSING IN THE NOW

We know that working with the material in this chapter can be quite heavy. It's hard to face the barriers, let alone the costs. But it is important not to lose sight of why we're inviting you to do this. This isn't some subtle manipulation exercise. It's also not about making you feel bad about yourself. No. Contacting the costs is about finding what works and seeing clearly what does not serve you well. Unless you do that, you'll continue to repeat what you've always done.

Before we wrap up, we'd like to invite you to do another brief centering exercise. Remember that there's no right or wrong way to do this exercise. Just follow along as best you can.

EXERCISE: WEAKENING THE BLOCKING POWER OF BARRIERS

Go ahead and get in a comfortable position in your chair. Sit upright with your feet flat on the floor, your arms and legs uncrossed, and your hands resting in your lap. Allow your eyes to close gently. Take a couple of gentle breaths: in … and out … in … and out. Notice the sound and feel of your own breath as you breathe in … and out.

Now turn your attention to being just where you are. Just being. There's nothing to do but be in this moment, resting in an awareness of your breath as you breathe in … and out. Allow the sense of just being as you are to wash over you like a warm summer breeze.

When you're ready, expand your awareness just a bit and make contact with why you're here, working with this program. Notice the investment you're making in your life. Become aware that many other people, just like you, are also making similar investments in their own lives. Notice that you are not alone in this. What you're doing in this moment is an act of courage, integrity, and self-love. This courageous act of yours is united with many other people from all walks of life who are doing the same.

Notice any doubts, reservations, fears, and worries. You don't need to make them go away or work on them. With each breath, imagine that you are creating more and more space for them, more space for you to be you, right here where you are.

Now see if for just a moment you can be present with any anxiety barriers that come to mind. If your instinct is to struggle with them, just notice that, without getting tangled up in the struggle. See if you can allow those thoughts, and other aspects of your experience, to just be. Open your heart to them, and as much as you can, welcome them as part of your experience.

And as we get ready to close this centering exercise, gently ask yourself this: Am I willing to learn how to change my relationship with my barriers and accept them as part of myself? And, are my life and my values important enough to me to be willing to do this now and perhaps again and again?

Then, when you are ready, gradually widen your attention to take in the sounds around you and slowly open your eyes with the intention to bring this awareness of just being as you are to the present moment and the rest of the day.

LIFE ENHANCEMENT EXERCISES

For this week, we recommend that you do the following:

- Commit to making a centering exercise part of your daily routine.

- Continue to practice exercises we covered early, especially ones that resonate with you.

- Don't rush through this chapter—give yourself time to fully lay out the costs of all the things you do to manage your WAFs.

- Remember that small changes, including all the work you've done with this workbook so far, will add up. You just don't know where it will take you. And that's okay.

THE TAKE-HOME MESSAGE

You likely opened this book with the hope of finding a better way to manage and control your WAFs so that you can get on with living your life the way you wish. This makes sense so long as you, just like so many anxiety sufferers, continue to see your WAFs as *the problem*.

Our intention in this chapter was to help you connect with another possibility, however hard that may be for you to wrap your head around at the moment. That possibility is this: Everything you've done and continue to do about your WAFs has cost you much more than the WAFs themselves. The struggle itself is a trap, one that will ensnare you when you actively resist and avoid your own experience. We'll show you a way out.

Assessing the Costs of My WAF Struggles to Take Back My Life

Point to Ponder: Life is a journey, not a destination. It is built one small step at a time by what I do. Managing anxiety has cost me dearly.

Questions to Consider: What have I given up as a consequence of managing my WAFs? What has cost me more—the WAFs themselves *or* all my efforts to control and avoid them? How have those efforts impacted my life? What would I do with my time and energy if it were not spent trying to manage anxiety, fear, unsettling thoughts, memories, and the like?

CHAPTER 7

What Matters More to You: Managing Anxiety or Living a Good Life?

We look for happiness in all the wrong places. Like a moth flying into the flame, we destroy ourselves in order to find temporary relief. Because we often find such relief, we continue to reinforce old patterns of suffering and strengthen dysfunctional patterns in the process.

—Pema Chödrön

What matters to you? This is one of the most profound questions we'll ask you to consider and reconsider throughout this book and for the rest of your life. Most people don't think about it until it's too late to do something about it. We don't want to see that happen to you.

Here we're going to walk you through two exercises that'll help you connect with what you want to be about in this life: a funeral meditation (adapted from Hayes et al., 2012) and writing your own epitaph. These exercises are very powerful and even a bit frightening. The payoff for doing them is a clearer vision of what you want your life to stand for. The exercises also reveal what struggling with WAFs has cost you.

We all know that death is inevitable. Sometimes we can delay death, but we can't avoid it. Although we can't control when or how we'll die, we can control how we live from this day forward. We know from firsthand accounts that something profound happens when people have been near death and have survived to live another day. Their lives change in dramatic ways.

Facing death forces people to take stock. And when they do that, many people end up radically changing what they've been doing and begin spending more time doing things they really care about. Old habits and activities that once seemed so important become trivial.

In short, contacting the precipice between life and death wakes people up. Something clicks. People change what they do and how they live in ways that are richer and more vital and meaningful than before. They make a choice to spend their remaining time on this planet doing things that matter. These activities are what they (and you) will be remembered for. The following exercise will help you make contact with this simple truth in a deeper way.

EXERCISE: FUNERAL MEDITATION

Go ahead and get comfortable. Imagine that you're observing your own funeral. Visualize yourself in an open casket. Smell the fresh flowers. Hear the soft music in the background. Look around the room. Who do you see?

Perhaps you can see your loved ones, family, friends, relatives, coworkers, and people you've met at one time or another. Listen closely to the conversations and what they're saying about you. What's your partner saying … your kids … your best friend … your colleagues … your neighbor?

Listen carefully to each of them as they say the words that, in your heart, you most want to hear about yourself. This is how you want the people that you care about to remember you. Your wisdom will let you pick and choose exactly what you want and need to hear from them.

Now just pause for a moment and keep imagining this situation. Go ahead, sit back, and close your eyes. Stay with this image for a few minutes. Then come back to reading.

Remember the comments you heard. In your heart of hearts, what did you want to hear about your life? Take a moment and jot down what you heard and wanted to hear said about you in the lines below.

What I heard people say about me was …

_____

_____

_____

What I wanted to hear people say about me was …

_____

_____

_____

There's something critically important in what you heard and wrote down a moment ago: each utterance reflects your values and gives you an idea of what you really want your life to be about. And what you heard others say about you was based on what they see you doing. Some of what you heard may have left you feeling disappointed. Perhaps one person said, "He was always so anxious and uptight … I wish he'd done more with his life" or "She had a tough life, never getting past her fears and worries."

The good news about this exercise is that your life isn't over yet. Your eulogies haven't been written. You still have time to do things to be the type of person you want to be. You can start living the way you want to be remembered later on.

There's another reason for doing this exercise. This reason is more practical and has to do with gaining perspective on your life and your actions. You won't be able to see the costs of the anxiety struggle in your life unless you can see what you want to be about. Anxiety is costly precisely because it gets in the way of what you want to do. If this weren't so, you wouldn't be reading this book. You'd be just like the millions of other people who have their share of WAFs, along with other sources of hardship and pain, and yet march on doing what matters to them.

The next exercise builds on the previous one. It'll help you to connect with what you truly care about in life and where you'd go if your WAFs weren't ruling the roost.

This may seem like another strange and somewhat scary exercise. If you stick with it and complete it and feel a bit upset, then you'll get in touch with what you want your life to stand for. So don't rush. Find a quiet place to reflect, openly and honestly, about what it is that makes your life worthwhile. If you need to do this exercise in several sittings, then do that.

EXERCISE: MY ANXIETY MANAGEMENT EPITAPH

Your task in this exercise is to write your epitaph (the inscription on your gravestone) as it would be written if you were to die today. What would it say if it was about what you've been doing with your anxiety management? What have you become by living in the service of your WAFs? Bring to mind all of your WAF coping-and-management strategies and be mindful of how they've gotten in the way of what you want to do. Think of everything you say aloud, think to yourself, or do with your hands or feet before, during, or after the WAFs show up to keep them at bay. List them all.

Here is what Joan, a woman with a fifteen-year history of struggle with panic, wrote for her Anxiety Management Epitaph.

HERE LIES

Joan Parker

Spent last 8 years homebound for fear of panic.

Avoided crowds, unfamiliar places, and driving.

Unable to work and had few friends.

Hadn't gone to the beach or mountains for decades.

Spent all her time working on her anxiety problems.

Now, when you're ready, go ahead and write your Anxiety Management Epitaph. Print a copy of the blank tombstone from the workbook companion website (http://www.newharbinger.com/33346) and work off that. Make it realistic by putting down your actual full name, and use short phrases, as Joan did, or bullet points.

The exercises up until now were probably difficult to do. We asked you to face squarely what your life has become in the service of anxiety and its management. The next exercise ought to be more uplifting.

We'd like you to do another epitaph-writing exercise, but with a twist. This time, write your epitaph as you'd really like it to read, without the stains of anxiety and fear having taken up all of your time and energy. You can think of this epitaph as representing the things you truly care about and wish to be known for. Rather than your Anxiety Management Epitaph, this is your Valued Life Epitaph!

EXERCISE: MY VALUED LIFE EPITAPH

Imagine that you could live your life free of any worry, anxiety, or fear. Wouldn't that be something? What would you do? What would you want to be about?

As you connect with this, imagine that one day the headstone in the drawing that follows will be on your grave. Notice that the headstone is blank. Your epitaph (words describing your life) hasn't been written. What inscription would you like to see on your headstone?

Think of a phrase or series of brief statements that would capture the essence of the life you want to lead. What is it you want to be remembered for? If you could somehow live your life without WAFs looming over your head, what would you be doing with your time and energy?

Give yourself some time to think about these really important questions. If you find an answer—or more than one—just write them down on the lines on "your" headstone. Think big. There are no limits to what you can be remembered for.

This isn't a hypothetical exercise. What you'll be remembered for, what defines your life, is up to you. It depends on what you do now. It depends on the actions you take. This is how you determine the wording of your epitaph.

Now, we make no promises that people will build a Lincoln-type memorial for you at the end of your life. Yet if you persistently move in your valued directions, chances are that people will write things on your tombstone other than "Here lies Tom: he devoted his life to coping with his fears" or "Here lies Mary: she spent most of her life struggling with panic."

When you're finished, compare your Valued Life Epitaph with your Anxiety Management Epitaph. If you need to, print copies of the worksheets for both exercises from the website and then transcribe what you wrote for each exercise. Next, place each epitaph side by side in front of you and really look at them carefully. As you read each of them again, ask yourself the following questions (in no particular order):

> *People will know you by what they see you do, not by what you think and feel about what you do.*

- What epitaph do you want to be known for?

- Which one is more vital to you?

- What epitaph best fits your life now?

- Is your life about anxiety management or life management?

- Are your WAF monsters ruling the roost? And is this what you want to be about?

- What have you become in the service of your WAFs?

- Are you living better?

- Must you be free of WAFs to live the life you want?

We understand that getting a handle on anxiety is important to you. Then again, would you really like your tombstone to read, "Here lies Harry: he finally got rid of his anxiety disorder"? If that inscription doesn't excite you, we can tell you that you're not alone. We've done this exercise with many people just like you. And we've never seen anyone write something like that.

What does it mean that people never mention WAFs in eulogies and on tombstones? Perhaps getting rid of your WAFs—a goal you've been working so hard to achieve—isn't going to matter much in the grand scheme of things. Think of it this way: every sixty seconds you spend trying to get a handle on your WAFs is a minute away from doing something that matters to you.

In short, the WAF struggle pulls you out of your life. If you're not doing things to be the type of person you want to be, *now* is the time to live the life you want and do the things that are most important to you. To start doing that, you'll need to make a choice to do something radically different than you've been doing up until now.

TAKE STOCK OF THE TIME YOU DO HAVE

Earlier, we walked you through an exercise where we asked you to imagine your life as a book. Some of it is already written, covering everything you've lived through up to this point. But much of it has yet to be written. You don't know when it will end and how. Yet even with that awareness, you may still be thinking you'll always have more time. There's always a tomorrow, another day, for your life to really begin. But that tomorrow may never come. You don't know, but you act as if you do. This too is a trap and a great setup for procrastination, for putting off living your life.

Right now, you can estimate how much time you have left on this planet. Not long ago at a training retreat, both of us introduced this exercise and did it ourselves. It was a huge eye opener and an experience that strengthened our resolve to make the most of the time that we do have.

Now, we invite you to do the same. The exercise is simple and requires a bit of math and a calculator. At the end of this exercise, you'll end up with an estimate of the number of days you do have left on this planet and be positioned to ask yourself, *How do I want to use the time I have left?*

Estimates by the World Health Organization (2015) suggest that the average life expectancy is about eighty years in the United States and a bit higher in some other Western countries around the world, based on data from 2013. Though we know that women tend to have a longer life expectancy than men, to keep this exercise simple, we'll assume that we all have about eighty years on this planet, or approximately 29,200 days to live our lives.

Now, go ahead and calculate how many days you've already lived by multiplying your current age in years by 365. After you get that number, subtract it from 29,200. This new number is an estimate of the number of days you likely have left to live.

What number did you come up with? This number may be alarming to face, but it is important that you do so. It reflects the time you likely have to write the story of your life from this point forward. So, we'll ask you once more, "How do you want to use the time that you have left?" This is a choice that you can make and something you can control.

I'M STUCK AND AT MY WIT'S END—NOW WHAT?

This is a watershed moment. There's a lesson here that can change your life. Knowing in your mind and heart—with absolute certainty—that the things you've done because of anxiety don't work is the first step on a new road.

Admitting and accepting that your WAFs are stronger than your efforts to stop them creates a paradoxical new freedom. You can do something new—because all the old, tried-and-true ways to cope aren't working and will not work. But how?

It starts with acknowledging that your experience is your best guide. What does your experience with your WAFs tell you? Go ahead and look back at your responses to the earlier exercises. The situation probably looks hopeless, and the old ways really are hopeless. All the ways you've dealt with anxiety up until now have gotten you to this place where you feel stuck.

Doing something radically new is hopeful. For in doing something new, you risk getting something new. To get that kind of hope, you must first *give up on and stop all the old WAF management-and-control efforts*. They haven't worked in the past and will not work in the future.

Everything you'll learn here rests on this understanding: All the old strategies for *managing* worry, anxiety, and fear lead to a dead end. They hurt you. This is why you need to stop them. Your mind will tell you otherwise, so you need to look to your experience here for guidance. It's time to let go of old, unworkable strategies. We know this sounds easier said than done, so we'll talk more about that at the beginning of the next chapter.

EXERCISE: ENHANCE YOUR LIFE WITH THE LIFE WORKSHEET

We've said that this book is about something much bigger than your WAFs. That "something" is your life and nurturing your capacity to live it, each and every day, without getting bogged down in the snares of your judgmental mind and the needless struggle with your emotional mind and body.

To help you, you'll need to learn how to see the struggle and its costs as they unfold, moment to moment, day in and day out, in real time. This is a skill that you can learn, and we've created a simple worksheet—Living in Full Experience (LIFE)—to help you do that.

The acronym LIFE is not accidental; it's our deliberate intention to frame this exercise in terms of what really counts: you living your life. A blank copy of the worksheet is at the end of this chapter and on the book website, http://www.newharbinger.com/33346. Be sure to print or make several copies of the worksheet for this week and carry them with you. You'll need them.

The purpose of the LIFE Worksheet is to help you get a better sense of where and when WAFs show up and, most importantly, what you do about them when they show up. You'll see that the LIFE worksheet can be used to monitor and track situations where your WAFs show up, related experiences you might have (thoughts, physical sensations, and behaviors), your willingness to have those experiences, and how your reactions to them get in the way of, or diminish, your capacity to engage in activities and experiences that you care about.

This worksheet should be filled out shortly after unwanted WAFs show up. If you put it off until much later or the next day, you'll almost guarantee yourself inaccurate information. And if your life depended on getting accurate information about your experience—and, in a sense, it really does here—then you ought to do the exercise as intended. Inaccurate information won't help you.

The LIFE Worksheet is short. You're asked to fill in the date and time of an unwanted WAF episode, check the sensations you may have experienced during an episode, and then check whether the emotion was more like fear, anxiety, depression, or some other feeling and rate how intensely you felt that emotion.

The next question asks you about your willingness to have what you were having without acting on your WAF experiences in any way. "Willingness" is a topic that we'll cover in detail shortly, but for now, you can think of willingness as allowing your WAF thoughts and feelings to be just as they are rather than struggling with them.

The last section has fill-in questions about the sensations and feelings you experienced and your responses. Take your time with them because they'll give you a clearer sense of what you're trading in, each moment of every day, in the service of controlling your WAFs.

Completing the LIFE worksheets throughout this week is a commitment. Don't do the worksheets because we said they're a good idea. Do them because you want a different outcome in your life. Make it a choice. Are you willing to do that?

If so, then start each day with the intention to complete the LIFE worksheets, as necessary, throughout the day. When you do that, you'll be doing something new and different.

Here's how Laura, a real estate agent and mother of two, completed one of her many LIFE worksheets for the week. She's been struggling with anxiety and worry for several years.

LIVING IN FULL EXPERIENCE—
THE LIFE WORKSHEET
A Life Enhancement Exercise

Date: <u>3/18/14</u> Time: <u>7:15</u> A.M. (P.M.)

Check off any sensations you experienced just now:

☐ Dizziness	☐ Breathlessness	☑ Fast heartbeat	☐ Blurred vision
☐ Tingling/numbness	☐ Unreality	☑ Sweatiness	☐ Hot/cold flashes
☑ Chest tightness/pain	☑ Trembling/shaking	☐ Feeling of choking	☐ Nausea
☐ Feeling of choking	☑ Neck/muscle tension	☐ Detached from self	

Check what emotion best describes your experience of these sensations (pick one):

☑ Fear   ☐ Anxiety   ☐ Depression   ☐ Other: _____

Rate how strongly you felt this emotion/feeling (circle number):

0 ------- 1 ------ 2 ------ 3 ------ 4 ------ 5 ------ 6 ----(7)---- 8
Mild/Weak   Moderate   Extremely Intense

Rate how willing you were to have these sensations/feelings without acting on them (e.g., to manage them, get rid of them, suppress them, run from them). If willingness were put as a "yes" or "no" question would you be 100%

YES---(NO)
Extremely Willing   Completely Unwilling
(arms wide open)   (arms closed)

Describe **where you were** when these sensations occurred: <u>I was running around the house frantically trying to get the kids ready for school and myself ready for a number of appointments with clients and errands I had to run, including a parent-child conference at the school.</u>

Describe **what you were doing** when these sensations occurred: <u>I was going through my planner trying to figure out how I was going to get everything done.</u>

Describe **what your mind was telling you** about the sensations/feelings: <u>I have so much to do and can't stand the uncertainty of this business. I wish I had more help with the kids. I get so anxious meeting new clients and worry that I'm going to lose it. I need to focus. Feeling exhausted.</u>

Describe **what you did** (if anything) about the thoughts/sensations/feelings: <u>I tried to take some deep breaths and use some positive affirmations that I picked up from another book I have. I grabbed some herbal tea. Turned on the radio.</u>

If you did anything about the thoughts/sensations or feelings, **did it get in the way of anything** you really value or care about? If so, describe what that was here: <u>I couldn't get out of my head. I was a wreck driving into the office and had to pull over because I thought I was going to pass out. Was late to the client appointment I had in the morning. The rest of the day spiraled out of control from there. I cancelled my afternoon appointment because I was too jacked up, and barely made it to the parent-teacher conference. It was like I was panicking all day long.</u>

LIFE ENHANCEMENT EXERCISES

You've reached a point in the book where you are becoming more aware of the costs and what it is that you truly want to be about in this life. For this week, we invite you to continue to stretch and grow by doing the following:

- Commit to making a centering exercise part of your daily routine.

- Take stock of the costs of your efforts to deal with your anxieties, fears, worries, rituals, and/or painful memories.

- Don't rush through this chapter—give yourself time to fully lay out the costs and all the things you do to manage your WAFs.

- Work with the LIFE Worksheet this week and learn where your struggles with WAFs get in the way of the life you wish to lead.

THE TAKE-HOME MESSAGE

Every strategy, every failed attempt, every plan or effort at WAF control has gotten in the way of what you want to do with your time and energy. You're living your Anxiety Management Epitaph much more than your Valued Life Epitaph. This needs to change. You can liberate yourself from the struggle. The answer lies in a place you've never looked before. It will be difficult, it will feel backward, it will mean heading *toward* what you instinctively rush away from. All that said, we promise that you can do it. What you learn in this workbook will work as long as you're willing to be open to what you experience rather than fight it. And this new path will give you relief from the struggle, the losses, and the failures. All you need to do now is to keep reading … *and* do the work.

What Matters Is Living a Full Life

Points to Ponder: My life is created by what I spend my time doing. I can choose to live my Anxiety Management Epitaph or my Valued Life Epitaph.

Questions to Consider: Have I (and others) suffered enough from the effects of controlling my anxiety? Do I want my life to be about much more than getting rid of my WAFs? Am I willing to give up being an anxiety manager and go down a different path?

LIVING IN FULL EXPERIENCE—
THE LIFE WORKSHEET
A Life Enhancement Exercise

Date: _____ Time: _____ A.M./P.M.

Check off any sensations you experienced just now:

- ☐ Dizziness
- ☐ Breathlessness
- ☐ Fast heartbeat
- ☐ Blurred vision
- ☐ Tingling/numbness
- ☐ Unreality
- ☐ Sweatiness
- ☐ Hot/cold flashes
- ☐ Chest tightness/pain
- ☐ Trembling/shaking
- ☐ Feeling of choking
- ☐ Nausea
- ☐ Feeling of choking
- ☐ Neck/muscle tension
- ☐ Detached from self

Check what emotion best describes your experience of these sensations (pick one):

- ☐ Fear
- ☐ Anxiety
- ☐ Depression
- ☐ Other: _____

Rate how strongly you felt this emotion/feeling (circle number):

0 ------ 1 ------ 2 ------ 3 ------ 4 ------ 5 ------ 6 ------ 7 ------ 8

Mild/Weak   Moderate   Extremely Intense

Rate how willing you were to have these sensations/feelings without acting on them (e.g., to manage them, get rid of them, suppress them, run from them). If willingness were put as a "yes" or "no" question would you be 100%

YES---NO

Extremely Willing   Completely Unwilling
(arms wide open)   (arms closed)

Describe **where you were** when these sensations occurred: _____

_____

Describe **what you were doing** when these sensations occurred: _____

_____

Describe **what your mind was telling you** about the sensations/feelings: _____

_____

Describe **what you did** (if anything) about the thoughts/sensations/feelings: _____

_____

If you did anything about the thoughts/sensations or feelings, **did it get in the way of anything** you really value or care about? If so, describe what that was here: _____

_____

_____

CHAPTER 8

Ending Your Struggle with Anxiety Is the Solution

Experience has shown that, ironically, it is often our very attempts to solve the problem that, in fact, maintain it. The attempted solutions become the true problem.

—Giorgio Nardone and Paul Watzlawick

When you look at anxiety as a problem, it will naturally require a solution. But what if the solutions you've tried are actually the real problem? Let that possibility sink in for a moment.

The exercises in the previous two chapters have shown you that all your attempts to fix your anxiety problem haven't solved anything. Each so-called solution—each attempt to stop or at least stem the tide of your WAFs—has gotten you to this place. And your WAFs still feel out of control.

We know that most seemingly sensible solutions to anxiety problems are really about control. Remember the myths we talked about in chapter 4. The voice in your head tells you to get a handle on your WAFs: *Breathe slowly, Take a pill, Watch TV, Go to bed early, Take it easy,* and so on. This voice comes from the well-established and recycled belief that WAFs are dangerous, that it's impossible to feel anxiety and still live a good life, that managing and controlling anxiety is the way out of misery and into happiness.

The voice is fooling you. Controlling anxiety doesn't work in the same way that control works in other areas of life. In this chapter you'll learn why. You'll also learn to recognize when and where control works well. And you'll learn how to start letting go of the anxiety-management agenda and get on with your life-management agenda.

ENDING THE TUG-OF-WAR WITH ANXIETY

You've already taken the first step toward understanding the struggle. You've examined the costs. You've faced all your past attempts to manage and control intense physical sensations, nervousness, worries, disturbing thoughts and images, urges, and other unwanted thoughts and feelings.

And, if you're still reading, then you've faced the difficult truth that nothing has really worked. No matter how hard you've tried, no strategy to manage anxiety has helped long term. On top of that, the costs of the struggle are still there.

So what can you do instead? Must you go on fighting the good fight until you win (or the WAFs win!)? The good news is that there's another way: you could give up the struggle with anxiety—and surrender.

We can almost guarantee that your mind is feeding you all kinds of messages right now. The alternative we just suggested cuts against all the old programming about what your mind has told you needs and ought to be done as far as your WAFs are concerned. So take a moment to observe what your mind is doing—without getting into an argument with your mind—and then read on.

Here's what letting go of the struggle agenda is about. It means allowing yourself to feel anxiety just as it is, just as it comes, instead of trying not to feel anxiety. You can learn to have those unpleasant thoughts and feelings *and* learn how to distance yourself from them just enough so that you can keep doing whatever you want to do—go to a party, meet new people, drive on the highway, take an elevator, see a movie, and so on.

The list of vital life-affirming actions has no limits, no borders—that is, so long as you let go of the struggle and stop fighting against your experiences. When you lay down your arms, you are in a sense admitting defeat. But admitting that doesn't mean you've lost something. It makes no sense to continue fighting an adversary that cannot and need not be defeated in order for you to have what you want in life. This is a smart and enormously vital move on your part.

By surrendering, you're really doing four things: First, you're acknowledging the struggle itself. Next, you're allowing yourself to experience how futile and exhausting that struggle has been. Third, you're facing the fact that the struggle has kept you stuck in the same place with nowhere to go. And lastly, and most importantly, you're regaining your freedom. Let's have a closer look at this process.

THE EXHAUSTING FIGHT WITH WAF MONSTERS

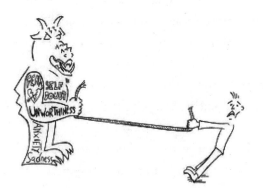

It may seem like you've been fighting a tug-of-war with a team of WAF monsters pulling at one end of the rope and you pulling at the other end. Yet no matter how hard you've pulled to defeat the WAF monsters, they've always come back stronger, pulling harder.

It may look like there's nothing else you can do while you're engaged in this sort of battle. You've got both hands firmly clenching the rope, and your feet are dug in, stuck in the same position. Back and forth it goes.

And as this battle plays out, you're getting more and more worked up—your chest tightens, your breathing becomes shallow, your teeth are clenched, your face is red with pearls of sweat welling up on your brow and forehead, and you can see the whites of your knuckles. Your hands are not moving and your feet aren't going anywhere. You're stuck in an endless and exhausting fight for your life, or so it seems.

Your options may appear limited in this situation. Yet you do have other options. What else could you do in this situation? Take a moment to jot down a few possibilities that come to mind.

_____

_____

You may have come up with only a few options here. That's okay. Your mind may have suggested that you pull harder, try harder, or dig in more. Maybe your mind suggested that there's a better medication or a new coping strategy that'll give you the strength to win. Yet isn't all of this more of the same—old wine, new label?

Here's another option: you don't need to win this fight. This may seem like another wacky idea—*and* it's a potentially vital idea too. It'll allow you to consider this: What would happen if you decided to stop fighting?

Think about that. Suppose you just decided to give up fighting and drop the rope. As you connect with this possibility, notice what happens to your hands and feet. They're free, right? And you've regained some space and options that were impossible while you were in the middle of the battle: you're now able to use your hands, feet, and mind for something other than fighting anxiety.

To help you see how this might play out in your life, imagine that something or someone you care deeply about was on the sidelines next to the battle, watching and waiting for you and the fight to finish.

Suppose it was your child waiting for a hug or a friend wanting to spend time with you. Or perhaps it was a project, a vacation, or something spiritually uplifting. See if you can visualize that important thing in your life that is just waiting … waiting for you to finish fighting. Would you just keep at it? Or, would you drop the rope and give your time and energy to whatever or whoever was waiting, hoping for you to spend time with them?

Now, let's have a closer look at what happens when you drop the rope. The WAF monsters haven't gone away just because you've stopped fighting. They're still there, taunting you with the rope, hoping that you take the bait and grab hold for another round. And you could certainly do that; sometimes you will, mostly out of habit. But the important thing is to notice when you've grabbed the rope and make a choice to let go. Making this choice will give you the space and energy to attend to something you care about—those people watching and waiting on the sidelines.

> *I can drop the rope and end the fight with myself.*

Dropping the rope and ending the struggle creates an opening and room to do something else in your life. If you aren't consumed with reducing and controlling anxiety, avoiding the next panic attack, stemming the tide of another painful memory, or extinguishing disturbing thoughts or worry, then you create a window of opportunity. You create space to move toward the life you've put on hold. One of our clients captured this moment very well when he told us, "When I drop the rope, I'm free."

Remember, your epitaph is written based on what you spend your time doing. If you need to, go back to chapter 7 and remind yourself of what you want your life to stand for. Put your Valued Life Epitaph on the sidelines if that helps you let go of the rope.

WHERE ARE YOU IN CONTROL?

So why are so many people reluctant to drop the rope? Why do we keep struggling with anxiety, hurt, and pain when it hasn't really worked well and has cost us so much? The answer has to do with what we've learned about struggling for control.

Below is a little story about two mice who both got caught in difficult and quite frightening situations. Have a look at their different ways of dealing with the situation.

The Struggle of the Two Mice

Two little mice were happily scurrying around a farmer's kitchen and pantry, looking for tasty snacks. The first mouse was on the kitchen floor sniffing for scraps from that night's dinner. All of a sudden the farm's tomcat entered the kitchen. When he saw the little mouse, he immediately went after it, and the little mouse ran for her life. She frantically ran around the kitchen floor looking for places to hide but couldn't find any at first. The cat's pursuit was relentless, and he had come awfully close to pouncing on the little mouse when she finally discovered a small hole in the floorboard. The mouse slipped into it and was safe. The cat was still trying to get her with his paws, but he couldn't. The hole was too small. The little mouse had saved her own life through her persistent efforts.

Meanwhile, the second little mouse from the pantry next door was looking for snacks up high on the countertop. Her eyes were fixed on a bread crumb at the edge of the counter, and so she went over to have a look. As she approached the bread crumb, she lost her footing and fell right into a bucket of cream on the floor below. At first, she struggled frantically to get out. Around and around she went, looking for a way out. The situation looked quite hopeless, and the little mouse was growing tired. Every minute of struggling sucked more energy out of her. Deep down inside she knew she would end up completely exhausted and drown if she continued like this. So she did something counterintuitive and courageous. She decided to slow down and take a closer look around at where she was and what was happening to her. That's when she realized, *I am in a bucket filled with tasty cream.* She started to take a few sips and continued to move around just fast enough to stay afloat—all the while taking sips of cream. This went on for quite a while. The little mouse wasn't happy to be caught in a bucket. At the same time, she noticed that if she didn't do too much and just kept on sipping away at the cream, she might eventually be fine. She wouldn't run out of energy, and sooner or later the cream would be gone—no more danger of drowning.

We're all just like the first little mouse in many ways. We've learned that effort and struggle *is* the way out of life's hardships. And there's some truth to this too. Human beings and animals will quite literally fight for their lives when faced with *real* danger in the world around them. In these situations, you ought to exert effort and struggle because both help to keep you safe from harm, or even death.

And you don't need to have experienced a life-threatening situation, either, to pick up on this idea. From a very early age, you've learned that success and happiness never come easily, and never come at all for those who wait, give in, or do nothing. This basic idea has been repeated and repackaged over generations.

Under many circumstances, this is a highly adaptive and workable strategy. It often produces desired outcomes. For instance, if you can do something to reduce the chance of real pain and suffering, then it makes sense to do so. Your experience tells you as much, and extensive psychological literature supports exercising effortful control for better psychological health and physical well-being. There's comfort in knowing this and acting in kind. Life may not always be fair, but we can and should do something to make things right.

As a person suffering from anxiety, you're all too familiar with the mantras of struggle and effortful control: *Pull yourself together*, *Where there is a will, there is a way*, or *Try harder*. Yet some of the exercises in the previous chapters show that these strategies don't work when it comes to anxiety.

Like the second mouse in the story, you're still stuck in a bucket. Your bucket is not filled with something that can actually hurt or kill you; your bucket is filled with WAFs, and you're desperately swimming around trying to find a way out. The struggle, in short, is with you. Your WAFs may not taste like cream, but if you slow down, look, and listen, you may notice that you can move and swim with them. You will only run out of energy and feel like you're drowning if you keep struggling with them. If you stay with the energy your WAFs provide, you might even be able to use that energy in a way that is helpful to you.

The key point here is that the same effort you might exert to keep yourself safe and protected from danger in the outside world can be overextended and applied to your inner emotional life where it doesn't work and actually hurts you. You'll only end up feeling exhausted and drained of energy.

Go back to the costs of anxiety management you worked up in chapter 7 and see if all the effort and struggle you've put into getting out or away from your anxiety has made you safer and moved you closer to the life you want. What does your experience tell you? The answer ought to be a resounding "no"!

Here's a thought: It may be possible to have anxiety and not be drowned by it if and when you decide to willingly experience anxiety just as it is and give up your struggle with it. For now, hold this idea lightly because we'll expand on it in the chapters to come.

You may wonder why control can work so well with the demands and strains of the world and yet be so ineffective with anxiety and other forms of emotional pain. The answer is that anxiety differs in important ways from other problems in life that can be controlled quite effectively. Being able to see this difference is critical, and it's a skill you can learn. You'll find exercises in this chapter and the next to help you discover when control works, when it doesn't work, and how to tell the difference.

When Control Works

Action—what you do with your hands and feet—is a great litmus test for knowing when control may work. You just need to ask if you or others could see what you're doing and the results of what you do. For instance, if you'd like to clean up your yard, you can get a rake and get started. Here are some other examples of situations where control works:

- If you want to change the color of the walls in a room in your home, you can go out and buy new paint and then paint the walls.

- If you no longer like some of your clothes, you can simply throw them away or pass them on to someone who may actually wear them.

- If you're in a job you don't like, you can quit that job, seek out a new employer, and work there instead.

- If you miss an old friend, you may decide to reconnect by picking up the phone and calling or sending an e-mail.

- If you want to perform an act of kindness, you can give a person a gift, a compliment, or a hug.

- If you want to promote your health and well-being, you can exercise regularly and watch what you eat and drink.

The common thread in these life examples is this: they all involve behavior—things you do with your hands, your feet, and your mouth. All are controllable because they tend to involve objects or situations in the world *outside* your skin. Changing things in the world around you often *is* possible and works well.

This strategy works so well in so many life areas that it only makes sense to want to apply it to manage emotional and physical pain happening *inside* you. And, at times, control does work to manage pain. For instance, you may take an aspirin for a headache, see a doctor for an illness or injury, take time to relax to feel more energized, or exercise regularly to maintain emotional balance.

You can also avoid or manage situations that may result in physical injury or death by acting to escape from them when and if they occur. We talked about these kinds of extreme situations a bit in chapter 2, mostly in the context of traumatic events. And you need the capacity for this kind of control in less extreme circumstances too.

As an example, suppose you're unlucky enough to be walking across the road and suddenly you see a car dart out from nowhere and approach at a high rate of speed. In this situation, the obvious response would be to run or jump out of the way. If you didn't act, you'd end up dead or severely injured. This type of fear-motivated behavior is highly adaptive and often works to everyone's advantage. There's nothing problematic about this form of control.

> *I can control what I do with my hands and feet.*

The problem is that what works well in the external world just doesn't work well when applied to things going on inside you. You may try to deal with your thoughts and feelings in the same way you deal with clothes you don't like. Now look at your experience to see what happens when you do that. Can you give away or throw out your unpleasant thoughts and feelings—has that ever worked for you? Can you replace an old painful memory or a reminder of your past with a new one—have you ever been able to do that?

133

Remember the exercise in chapter 4 where we asked you *not* to think of [what was it?]. This is pretty much impossible, because the thought, *Don't think about the PINK ELEPHANT!* is itself, obviously, a thought about a pink elephant. The more you try not to have this thought, the more you'll have it. The same is true of unpleasant thoughts, feelings, and bodily sensations.

The take-home message here is this: You can't win a fight against yourself. One part of you will always lose. And, as much as you may want to throw out your WAFs, there's simply no way to take them in your hands and out to the dumpster. Your WAFs can't be removed in the same way that you can swap out a chair you don't like in your living room. Your WAFs follow you wherever you go because they are part of you, part of your unique history.

If you can allow yourself to come to terms with this basic truth, then you'll be faced with the stark and sobering reality that more effort and muscle power isn't going to help you one iota. In fact, if you look back and review chapters 6 and 7, then your experience ought to be screaming this message loudly at you.

Let's examine more closely when control doesn't work and why this is so.

When Control Doesn't Work

Anxiety is, in many respects, an unpleasant emotional state. So it's understandable when you say, "I don't like anxiety" or "I want to get rid of it." Most people without anxiety problems don't like anxiety either. Yet you'll recall that not liking anxiety doesn't make it a problem. If that were true, then most people on this planet would suffer from anxiety disorders.

Problems arise when "not liking" gets mixed with control strategies that are taken to the extreme—when they become overly intense and rigid and when they're applied in situations where they're unnecessary and don't work. In short, the strategies don't produce the anxiety reduction you were hoping for, or the temporary relief they offer restricts your life. Consider Roger's story.

■ *Roger's Story*

Roger had been battling social anxiety for as long as he could remember. Much of his anxiety and panic centered on his job. He worked hard to prevent his anxiety and panic at work. Situations where he had to talk in front of small groups of businesspeople were downright nasty for him—lots of anxiety, sleepless nights beforehand, dread about the possibility of screwing up, making a fool of himself, being judged. Nothing seemed to work. This led Roger to quit his well-paying and interesting job. He ended up taking a back-office job where he didn't have to interact with other people. He also earned much less money and felt bored and isolated.

In this example and in many others we've seen, control efforts are life constricting, not life expanding. You probably feel this way too. You may even beat yourself up for not being able to control your

WAFs. You're not alone. From an early age, most of us are taught that we *should* be able to control them. And, this message is perpetuated by our culture in many ways.

One problem with control strategies is this: they often work just enough to keep your WAFs at bay. In fact, every effort, every moment of struggle and avoidance, will often buy you a brief honeymoon from the pain and its source. But they key word here is brief. None of this really works in the long run.

You pay a high price for each brief honeymoon, each moment you act to engage or move away from your anxieties and fears. And, over time, you're left feeling more anxious, anticipating and preparing for the next WAF attack. As Roger learned, once this cycle of struggle and control is set into motion, it can take over and become your life.

Anxiety Is Not a Hot Stove: Even When You Pull Away, You Still Get Burned

Life has taught you how well control works. As a child you probably avoided touching a red-hot stove because it hurt to touch it. You may have learned this the hard way or by listening to your parents or caregivers warning you about the consequences: "Don't touch _____ because you'll get hurt." Keeping your hand away from hot things kept you safe and prevented injury.

This sensible avoidance strategy has repeated itself in both obvious and subtle ways in your life— because it often works to keep you alive and unharmed. Take a moment to think about a situation or two where this has been true in your experience and write them below.

_____

_____

What you've learned over and over again is that control works to help you avoid and reduce external sources of pain and harm. Naturally then, it would seem that these strategies ought to work when you apply them to internal sources of pain and hurt. It's vitally important that you begin to understand this external versus internal distinction.

People get into trouble when they act to avoid their emotional pain and hurt (inside) in the same way that they would act to avoid sources of real harm and danger in the world around them (outside). Look at your experience here—you've been down this road too.

You've treated your WAFs, and responded to them, much like when faced with a red-hot stove. You try to pull away, get away, and avoid them because anxiety, like the hot stove, seems dangerous. When WAFs show up, you feel you must do something. And yet you keep getting burned.

Anxiety is one type of emotional pain. When people act to get rid of emotional and psychological pain, they end up, instead, with more of it. All of what we know about emotional pain boils down to this simple fact: you can't keep your unpleasant thoughts and emotions from burning you the way that you can pull your hand back from a hot stove.

Why might this be? The next exercise will help you experience part of the answer.

EXERCISE: THOUGHTS AND EMOTIONS HAVE NO "ON/OFF" SWITCH

Start by getting in a comfortable position. When you're ready, we'd like you to do the following: make yourself feel happy. Go ahead and try it now. Just make yourself as happy as you know how to be. Really work at it. Can you do it?

If you were successful, then you likely brought on the feeling of happiness by thinking about something else. For instance, you may have conjured up a memory of a beautiful experience from your past, visualized something you like, or thought of an event you are looking forward to. Yet this isn't what we were asking of you. We want you to just flip the switch and be super happy for the sake of it, not as a response to something that may help make you feel that way.

Now, try to make yourself feel really anxious or afraid. Do it without thinking of something really scary or painful. We want you to try really hard. Just turn on the switch. Can you do it?

If your experience is not convincing you how impossible this really is, then you can go on to try one of the following:

1. Make yourself fall madly in love—meaning genuine, deeply felt love—with the first new person you see.

2. Go ahead and make your left leg numb, so numb in fact that if it was pricked with a sharp needle you wouldn't feel a thing.

We hope that this exercise helped you learn that emotions have no on/off switch. It's next to impossible for anyone to feel one way or another just because they want to. Emotions just happen as we engage in the world. They're not something we deliberately do apart from that world.

Emotions aren't something you can choose to have more or less of either. When you think and behave otherwise, you'll activate every aspect of your nervous system that keeps you feeling anxious and afraid. And you'll do things that end up keeping you stuck and miserable. You'll get more of the very thing you don't want to feel and think.

This happens because your body is a system with built-in feedback loops—your brain and nervous system. When you act against parts of this system—avoiding, suppressing, or escaping—it sends out reverberations to all other parts of the system. This mind-body connection is like a sensitive spider web in this respect. Everything is connected. Trying to run away from unpleasant experiences—be they feelings, thoughts, memories, or bodily sensations—amplifies your pain. And your life will seem to be passing by too.

The next exercise (adapted from Hayes et al., 2012) will help you experience why struggling with unpleasant feelings and thoughts can make them worse. To begin, find a quiet place where you can sit and get comfortable.

EXERCISE: YOU'RE WIRED TO A PERFECT POLYGRAPH AND ... ZAP!

Imagine that you're connected to the best and most sensitive polygraph machine that's ever been built. This polygraph is super effective at detecting anxiety. So there's no way you can be aroused or anxious without the machine noticing it.

Now here's your task, which sounds quite simple: all you have to do is stay relaxed—just stay calm—while thinking about a recent episode where you felt anxious. Just think about an episode where you were anxious ... without getting anxious now. If you get the least bit anxious, this machine will detect it.

We know how important it is to you to be successful here, so we're going to give you a special incentive. If you can stay completely relaxed while you imagine the WAF scene, then we'll give you $100,000! (Imaginary money, of course, but pretend that you'd get that cash payout.)

The catch is that the polygraph is designed to give you a deadly shock if you show the slightest bit of anxiety or arousal. As long as you stay relaxed, you won't die. But if you get the least bit anxious or aroused—and remember this perfect polygraph will notice that immediately—the machine will deliver the shock and kill you. So just relax!

Take a moment to jot down what you think would happen in this situation.

_____

_____

Did you stay perfectly calm and get the payout? Or did you end up dead? We think you know the outcome and so do we—dead as a doornail. The tiniest bit of anxiety would be terrifying for you, and for any other person in this situation.

Every day you wake up with your life at stake. You need to be calm, not panic, and avoid the thoughts and worries because your life seems to depend on it. And of course, there it comes: *I need to be calm at this social event ... Oh, no! I'm getting tense and anxious—zap ... zap ... zap.* And there's another vital aspect of your life, missed or ruined.

There's no way to stay calm when you're connected to the perfect polygraph: your nervous system. This system is better than any lie detector at detecting anxiety. When the WAFs show up, you struggle to keep them at bay because everything you want in life seems to hang in the balance. As you do that, your nervous system kicks in. The web reverberates. And guess what you get: more anxious and panicky. And you get zapped too!

137

Take Annie, who was diagnosed with obsessive-compulsive disorder.

■ *Annie's Story*

Annie feared that she'd shout out profanities in public. She was truly horrified about the possibility of shouting out profanities during a church service. So she spent lots of time trying to figure out how to prevent that from happening. She tried really hard not to think about shouting profanities during church. And here's what ended up happening—she ended up consumed with thoughts about profanities, was extremely anxious, and eventually stopped going to church.

Here the very act of trying to suppress the thought brought about the unwanted thought and emotional experience. And it led Annie to act in ways to control the problem that ended up getting in the way of something that she greatly enjoyed doing. This is how it works with your brain and body too. It's all one big interconnected web that grows and grows as you age and develop new experiences. The more you act on your WAF web, the more it'll reverberate and spread into all areas of your life.

The way to stop the vibrations is to go after the source, the fuel, driving the WAF struggle-and-control machine. That source is unwillingness—your unwillingness to make space for *every* aspect of your experience and identity. The fuel for unwillingness is your judgmental mind talking to you, baiting you, and feeding you messages like *You can't have WAFs and be happy and live life fully. To have the "good life" means that you must be free of WAFs.*

So long as you buy this message, you'll be unwilling to allow your WAFs into your life. This unwillingness will add fuel to the fire driving more struggle and control. At this point in the workbook, you should have a good sense of what your time spent struggling has bought you. And we're almost certain that very little of it is vital and life expanding.

The good news is that living well doesn't require that you first start feeling and thinking well. Many people live with enormous pain and hardship and with every reason to cave in and give up on life. And yet, they continue to move forward in life with meaning, dignity, and a sense of purpose. You may wonder what secret they know that enables them to do that.

Their secret is this: they don't take the bait. They don't spend their valuable time on this earth struggling and fighting with their physical, emotional, and psychological pain. These individuals experience pain just like every other human being on this planet, and they've learned how not to get stuck in that pain. You too are on this path right now, and we'll be showing you how to do more of that in the next chapter.

The simple lesson here is this: control works against you when applied to unwanted and painful aspects of your private world. To get out of this cycle, you'll need to first come to terms with the fact that deliberate control isn't a solution. It's the *problem*.

YOU CAN RUN, BUT YOU CAN'T HIDE FROM YOURSELF

There's another reason why you can't avoid and run away from feelings of anxiety and fear in the same way that you might run from or avoid dangerous objects or situations. That reason has to do with the source of the WAF emotional pain. That source is you.

Imagine that a vicious dog or a car is coming toward you. You can take quick and decisive evasive action by literally running for your life to avoid potential harm and danger. Running away from this external source of danger gets you to safety. Here you're in control with your hands and feet because the source of danger is outside you.

Now picture this scenario: you've experienced a trauma, like a violent sexual assault or a terrible car accident. Memories of the event can pop up in your mind at any time—no matter where you go or what you do. If you're prone to having recurrent obtrusive thoughts (obsessions) such as *I could have contaminated myself*, your experience will tell you that these thoughts can occur no matter what you happen to be doing or where you happen to go.

Or if you've experienced panic attacks, you know that they can show up in many different situations. Sure, some types of situations seem to make panic more likely, but many people who experience frequent panic attacks know that panic can happen any time or any place, even while sleeping in bed.

The bottom line is that your thoughts and feelings—the good, the bad, and the ugly—always go with you wherever you go. You cannot escape or avoid your feelings of anxiety, apprehension, and insecurity by going somewhere else for one simple reason: they are part of you. You take them with you everywhere, along with everything else going on inside your mind and body.

If this is true of your experience, then trying to run and hide from your WAFs is akin to trying to run and hide from you. There's really no way to do it. Your WAFs are part of a larger package that helps define what is uniquely human about you. You cannot escape or avoid them so long as you're alive. To act against them is to act against your very being. To act against them also means that you'll remain stuck or that things might even get worse.

You Can't Argue Away Your WAFs

Like many people, you've probably tried getting a handle on your feelings of anxiety by changing your thoughts about what you're afraid of. And, like most people, your experience probably tells you that it doesn't work well. Your experience is right. So, why can't you just talk your emotions away?

The main reason has to do with the way the brain has evolved over time. The oldest part of the brain controls emotions such as fear and panic. This part of the brain doesn't respond very well to words and reasons such as "No need to be frightened" or "Just calm down."

In fact, the oldest part of the brain is very similar to the brain structure of more primitive creatures, like snakes and crocodiles. Have you ever tried arguing with a snake or a crocodile? Probably not because if you had, you wouldn't be sitting here reading this book. It wouldn't have worked. You'd be dead! You can't talk a snake or crocodile into doing anything. Likewise, you can't change your unpleasant emotions by arguing them away.

Another reason why you can't think your way out of feeling anxious or afraid has to do with the way the mind works. Each thought you have is part of a web of connections. When you try to think yourself out of a thought, a memory, or a feeling, you must contact the very thought or feeling you'd rather not have.

Even if you try distraction, your mind will be secretly working in the background figuring out what you're not supposed to be thinking about (the pink elephant …). And this will bring you right back to the very thing you don't want to have. That's how the mind works. There's just no way to think yourself out of anxious thoughts or feelings without conjuring up the very thing you don't want to have.

You Can't Control Anxiety by Talking Yourself Out of It

Here's a story from our experience that nicely illustrates the impossibility of trying to talk anxiety away.

The story takes place in a small town in a tropical part of Australia where every year at the beginning of the rainy season, the whole town becomes infested with frogs. The frogs are everywhere. And sometimes when people get in the way, the frogs jump up at them. These unexpected "frog attacks" startle and scare some people so much that quite a few residents develop frog phobias. The fear is that intense. Many people don't want to leave their homes. The possibility of an encounter with one of these "disgusting" creatures can be crippling.

Some people try to talk their fear away. They tell themselves something like *These little green frogs are absolutely harmless and couldn't hurt me.* What they are really doing though is replacing one type of thought in their heads (frogs are disgusting) with another type of thought (frogs aren't really dangerous and actually look quite cute). These mental gymnastics don't make a bit of difference. The fear and the disgust are still there and so too are the frogs. They can't talk themselves out of what they were feeling.

The Australians can run away and stay away from frogs but at a significant cost to their personal freedom. What they can't do is run away from their "froggy" thoughts and feelings. Their thoughts, feelings, and apprehensions about frogs follow them everywhere.

In the end, these individuals are faced with a choice, and many end up choosing to go nowhere and stay in their homes with their fears and apprehensions. It is often at this point of sheer frustration and despair that people finally seek help.

EXPERIENCING IS THE ANSWER

The oldest part of your brain doesn't respond well to words and reason, but it can learn from direct experience. You can teach your old brain something new if you give it something new. This is how our brains work—what goes in stays in. This means you can alter the mix. Doing something new adds something new. This can happen if you're willing to give up rehearsing old strategies—like running away from the thoughts and feelings you don't like—and instead do something new, like experiencing your WAFs for what they are.

EXERCISE: HOLDING ANXIETY GENTLY

This exercise will give you a small taste of what we mean by doing something new. Find a place where you can sit comfortably without being disturbed for about five minutes. Get yourself settled with a few rich deep breaths in … and out … in … and out.

Once you're settled, take both of your hands and cup them to make the shape of a bowl, palms facing up. Allow them to rest softly in your lap. Notice the quality of those hands and the shape they are in. They are open and ready to hold something. As you get in touch with that, become aware that those very hands have been used by you in many, many ways.

They have been used for work, for love, to touch and be touched, to hold and let go, to express yourself in writing or when speaking with someone, and to comfort, to heal, and to share kindness. Allow yourself to sink into the goodness contained in your hands.

And from that place of goodness, see if you can allow, even if just for a moment, a small, tiny piece of your anxiety concerns to settle there. Like a feather floating down, imagine that piece of your anxiety gently comes to rest in the middle of your kind and loving hands. Just something small—a part of yourself that you might be willing to let rest in your hands.

Take a moment to settle into that—this piece of your anxiety is now resting within the goodness of your hands. What is it like to hold a piece of your anxiety and yourself this way? Simply notice, breathe, and sense the warmth and goodness of your hands. There's nothing else to do here.

You can stay with this experience as long as you wish. When you're ready, go ahead and release that piece of your anxiety, much like you would if you were holding a dove and releasing it to fly away. And then, before moving on, take a moment to pause and reflect on what you may have learned from this exercise. Remind yourself that you can hold anxiety in a kind way and experience something new.

The exercise you just did may seem a bit silly or odd. That's perfectly okay. But don't allow your mind to derail you from what you learned just now. Instead of arguing with your feelings and thoughts, allow yourself to appreciate what it's like to observe and stay with them, openly, with kindness, and dare we say, with love. Each time you consciously meet your WAFs in this way, you'll be adding something new to the mix and things will really start changing in your life. This is one of the most important steps to leading a life no longer ruled by your WAFs.

In the next chapters, we'll cover other skills to help you experience your unpleasant thoughts and feelings without picking up the rope and fighting and defeating them. This, by the way, is exactly what helped the residents of tropical Australia get on with living their lives, even without overcoming their fear of frogs. You can do this too.

LIFE ENHANCEMENT EXERCISES

You're continuing to make important changes by reading and doing the exercises we've covered so far. For this week, we invite you to continue this important work and do the following:

- Commit to making a centering exercise part of your daily routine.

- Work with the material in this workbook—be active, do the exercises, and pause to reflect on what you've learned.

- Practice holding a piece of your anxiety in your kind and loving hands and notice what happens when you choose to do that.

- Enlist the support and encouragement of someone close to you and share what you're doing to make significant changes in your life. Ask this person to help you notice when you're picking up the rope and struggling or trying to control or avoid your WAFs.

THE TAKE-HOME MESSAGE

You cannot control your anxiety by running away from, avoiding, or suppressing unwanted sensations, feelings, thoughts, worries, or images—as much as you may want to. This only buys you more anxiety, frustration, and a sense of helplessness. When your WAFs show up, acknowledge feeling stuck, drop the rope, and make room for something new.

As Steve Maraboli (2014) reminds us, when you choose to take control over the things you *actually* have control over instead of the things you don't, amazing changes occur. Don't forget that. Stick it on your fridge. Focus on what you can control to keep moving forward in directions you care about. Be mindful of this important point when WAFs show up in your daily life.

Trying to Control the Uncontrollable Is the Problem

Point to Ponder: Trying to control my WAFs makes my life worse, not better.

Question to Consider: Am I willing to give up trying to control what I cannot control so I can move forward with my life?

CHAPTER 9

You Control Your Choices, Actions, and Destiny

You are the master of your own destiny. Use your strengths well. They are the keys to your destiny and your success in life. Once you know yourself and take action to realize your dreams, you can unlock the doors to your own potential.

—Neil Somerville

The epigraph from Neil Somerville above reminds us of a simple truth—we are all the masters of our own destiny. Nobody else can create your life for you. Blaming others or your anxiety for keeping you stuck won't help you either. You have to decide that enough is enough. You'll need to draw a line in the sand. There is no undoing your past or making it go away. What was done is done. The most important question to ask yourself is how you want to live your life from this moment forward. To be successful, you'll need to be clear about what you can control.

So far, you've learned that conscious, deliberate, purposeful control works well in the external world, outside your skin, where the following rule applies: *If you don't like what you are doing, figure out a way to change it or get rid of it using your mouth, hands, and feet. Then go ahead and do it.* You also learned that this rule doesn't work well when applied to the things you don't like that are going on inside your mind and body.

But understanding this distinction is not enough. Most people get it quickly, and then fall right back into the trap of trying to steer their lives forward by working hard to control things that they have absolutely no control over. This only leads to frustration and despair. You'd be much better off refocusing your attention and expending your energy on the three areas where you *do* have control: your choices, your actions, and your destiny. Let's have a look.

YOU HAVE CONTROL OVER THE CHOICES YOU MAKE

Every moment in life is about choices. Do I eat or not? Do I brush my teeth or not? Do I share a story with a friend or not? Do I work out or not? Do I show love or not? You get the idea. The universe of possible choices here is endless.

You have full responsibility for the choices you make. Coming to terms with this can feel both sobering and liberating. Deep down you know that you cannot choose whether or not to feel panic, anxiety, or worry. If anxiety were a choice, we can guarantee that nobody would chose to feel it.

But here's what you can do. You can decide what you do with those feelings and thoughts when they show up. You can choose the kind of relationship you wish to have with your emotional life. To get a sense of what we mean, go ahead and think of your anxiety as a person. Give it a name. Imagine how it looks, how it dresses, its voice, personality, gender, and how it speaks to you.

Once you have this character clearly in your mind, imagine that she or he shows up on your door step one day uninvited. As you open the door slowly, ask yourself this—what is my reaction to seeing this character? Am I choosing to greet her or him in a loving way, perhaps as a dear friend or family member? Or, do I choose to greet the anxiety character as an enemy or unwelcome guest? You might be ambivalent. Notice here that treating anxiety with ambivalence or as an enemy would not be something you would hope for in a healthy relationship with another person in your life. This is where things need to change.

The choice here is to practice a more inviting and welcoming relationship with your anxiety. Instead of choosing to treat it as an enemy, you can learn to treat it as a friend. It doesn't mean that you like everything about anxiety, but that's true of your dear friends and family members too. The main point here is that you're free to choose how you respond and what you do with your emotional upset and pain when you feel it.

It's your choice whether you stay with your WAFs, acknowledge their presence, let them be, and observe them with a sense of curiosity and kind acceptance, or whether you do as they say, pick up the rope, and give in to the impulses to act by choosing avoidance, escape, suppression, or other ways to try to get rid of or control the WAFs.

Let's take a look at some specific situations where you have the power to choose what you do when your WAFs show up:

- Observing what my mind says without further action versus doing what my mind says

- Meeting my WAFs with compassion and allowing them to be there versus struggling with them or trying to make them go away

- Observing what my body does versus listening to what my mind tells me about what my body does

- Doing nothing about the WAF feelings and thoughts versus distracting myself, taking pills, and running away from them

- Practicing patience with myself versus blaming and putting myself or others down for having WAFs

- Moving forward in my life with WAFs versus struggling with them and remaining stuck

YOU CAN CONTROL YOUR ACTIONS

Your actions are what you do with your hands, feet, and mouth when WAFs show up. How you respond to the unpleasant thoughts, memories, physical sensations, and feelings dished out by your body and mind is very much within your control. Learning to respond differently than you've done in the past is the key to getting unstuck.

Let's say you're in the mall and feel a panic attack coming on. Then you act on it: perhaps you take one of the pills you carry with you at all times; then you head for the exit. These are both actions. Alternatively, you might do nothing about the panic attack and simply notice it for what it is, not for what your mind says it is. You stay in the mall and focus on doing what really matters to you, even if that means taking the panic along for the ride. If you're really shaky, you could sit down or lean against a wall, observe what's going on, and wait until you're not quite as shaky anymore. Then you get up and buy your daughter the shoes you promised her. In both scenarios, you're doing something. And your choice of actions, in a very real sense, helps define who you are and what your life is about.

Looking at your experience will tell you how difficult it is to get a handle on the feeling part of your WAFs—the bodily sensations, nervousness, or sense of dread. Your experience will also tell you how hard it is not to give in to the action part of your WAFs—the impulse to do something to make it go away and feel better.

Remember that the purpose of anxiety is to make us act. So when WAFs show up, the impulse to act on them is very strong. We understand how easy it is to feel overwhelmed by WAF-driven impulses.

EXERCISE: FINDING FRESH ALTERNATIVES TO THE SAME OLD WAF IMPULSES

Even an impulse to act is a feeling. But the action is not inevitable. There's a split second between every impulse and every action. In this gap you can intervene to determine what you're going to do and how you're going to respond.

To help you get a sense of this, pull some of your completed LIFE worksheets from this past week. Select one episode where the impulse to act on your WAFs was strong and where the action kept you away from, or pulled you out of, something that was important or potentially vital for you.

Below, list the WAF feeling, what you did in response to it, and the costs of your actions.

WAF feelings (my thoughts, feelings, sensations): _____

_____

WAF impulse (my WAF coping actions): _____

_____

Consequences of my WAF response (what I lost or missed out on): _____

_____

How would you describe how you treat your WAF feeling and impulse? (e.g., as an enemy, stranger, unwelcome guest)

_____

Lastly, how would you describe the tone of your relationship with your WAFs? (e.g., uncaring, unloving, unkind, loving, friendly, caring, supportive, kind, compassionate)

_____

Step back and ask yourself, "Is it really necessary to act on these feelings (or this thought)?" What else might you have done instead? Brainstorm some life-affirming alternative actions and write them down below.

Other life-affirming WAF responses: _____

_____

Potential consequences of these new responses (what I would have gained in my life):

_____

How would you describe how you treat your WAF feeling and impulse? (e.g., as an enemy, stranger, unwelcome guest)

_____

Lastly, how would you describe the tone of your relationship with your WAFs? (e.g., uncaring, unloving, unkind, loving, friendly, caring, supportive, kind, compassionate)

_____

The point of this brief exercise is to show you that you do have control and choices in this moment, no matter how powerful the anxiety feelings and impulses to act are.

It would be helpful at this point for you to go back and review the material in chapter 6, and ask yourself again what has cost you more: your anxious thoughts and feelings or how you've responded to those thoughts and feelings.

The costs we covered in chapter 6 are created by your actions. Acting on your WAFs got you into trouble. This is where you need to take charge and make changes.

YOU CAN CONTROL YOUR DESTINY

The cumulative effect of your choices and your actions will determine what your life will become—in other words, your destiny. This is the prize!

This doesn't mean that the outcome of your choices and actions will always be what you want. Many events in life, both good and bad, will happen outside of your control. Nobody knows what the future will hold. What most people hope for is that the cumulative effect of their choices and actions will yield a sense that their life was lived well. Everything you do from here on out adds up to that. Choice is destiny.

EXERCISE: CHOICES AND ACTIONS—MY LIFE AND MY DESTINY

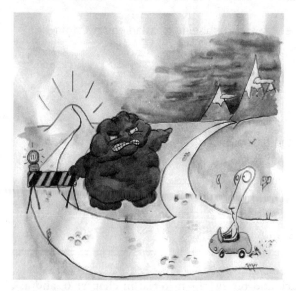

Imagine you're driving through life on a long road toward a mountain—your "Value Mountain." It stands for everything you care about in life, and what you want to be about as a person. This is the place you want to go. You'll see it in the distance, as in the illustrations below.

You're driving happily along the road toward your Value Mountain, and suddenly anxiety jumps out and blocks the road. You slow down and try to avoid hitting the WAF. You quickly turn right and find yourself on the "emotional avoidance" detour. This detour has its own road. It simply goes round and round in circles. You stay there because the WAFs are still blocking the road. So you go round and round, waiting, hoping, but going nowhere. You feel bad about going in circles. You feel mad at the WAFs for blocking the road. Your life ticks by.

This is what happens when you engage in a struggle with your unpleasant thoughts and feelings. You feel stuck, going around in circles, to nowhere. You don't want your life to be about driving on the control-and-avoidance detour. And yet it's so easy to get stuck on this detour when WAFs show up.

You're not alone on this detour. The illustration doesn't show how congested it actually is. Many people just like you are traveling on this road to nowhere. But there's an alternative.

You can take the WAFs—all those unpleasant feelings, physical sensations, thoughts, images, and worries—with you on your ride through life, without acting on them. You can choose to drive forward with them because choosing the old alternative costs you.

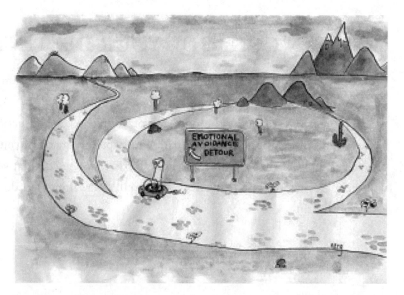

The first and most important task here is to make a choice to do something different when your WAFs show up. The second part requires that you be willing to take what you're thinking and feeling with you as you move forward. Unless you do, you'll continue to feel stuck.

LETTING GO OF THE STRUGGLE FOR CONTROL

Letting go of the struggle for control isn't as hard as it may seem. It begins with you making a decision to do so. The hardest part is putting your decision into action.

One of the chief barriers to action is failing to spot places where you have control and places where you don't have much control. Falling back into the old control agenda, where control isn't possible, is a surefire way to stay stuck.

To get and remain unstuck, you'll need to develop greater ease in the early detection of situations where control is possible in your life: those are the places where you need to expend your time and effort. The exercise below will help you do just that. You can think of it as a preparation for the important work to come.

EXERCISE: THE DIFFERENCE BETWEEN WHAT I CAN AND CANNOT CONTROL

Read each statement and then, without much thought, circle the number next to each situation you believe you can control. Don't circle numbers for situations that are outside your control.

1. What someone else is thinking	9. How others respond to my choices, expressed thoughts, feelings, and actions	17. What other people do
2. The choices I make	10. How I behave with respect to other people	18. Whether I follow certain rules or standards
3. How nervous I get	11. The choices others make	19. Other people liking me
4. How I respond to other people	12. What I do when I get anxious	20. Whether I prepare for tasks and do my best
5. What other people value and care about	13. How often the same thoughts or images come back into my mind	21. What I feel at any point
6. What I say and do in a situation	14. How I respond to my thoughts and feelings (positive or negative)	22. What I do with my precious time on this earth
7. Worries I have from time to time	15. Other people following rules or standards	23. The thoughts I have from time to time
8. The direction I want my life to take	16. Whether I follow through with commitments	24. My values and what I care about

Now go back and look at the numbers you circled. All the odd-numbered items represent situations where you have absolutely no control. You may think otherwise, but if you go back and reflect, you'll see that you truly don't have control in any of the odd-numbered scenarios.

Part of the problem is that your mind tells you that you do or *should* have control when you don't. Remember, when you struggle to control what you cannot control, you'll only end up feeling more anxious and disappointed. WAFs need this struggle to stay powerful. When they show up, you need to recognize them for what they are, stop, and then look for places where you can exert control over your choices and actions with an eye on what you want your life to be about.

The even-numbered situations represent a sampling of life circumstances where you do have control. They share one thing in common: they represent your actions, what *you* say or do.

THE BIG QUESTION: ARE YOU READY FOR A CHANGE?

Perhaps your fear is that anxiety will finally win and all the catastrophic events you've been trying to avoid will finally come to pass. So you do what you can to stay safe—protected from those strong feelings, scary thoughts, and worries. You remain vigilant, on guard, and anxious.

Here's an idea, one that we've hammered on throughout this chapter and those that came before: What if all this protecting and avoiding and hiding were the problem? What if there's no need to run away from anything? What if letting the WAFs be what they are—physical sensations, feeling, thoughts, or images—without doing something about them were the beginning of an answer?

You've tried the old ways long enough. They haven't worked. Instead, what they've done is created many more problems. The struggle just keeps playing out in your life. Are you ready for a change? What if you stopped struggling and dropped the rope?

Dropping the Rope: The First Step in Becoming a Life Manager

You may wonder how you can drop the rope to end your tug-of-war with WAFs. The first thing you'd need to do is give up your job as anxiety manager at WAFs "R" Us. If you haven't done that yet, are you willing to do that now? If so, make it a commitment by signing your resignation statement below.

I, _____ [print your name], have worked as anxiety manager at WAFs "R" Us for _____ [insert number] months/years [circle one]. This position has been enormously challenging in many ways. I am no longer willing to continue with it. I am at a point in my life where I am ready for something new—ready for a position that makes room for *aspects of my life that have been diminished or put on hold because of my job with this company. Thus, I formally resign from my current position, effective immediately.*

Sincerely, _____ [sign your name here]

Once you've committed to giving up the old path, you're positioned to take up a new job of "life manager." This workbook is a job-training manual of sorts for this position. Taking charge of your life is a skill that you can learn, beginning with learning how not to get hooked by your judgmental mind and by the urge to pick up the rope and fight the WAF war.

Still, you need to be prepared for what you're getting into. Being a life manager means that you'll experience life's ups and downs. And sometimes you'll slip back into old habits—your old training at WAFs "R" Us. In fact, we can almost guarantee that you will. Anxiety is a powerful emotion. It won't just play nice because you've decided not to play.

When you decide to drop the rope, your WAFs will yell at you, be right in your face, and dangle that rope right in front of your eyes. WAFs need the fuel that comes from a good fight with you. It's not simply that struggling with WAFs drains you, but that WAFs themselves actually feed off and grow stronger because of your struggle with them. This is why dropping the rope and becoming an observer, not a player, can be so powerful.

Up until now, you've probably felt like you've had few choices apart from your old methods and perhaps just using them with more effort. Here, we're stressing that your old methods and newer ones like them are actively making things worse. And we're not asking you to just believe us. Look at your own experience up until now and learn from it. So the choice you have now is really about dropping the old methods to make way for something new. This is how you'll make your life better.

Many people have successfully let go of the struggle by learning to watch their sensations, thoughts, and feelings as they are, and not as what their mind says they are. Simply noticing what you feel means beginning to acknowledge and allow those feelings to be present. It doesn't mean liking what you feel or agreeing with what somebody has done to you.

It only means being aware of your anxiety, acknowledging it for what it is—a thought, a feeling, a sensation, a memory, an image—without taking sides or doing anything about it. And it means recognizing that you and you alone have choices in how you respond.

We know that dropping the rope is easier said than done. It's probably radically different from what you've done in the past. So in the coming chapters, we'll provide you with simple and powerful exercises that will help you drop the rope and expend your time and energy more wisely. You'll become an expert observer of anxiety—not a participant with a stake in the outcome. You'll also nurture a deeper capacity for kindness and compassion for yourself. It's like building a new relationship with your anxiety. When you do more observing than fighting, you'll find that you're freer to exercise your capacity to choose, take action, and create your destiny.

You Are Response-Able!

Responsibility means that you are able to respond, or "response-able." As you choose to take control of areas in your life where you have control, we can almost guarantee that your judgmental mind will come up with thoughts like *You're too weak, Nothing will ever change,* or *You've never succeeded in the past; why should things be different now?* Heaping negative energy on top of negative energy by blaming and beating up on yourself isn't helpful; neither is arguing back. Blaming yourself and arguing with your mind only feed anxiety and create more worries.

These and other thoughts are simply more old rusty hooks that are trying to snare you and keep you from doing something radically different from what you've done before. The way not to get hooked is to not feed them. You do that by simply thanking your mind for those old thoughts and ceasing to dignify them with a response, giving them more value and importance than they deserve. Then, and only then, are you on the way to dropping the rope. No need to argue back.

Instead, ask yourself this: who has response-ability for the WAFs showing up or not? It's not you! That's just your old conditioning history talking.

Now ask yourself this: Who can choose and is truly *able* to respond differently than in the past when WAFs throw you the rope? Who has the power to persist in making life changes when your judgmental mind is trying to steer you off course? Like it says in the Cole Porter song, "You, you, you!"

WILLINGNESS IS ABOUT DOING

Willingness means making a choice to experience anxiety for what it is—a bunch of sensations, feelings, thoughts, and images—it's not the unacceptable stuff your mind tells you it is. It's not about liking, wanting, putting up with, or tolerating. It's also not about enduring anxiety with brute force of will.

In this sense, willingness is a leap of faith. It's like jumping off a diving board into a pool, not knowing exactly what the water temperature will be or what the experience will be like. This is quite different than wading into the pool, testing the waters, seeing if it is too hot, too cold, too dirty, and so on. That wading isn't willingness. It's gradual and conditional, and so you are left making choices based on how you feel or might feel.

Willingness as a leap has a different quality to it and it's the opposite of control and avoidance. It means to show up and be open to experiencing everything that your mind and body may offer, not knowing exactly what you may find or experience from one moment to the next. This stance is arms open wide and the opposite of fighting anxiety with all you've got.

In fact, if you're willing, you can actually do it right now. Stand up for a moment (if you can), open your arms as wide as you can, and keep them like that for a while. And while you're standing like this, allow all your experiences to come and be just what they are—make no attempt to change them. Really feel them all and let them be. Assuming this posture is a great practice and can actually be fun. This willingness posture captures and symbolizes better than any other gesture or posture what we're doing in this book: opening up to our experiences and allowing them to be there.

We often find that people treat anxiety as their worst enemy. But what if anxiety isn't the enemy? What if you could learn to develop some kindness and compassion for all your experience—including anxiety—and for yourself? Struggling would no longer be necessary. You'd cut the fuel line for your WAFs, and new options would become available to you. This is why developing willingness is so powerful.

Willingness is both a stance toward life and an activity. It is about doing, and doing in the direction of what you value and truly care about. So when we encourage you to be willing, we're asking you to be ready for action. And we're asking you to open up to every aspect of your experience, fully, and without defense.

Doing so allows you to put the serenity creed into action: when you're willing to experience what is, and to accept what cannot be changed, you're positioned to change what can be changed.

WILLINGNESS MAKES GROWTH POSSIBLE

You may think it would be much easier to be willing if you didn't have the pain you feel, if you weren't experiencing all those intense feelings and thoughts. Yet it is not the absence of trauma, pain, and intense, unpleasant feelings and thoughts that keeps people healthy.

There is a difference between health and suffering. In fact, studies in many countries have found that the difference lies in whether people are willing to experience the totality of their psychological and emotional world and still do what matters most to them. Ultimately, willingness is about finding a way to live a meaningful and productive life *with* your pain. When you are willing to live such a life *and* take the totality of personal pains and joys along for the ride, you're on your way out of suffering.

We aren't saying this is easy. And yet this type of pain—having anxiety *and* doing what matters—is like a growing pain. Remember the story about the emperor moth in chapter 5. Being cut off from the experience of pain and struggle wasn't helpful to the moth; it never learned to fly. At times, your old knee-jerk reaction of struggling with WAFs will occur so fast that it'll take a moment to recognize that you're caught up in the tug-of-war again. When that happens, notice what's going on and then let go of the rope. You've just been sucker punched into struggling. Give yourself three seconds to recover. Pull yourself up and then exert your response-ability for what you do next. It's just a passing phase before you can take off and fly.

Always remember that you can make a different choice by adopting the stance of willingness—by opening up and softening to the experience of anxiety. You can live a vital and meaningful life if you're willing to have and experience anxiety.

EXERCISE: THE WILLINGNESS SWITCH

Imagine you have two switches in front of you. They look like light switches and both have an on/off setting. One switch is called "anxiety" and the other is called "willingness." It seems like both switches can be turned on or off. When you started reading this book, you were probably hoping to find a way to turn the anxiety switch off, but this turned out to be a false hope. The on/off toggle of the anxiety switch isn't working. This may even make you feel like you're a victim of anxiety, that you're helpless. And your mind says, *That sucks.* You're disappointed over and over again.

So we'd like to share a secret with you. The willingness switch is really the more important of the two because it's the one that will make a difference in your life. Unlike the anxiety switch, you can and do control the willingness switch. When it comes to willingness, you're not a helpless victim, because that switch is controlled by your actions. Remember, this is *the place where you are response-able.* It's your choice to flip the willingness switch on or off.

We're not sure what would happen with your anxiety if you switched the willingness on. We only know one thing: you really can switch it on if you make a choice to do so. And then things might start to happen in your life. You could start doing what you really want to do and start moving in the direction of your Valued Life Epitaph inscription.

In this metaphor, we're not talking about ignoring anxiety. We're simply encouraging you to turn your attention from what you cannot control to what you can control. You probably don't know what will happen to your anxiety if you don't attempt to control it. You may have a prediction. Yet, based on your experience, do you actually know? Have you ever approached anxiety with willingness to have it? What happens over time might surprise you.

WILLINGNESS IS DOING, NOT TRYING TO DO

"I'll try" is often the first response we hear when we talk to people about willingness: "Next time I'm anxious, I'll really try to be willing and not do what I usually do." And when things haven't worked out, we hear, "I've tried to go to work and face my fear of failure. I've tried *really* hard, but I just couldn't do it. My anxiety was just too high. So I stayed home."

The following brief exercise is a powerful way for you to connect with the fact that willingness is an all-or-nothing action: you do or you don't; it's not about trying to do something.

EXERCISE: THE TRYING PEN

To get a sense of what we mean, go ahead and have a seat at a table and place a pen in front of you. Now, we'd like you to *try* to pick up the pen. Try as hard as you can. Go ahead and *try* it. If you find yourself picking up the pen, stop! That isn't what we asked you to do. We want you to *try* to pick it up. After some effort, you're probably thinking, *Well, I can't do that. Either I pick it up or I don't.* You're right. There's no way to try to pick up the pen and at the same time actually pick it up.

You may have noticed that you hand was stuck hovering over the pen when you tried to pick it up. That's what trying gets you. You end up hovering over things in your life and not doing what you wish to do—like when you try to lose weight, try to get more exercise, try to do a better job, try to be a better lover, try to be a more responsive parent, try to be more organized, try to be a better listener, or try to be less anxious. Trying just leaves you hovering, in a state of paralysis, and stuck.

So trying is really a form of "not doing." This is why we never want you to try anything. You must first make a choice about whether you're willing to do something. If you are completely willing rather than just a bit willing, then go ahead and do it. And if you aren't willing, then don't do it. Remember willingness only has an on/off switch, not some type of dial you can move up or down a little. Just like a woman can't be a bit pregnant—either she is or she isn't—you can't be a bit willing.

Focus on the doing and not the outcomes. Even if you are 100 percent willing, you may not always get what you want. Doing is not about getting it right or meeting failure either. For instance, you could decide to pick up the pen and then find that it slips from your fingers and drops to the floor. Your mind might say, *You tried, but it didn't work.* Yet your experience tells you that you could still bend over and repeat the act of picking up the pen, if that's what you're committed to doing. Some activities in life simply require persistence: you may need to do them over and over again before you accomplish your goal. Failure is one of many subjective evaluations of what we like to call your *mind machine*, which comes up with a seemingly never-ending stream of judgmental thoughts. You can choose not to let your judgmental mind stop you from doing what's important.

So are you willing to go out with your hands and feet and take your anxiety with you? Remember, willingness is neither a feeling nor a thought. Willingness is simply a choice and a commitment to have what you already have. This frees you up to go where you want to go.

So, Are You Willing?

Responsibility for what you do begins with you. It's time to face this stark truth squarely. Your behavior is something you can control—even when you're in the grip of powerful emotions like your WAFs. Your behavior includes the kind of relationship you nurture with yourself and your emotional life. This is good news.

At times, it will feel as if you have no choice but to resort to your old patterns of avoidance and struggle. Your mind will tell you *It's too hard*, *There's too much anxiety*, and *I must get out of here*. When that happens, it's important to nurture willingness.

Up to this point, we expect that putting willingness together with your WAFs sounds nuts. In fact, it's likely you opened this book with a deep feeling of unwillingness toward your WAFs. You can get a sense of this yourself, by going back to your LIFE worksheets from the past week. Look at your willingness rating for each WAF episode and then count the number of times you answered "yes" (I'm 100% willing) or "no" (I'm 100% unwilling). If you haven't had WAF episodes in the past week, then give a best estimate of your willingness now with a yes or no answer.

The number of times you answered "yes" to willingness (e.g., I was 100% willing to have my WAFs without acting on them to manage, get rid of, suppress, or run from them) was _____.

The number of times you answered "no" to willingness (e.g., I was 100% unwilling to have my WAFs without acting on them to manage, get rid of, suppress, or run from them) was _____.

Willingness Isn't a Feeling

Many people think of willingness and unwillingness as feelings, but remember—willingness isn't a feeling. So when we encourage you to be willing, we aren't asking you to change how you feel. You can still think that your WAFs are unpleasant and you can dislike the discomfort.

With willingness, we're asking you to make a choice. That choice is to be with your WAFs when they show up and to stop your efforts to make them go away by acting in ways that hurt you and your life.

> *Your commitment is to do your best; it's not a commitment to succeed.*

If you're willing to make this commitment, then pick up a pen and sign your name on the line below. If you cannot sign the commitment, then it's best to stop, go back, and dig in to where you are in life with your anxiety before reading on. Look at the costs and the two epitaphs you worked on. See if you can connect with the life you truly want to lead. What's really holding you back now? You've already taken a bold step by opening this book and getting this far. You have everything you need to go on.

The Willingness Commitment

I am willing to take my WAFs with me as I use my hands and feet to move myself in the directions I want my life to take.

_____   _____

Signature   Date

LIFE ENHANCEMENT EXERCISES

We encourage you to do the following this week:

- Commit to making a centering exercise part of your daily routine.

- Continue to notice WAFs in your daily life using the LIFE Worksheet.

- Become aware of your relationship with your WAFs—is it friendly or hostile?

- Be mindful of your actions in areas where you really do not have control and practice dropping the rope, letting go, and being just as you are.

- Remember that change is a journey, not a destination.

THE TAKE-HOME MESSAGE

Instead of choosing to struggle with your WAFs, you can choose to drop the rope and be response-able. The idea of response-ability is a very positive and liberating one. You control your choices and actions, what you say, and what you do, including how you respond to your WAFs. All the remaining chapters are about fostering your willingness and ability to choose, take action, and move forward in your life. They are about maximizing control where you have it. This is how you create your destiny.

Response-Ability Is Control over My Choices, Actions, and Destiny

Points to Ponder: I can choose how I respond to my WAFs. Making different choices from those I've made in the past could improve my life. I am response-able. There's no try, only do.

Question to Consider: Am I willing to go out with my hands and feet and take my anxiety with me to move in the direction I want my life to take?

CHAPTER 10

Getting Into Your Life with Mindful Acceptance

Water is fluid, soft, and yielding. But water will wear away rock, which is rigid and cannot yield. As a rule, whatever is fluid, soft, and yielding will overcome whatever is rigid and hard.

—Lao Tzu (600 BC)

Take a moment and allow yourself to sit with the opening quote you just read. Then, when you're ready, insert the first noun that comes to mind as you consider each of the following statements.

My WAFs are like _____ (noun).

My responses to my WAFs are like _____ (noun).

Now, stop. Look at what your mind came up with to characterize your WAFs and your responses to them. Did you select nouns describing things that are soft, gentle, fluid, or yielding? We'd guess not. It's more likely that your mind came up with nouns describing things that are solid as rock and unyielding. When you put both statements together, what you are left with is something like this—rock against rock.

Your judgmental mind can readily turn anything that is normally fluid and flexible—like thoughts, feelings, sensations, and memories—into something hard and heavy that's pushing you around and seemingly ruining your life. Once your mind does that, it is natural to ramp up your efforts to alleviate the burden—the weight of the WAFs. The problem though is that resistance and struggle have a hard and weighty quality too. So there you are, carrying the burden of your WAFs and your unsuccessful struggles with them. Hardness begets hardness. This needs to stop.

Lao Tzu teaches us this simple truth: whatever is soft is strong. Allow this powerful message to sink in, for everything you are about to learn rests on this understanding. Packed in this pearl of wisdom is one of the most powerful antidotes to human suffering. The antidote is to soften when your tendency is to harden. To expand when you'd rather contract. To lean into life when your impulse is to turn away. Above all, you learn to nurture your capacity for gentleness, kindness, and compassion in relation to your mind, body, and world. These softer, more fluid, more flexible, and, dare we say, more vital qualities are wrapped up in two words—mindful acceptance.

Mindful acceptance is a stance toward life: watching the struggle without judging it, feeling the pain without drowning in it, and honoring the hurt without becoming it. It's not a feeling or an attitude. It doesn't come from crystals or insight. As Tara Brach (2004) teaches us, the practice involves a willingness to experience one's self and one's life just as it is. Mindful acceptance is a skill that will offer you moments of genuine freedom from suffering. But this skill, like any other, takes practice and some work to learn.

Before we show you how, we'd like you to go back to the two fill-in statements you completed at the beginning of this chapter. And, with your most troublesome WAF concerns in mind, we'd like you to do that exercise again, but with a slight twist.

EXERCISE: VISUALIZING THE SOFT-ROCK WAF SHUFFLE

This exercise is intended to help you connect with what a softer response can buy you in relation to your WAFs. Start by finding a quiet and comfortable place. And when you're ready, allow yourself a moment to think about your WAFs. Let all the words that come to mind pour forth, unedited. In the space below, write all of them down as quickly as they come to you. Reveal the hardness and negative energy.

Here's how Matt, who had a long history of suffering with panic, described his WAFs: My WAFs are *nasty, crippling, intense, overwhelming, gripping, painful, a burden, a wall, a knife, screwed up, exhausting, shameful, embarrassing.*

Now it's your turn. *My WAFs are* _____

_____.

Once you've got it all down, we'd like you to connect with the negative energy, the hardness in the words you used to describe your WAFs. Give yourself a minute to get into it.

Next, gently switch to the first word from the list below. Read it slowly and then close your eyes and sit with it. Imagine yourself doing what the statement says when your WAFs show up. Connect with the quality of each word in the list that follows. Let the quality of the word touch you. Try to become it. This is the softer response we're after.

We'd like you to repeat this exercise by shuttling back and forth between the *hard* words you came up with about your WAFs and each *softer* response option below. Continue this back and forth. Imagine yourself meeting your *hard* WAFs with each *softer* response. Give yourself at least one minute with each new response option.

I will meet my hard WAFs with these qualities:

Softness • *Gentleness* • *Kindness* • *Openness* • *Compassion*

Love • *Patience* • *Humor* • *Caring* • *Curiosity*

As you did this brief exercise, did you notice anything? Did the quality of your thoughts about your WAFs change, even just a little bit, as you cycled back and forth through each softer response option? This may be hard for you to detect. If so, ask yourself this: After doing the exercise, would you describe your WAFs using the same words that you used before? Or, even if you chose to use the same words, do you really need to buy in to them and do what they say?

Don't worry if you didn't notice anything dramatic here. The intent of this exercise is to reveal, even if only in a small way, what the softness of mindful acceptance can offer you. It can wear away the hardness of your WAFs and the very need to do anything about them. But to truly get that, you'll need to practice developing the skill of mindful acceptance. Remember, softness will wear away rock—the hardness that underlies your tendency to struggle, to fight, and to pick up the rope.

You have the capacity to choose this softer, skillful alternative. And as you'll see with time and practice, mindful acceptance can be used in many areas of your life, not solely in places where anxious pain and hurt tend to get you sidetracked from where you want to go. You'll be learning skills that go beyond your anxieties and fears. These skills will improve your life in many ways.

WHAT ACCEPTANCE IS AND CAN DO FOR YOU

Many people we've worked with have told themselves at some point, *I just need to accept my anxiety.* In fact, we hear this quite a bit. You may have told yourself that too. The problem is that many people do not have a good sense of what acceptance really means.

In fact, people often think of acceptance as just taking it. So, they give up and stop making efforts to change. The word "acceptance" also conjures up many other negative associations like succumbing to your pain, giving in, resigning, being weak, or behaving like a loser or a patsy. These are all passive forms of acceptance. This way of thinking about acceptance is unhelpful because it will keep you stuck—resigned to letting your WAFs (something you cannot control) guide your actions (something you can control). Giving up and bowing to your WAFs will lead you down the path of self-denigration and ultimately to more struggle and suffering.

Here's a more vital take on acceptance. The word itself literally means "to take what is offered." It is a choice to open up and be with whatever is happening anyway. With this type of acceptance, you're actively doing something new. You are choosing to open and be with what is, just as it is.

And as you do that, you can expect that your mind may not play nice. Your mind has fed you the message that your anxious pain is your enemy, and it has linked that pain to just about everything you want to be about as a person and with your life. And your mind tells you that your emotional pain stands between you and your life.

So it may seem that you are left with only two choices: sit and wallow with the emotional pain and do nothing, or struggle to get the pain out of the way while important aspects of your life slip away. The first is passive acceptance and the second is flat out nonacceptance. Both of them are bad for you. You know that already just by looking at your experience up until now.

Mindful acceptance is a third option that we want to explore further because it might just be good for you.

Mindful Acceptance Is Active, Soft, and Vital

Mindful acceptance is an active, fully conscious, softer stance toward your mind and body and your life experiences. It simply involves noticing what you think and feel and allowing those thoughts and feelings to be there—it doesn't mean liking or agreeing with them.

Acceptance is about acknowledging and experiencing what happened in the past and what's happening in the present moment without judging and getting all tangled up in that experience. This will help you wake up to reality as it is, not as your judgmental mind and past history say it is.

EXERCISE: "OH, WHAT A _____ ROSE"

To get a sense of that, do this: close your eyes and imagine a long-stemmed rose, freshly cut after a gentle rain, hovering in front of you. Look it over carefully. Notice all the details—the textures, smell, shapes, and colors.

See the light and shadows, the dew drops, and the stem. In your mind, simply notice the qualities of the rose and your experience of it.

As you did this exercise, did your mind throw in evaluations of the rose? You might have thought, *How beautiful* or *It smells really nice*. Your mind could have readily come up with more negative evaluations too, like, *That's an ugly rose*, *This exercise sucks*, or even *What a stupid rose*. It might have even brought to mind a memory of a loving moment, or a relationship that went sour.

Notice though that your evaluations don't change the rose one bit—the rose is a rose regardless of what your mind calls it. Notice also that your evaluations of the rose aren't the rose. The rose won't change because your mind calls it this or that. Mindful acceptance is a powerful way to notice when you're caught up in evaluations of your experience more than in the raw experience itself. Acceptance calls you to open up to life just as it is.

Mindful acceptance also has a welcoming and kind quality to it. We like to think about it as *compassion in action*. With that, you cultivate your capacity to meet the hardness of your judgmental mind and emotional hurts with softness and gentleness. When you do that, you also weaken the power of your judgmental mind to get you hooked by your anxieties, fears, hurts, shame, anger, or remorse—all the sticky negative energy that can pull you out of your life and keep you stuck.

Consider when you've been asked to go somewhere where you know your WAFs are likely to show up. One of the first things you'll notice is feeling yourself hardening. Some people experience hardening as a tightening, tensing, or sense of closing down. It can happen in an instant. As you harden more, all the things you'd like to do seem to wash away. Then, you want to run, withdraw, and be somewhere other than where you are. Your judgmental mind pulls you out of the present. And with that, the old habitual comfort-seeking actions kick in, and wham—there you are, stuck, holding the rope, and struggling with yourself.

> *Acceptance means noticing and acknowledging what you experience— not liking what you experience.*

Mindful Acceptance Can Get You Unstuck

Mindful acceptance is a powerful way to get unstuck, unhooked, and moving forward. It starts with cultivating your willingness to stay with the urge to act on your own discomfort—without doing what your mind and history compel you to do for another quick fix of temporary relief. You then get curious about what you're experiencing and make a choice to see things clearly as they are, softening to the urge to run from or avoid your worries, anxieties, and fears. The practice of seeing things clearly and softening creates space to make more vital choices.

There's no magic to this process. You decide to do it. And you do it by choosing to let go of the struggle with your inner painful and hurtful experiences, be they worries, anxieties, fears, or anger, hostility, or sadness. You let go by bringing kindness and gentle attention to unwanted WAF thoughts and feelings, by simply allowing them to be. Our colleague Jeffrey Brantley (2003) describes this process as one of becoming a friend to yourself and to your WAFs.

It's very easy for all of us to run through life mindlessly, on autopilot. Our heads are in the past or the future or elsewhere. Yet you know that your life is only lived in the present because that's where you are. The present is the only place where you can make a difference in your life.

And there are many times when you've gotten hooked, snared by what your critical judgmental mind is feeding you. Our minds are constantly adding unnecessary baggage to our experiences, creating an illusion of a reality that simply isn't so. Recall that a duckling is a duck, regardless of what your mind says about it—an ugly duckling is as much a duck as a cute duckling.

This is where mindful acceptance can make a real difference. It'll help you learn to recognize the mind game for what it is—a substitute reality, not reality itself. Mindful acceptance will position you to break your identification with the thoughts that fuel your struggle. You'll start to see your urges to act on your WAFs as urges. You'll learn to sit with them without needing to change them or do what they say. And as you start cultivating a softer response to your mind, body, and world, things will change. Suddenly there will be space to move. You'll see how this works when you get to the Chinese Finger Trap exercise in a moment.

Mindful Acceptance Is a Skill and a Valuable Choice

People often associate mindfulness with meditative religious traditions such as Buddhism. Though there's a resemblance, you need not ascribe to a religion to practice being mindful. Mindfulness is a skill of kind observing of your experience, day in and day out—what's happening on the inside and outside—as it is.

The problem is that we live a good portion of our lives in our heads—interpreting, evaluating, and judging ourselves, the past and future, others, and our world. As we're doing that, we're not focused on what is really going on right now. Mindful acceptance will put you in fuller and more honest and open contact with everything you experience. You'll see things more clearly, gain perspective, and start to notice that what's happening is just what's happening.

This can be difficult, for we all have a natural reaction to run away as we open up and begin to face squarely things that we don't like very much. Yet acceptance isn't about liking unpleasant feelings. It just means acknowledging them and no longer fighting them or denying them. This will free up energy you need to create the life you want to live.

What we're after here is playfulness and transparency of the kind that would allow you to notice more fully the displeasure, unease, discomfort, hurt, and even joy, goodness, and beauty. And we're after melding that with softer qualities of caring, compassion, and love. So as you develop the skills of acceptance, keep in mind that this isn't another clever fix to dull your WAF pain. If you find yourself using it this way, you're missing the boat. And you'll likely be disappointed with the results.

As you begin to apply mindful acceptance, you'll see that your WAFs are just a collection of thoughts as thoughts, images as images, feelings as feelings, and sensations as sensations. That's it. You'll also be able to recognize judgments, negative evaluations, and pesky urges while bringing to those experiences a quality of gentle curiosity, kindness, compassion, caring, and wholeness. This isn't easy to do. And it's next to impossible to do without learning how to be a compassionate observer of your experiences. This is why practice is an important part of active acceptance.

Initially mindful acceptance is best practiced at home, in a comfortable, safe environment. As you get more skilled at it, you can gradually expand to include more stressful, emotion-triggering situations, including those that involve your WAFs. A substantial body of research shows that this skill set can be enormously helpful in keeping you from getting hooked by your judgmental mind.

Mindful Acceptance Makes Space for New Solutions

We focus so much on acceptance because struggling with your WAFs hasn't worked and acceptance makes room for new beginnings, new ways of responding. It's the antidote to struggle. It's life expanding. It gives you space to control what you do. Acceptance is doing something new!

We're not saying that your mind is the enemy. Your mind isn't the problem—not even a critical judgmental mind that feeds you a stream of recycled scary thoughts and images.

Problems happen when you get hooked on thoughts and images, believing in them so strongly that you identify with them and allow them to pull you out of your life. At that point, you're completely caught up in your head. Mindful acceptance will help you to let go of the story line and just observe what's going on. It'll also help you see when your mind serves you well and when it doesn't. This understanding is key.

You cannot think yourself into a life. You cannot feel your way into a life. You need to get moving with your hands, feet, and mouth. Whenever your mind serves you well on this road—and sometimes it does—listen to it and do what it says. However, if listening keeps you stuck, then it's time to take stock: allow some gentle space between what your mind says works and matters and what your experience says works and matters. Then recommit to go forward with action because this is the only thing that matters. Mindful acceptance will help you gain the needed space to do just that.

EXERCISE: CHINESE FINGER TRAP

To get a sense of what we mean by creating space, imagine playing with one of those Chinese finger traps that you may have played with as a child. A finger trap is a tube of woven straw, about five inches long and half an inch wide. Perhaps you can find one in a novelty or party store and do the exercise for real. If not, just imagine doing it.

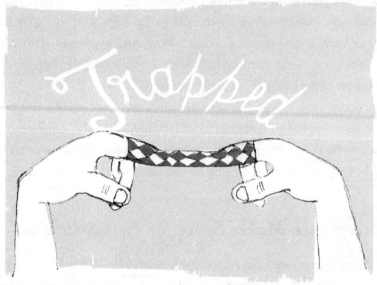

During this exercise, you pick up the finger trap and slide one index finger into each end of the tube. After you fully insert your fingers, try pulling them out. If you were to do that, you'd notice that the tube catches and tightens. You'd experience some discomfort as the tube squeezes your fingers and reduces circulation.

You may feel a little confused. Pulling out of the tube seems like an obvious and natural solution. Yet it doesn't work. The harder you try to pull out of the trap, the more stuck you become. That's exactly how the WAF trap works too.

The finger trap shows that our instinctive solutions to our emotional and psychological hurts and pain often turn out to be no solutions at all. In fact, these so-called solutions create even bigger problems. Pulling away from anxiety and fear may seem like a natural and logical way to free yourself from the WAF trap. But your experience with anxiety tells you that this struggle has only brought you more discomfort and life problems. You're *trapped*!

The good news is that there's an alternative that works and is supported by our research. To get there, you have to do something that goes against the grain. Instead of pulling out, you push in. This move will give you more space, more wiggle room. This is what acceptance offers.

Acceptance is doing something counterintuitive. As you practice leaning into pain and anxiety rather than pulling away, you'll be learning to stay with your experience. You acknowledge the discomfort and make room for it, allowing it to be, without doing anything about it and without trying to make it go away. This will give you enough room to move around and live your life.

THE FOUR QUALITIES OF MINDFUL ACCEPTANCE

Mindfulness and acceptance are difficult concepts to pin down for many people, including us. That said, there's a general consensus about four qualities that go into mindful acceptance. Jon Kabat-Zinn (1994), a noted mindfulness scholar and therapist, packs the essential qualities of mindfulness into the following definition: "paying attention in a particular way: on purpose, in the present moment, and non-judgmentally" (p. 4). Let's unpack each part before we go forward with the practice.

Paying Attention

Paying attention in the here and now is enormously challenging because we all live with two sources of distractions: those from the world around us and those emanating from within our heads. Both sources can pull you out of the present in a flash. If you've suffered a past trauma or relive painful memories, then you know this pull and spin quite well.

On top of that, your critical judgmental mind will often pull you out of the present too. So, you may spend your time thinking about your life, remembering the past, and contemplating your future. And you'll tend to react to people and situations based on old habitual patterns of thinking, feeling, relating, and behaving. These actions may have hurt you and others in your life. All of this activity pulls you out of the present moment—the place where your life is lived out—and can lead you in directions you don't want to go.

Learning to pay attention, fully and with as little defense as possible, can liberate you from these traps and put you in fuller contact with yourself and your world as it is, right where you are. Paying attention means more contact with yourself and the circumstances of your life. More contact means more potential vitality. More vitality means that you'll likely feel better and grow. There's no way to learn and grow if you don't pay attention.

On Purpose

To pay attention, you must consciously choose to do it, and do it again and again, over and over throughout your day and your life. This alone can be difficult to do. Yet when you do it, you are doing something different than you've done before. You're taking the reins and noticing, with a gentle curiosity, what's happening as it's happening. As you do more of that, you'll interrupt the mind machine that's feeding you the same old unworkable strategies that have kept you stuck. Instead of pulling out of your experiences, you'll be deliberately moving into them.

Sometimes you'll get pulled back into the same old automatic patterns that have kept you stuck. The skill is to recognize when this is happening, recommit to acting with purpose, and get back to noticing what's really happening. And when those old habits rear their ugly heads from time to time, just notice them. Don't put yourself down for having "failed." Instead, be glad and grateful that you've recognized the old dead ends. You might just say, *There's my old history again.* Then, after thanking your mind and body for that reminder, you can gently and purposefully return to what you'd really like to notice and do in the moment.

In the Present Moment

We all live in the here and now, but our minds can quickly take us elsewhere. You've had this experience too. If you pay attention you'll be amazed how often this happens on any given day. In fact, it happens more times than not. Taking a shower while thinking about what you're going to wear or the things you need to get done is a good example. Your body is in the shower, yet your head is elsewhere. You may have had the experience of reading a page of a book or the newspaper, only to find your eyes are at the bottom of the page but you don't remember a damn thing you just read. Or you may be driving while thinking about this or that, only to realize that you've gone five miles and can't remember a darn thing you've passed along the way. And you might have missed your exit too.

The point here is that we all can be readily pulled out of the present. And when that happens, you can and often will miss the here-and-now experience—the only place that is real.

Nonjudgmentally

Of all the qualities of mindful acceptance, this one is the most challenging to learn. And it will definitely be a gradual learning process. You'll remember from earlier chapters that we all have a tendency to evaluate and judge just about everything we do: good—bad, right—wrong, sour—sweet, should—shouldn't, and so on.

You know the ways you judge situations, other people, and your own thoughts, feelings and behaviors—often in a chain reaction of increasing judgment and distress: *This is horrible! What an idiot! How could I do that?! I can't take this anymore! Why can't I be normal?* or *Here I go again.* This is the fuel for the struggle with your WAFs. And, if you look closely, you'll see that none of it is helpful to you.

Positive judgment can be every bit as problematic: *I need ..., I want ..., I should have ...,* or *I deserve ...* All such judgments flow from thinking that you're missing out on something or that you must have something. When you hold on to these thoughts, particularly when they are automatic and intense, you can quickly lose focus, forget what's important, and get caught in cycles of struggle and self-blame.

The problem here is attachment to the judgments—taking them so seriously. We're not asking you to stop your mind from producing judgments and evaluations. It's impossible because that's what minds do, and there is no healthy way we know of to stop that process. The solution is to notice the judgments and not do as they say.

All judgment creates an illusion of a reality that isn't so. When you fuse with what your mind is telling you, you pull out of your experience and end up struggling to remove the unpleasantness or to get something you don't have. Perhaps that something is peace of mind, being relaxed, or even happiness. Your mind makes it seem like these qualities are something that you can have, hold, and keep. The evaluations seem real.

Stop here and check your experience to see if this is really the way it is: Can you get happiness and hold on to it like you can get a can of soda and keep it with you as long as you wish? Or does happiness tend to ebb and flow over time just like most thoughts and emotions? Are feelings something you can grab on to and hold like objects in the physical world? When you act as if you can hold on to them—and try to do what your judgmental mind says—you'll end up miserable.

Putting the qualities of acceptance—willingness, openness, compassion, kindness, and playfulness—into action is the single most powerful way to dilute the fuel that drives your WAF suffering. These softer qualities, when mixed with paying attention, on purpose, with as little judgment as possible, and in the present moment, will undercut the very need to struggle and will give you the freedom to do what matters to you.

You may have a hard time imagining bringing these nonjudgmental qualities to your experiences, particularly when unpleasant thoughts, memories, or feelings show up. And we can almost guarantee that your mind will continue to judge your experiences. Your task is to recognize judgments as products of your mind, and whenever they show up, you can just label them "thinking." There is nothing mysterious about learning to become less judgmental over time. You have a choice here.

You can choose to continue to react to your unpleasant experiences with hardness and negative energy. Or you can decide to be kinder and gentler with yourself, to create space between you and what your mind (based on old history) is telling you. This is one of the kindest things you can do for yourself. The choice here is entirely up to you. If you are willing to choose the softer path, then you'll be doing something new. It'll be a slow and gradual process with lots of setbacks on the path. The important thing is to keep going in a new direction.

MINDFUL ACCEPTANCE PRACTICE

Mindfulness exercises are a way of learning that we cannot choose what comes into our minds and what we feel. We can only choose *what* we pay attention to, *how* we pay attention, and what we *do*. The exercise below will help you do just that. It ought to take about fifteen minutes. You'll find an audio version of the exercise on the book website at http://www.newharbinger.com/33346.

In this exercise, we again focus on the breath because what's going on in your mind and body is constantly shifting and changing—just like your breathing. This exercise will help you develop the skill of paying attention to your breathing while allowing other internal activities such as thoughts, feelings, or sensations to come and go without getting tangled up in them. If you pay attention with a quality of openness and compassion, you'll see that all of this inside activity does change from moment to moment without effort on your part. With time, you'll also realize that no matter how bad an internal experience seems, it neither lasts forever nor can do any harm.

We'd like you to keep in mind that this exercise is not about making you feel different, better, relaxed, or calm. This may happen or it may not. The idea is to bring compassion and a kind awareness to *any* sensations that show up, including any thoughts or worries that come into your mind. It's about learning to stay with your WAFs with loving-kindness toward yourself, bringing as much warmth and compassion into the situation as you can. This is a concrete way of learning that anxiety isn't the enemy.

Remember that mindful acceptance is a skill that grows with practice. The goal is to develop the skill so that you can then apply it in your life, anytime or anyplace. There's no right or wrong way to practice. The important thing is that you commit to doing these exercises on the path of becoming a better observer and full participant in your life.

We suggest you simply select a quiet place where you feel comfortable and distraction is limited. Let's call this your peaceful place. The easiest way to do this exercise is by listening to and following the instructions on the website. If you read the exercise and decide to commit it to memory, just do it slowly.

After practicing with the audio recording for a week or two, you may prefer to practice at your own pace without the audio guiding you. At any time, you can go back and do the exercise while listening to the recording.

EXERCISE: ACCEPTANCE OF THOUGHTS AND FEELINGS

Get in a comfortable position in your chair. Sit upright with your feet flat on the floor, your arms and legs uncrossed, and your hands resting in your lap (palms up or down, whichever is more comfortable). Allow your eyes to close gently.

Take a few moments to get in touch with the movement of your breath and the sensations in your body. As you do that, slowly bring your attention to the gentle rising and falling of your breath in your chest and belly. Like ocean waves coming in and out, your breath is always there. Notice its rhythm … the changing patterns of sensations … the temperature of the air as it passes in and out of your nose … the movement in your chest and belly. Take a few moments to feel the physical sensations of the breath moving in … and out.

There's no need to control your breathing. Simply let the breath breathe itself. As best you can, bring an attitude of generous allowing and gentle acceptance to your experience, just as it is.

Sooner or later your mind will wander away from the breath to other concerns, thoughts, worries, images, bodily sensations, planning, or daydreams, or it may just drift along. This is what minds do much of the time. When you notice that your mind has wandered, just acknowledge that awareness of your experience. Then, gently, and with kindness, come back to the breath.

If you become aware of feelings, tension, or other intense physical sensations, just notice them, acknowledge their presence, and see if you can make space for them. Imagine with each in-breath you are creating more space inside of you for all of you and see if you can welcome that as you return to the breath.

You may notice sensations in your body and how they change from moment to moment. Sometimes they're stronger, sometimes they stay the same, and sometimes they grow weaker—it doesn't really matter what they do. Breathe calmly into and out from the sensations of any places where you feel discomfort, imagining the breath moving into, and out from, that region of the body. As you do, remind yourself that you are getting better at feeling and being with all that is you, as it is, in this moment.

Along with physical sensations in your body, you may also notice thoughts about the sensations and thoughts about the thoughts. You may notice your mind coming up with evaluations such as "dangerous" or "getting worse," or "bored." If that happens, notice those evaluations and return to the breath and the present moment, as it is. Thoughts are thoughts, physical sensations are physical sensations, feelings are feelings, nothing more, nothing less.

If you wish, you can name thoughts and feelings as you notice them. For instance, if you notice dwelling on the past, label that "a memory" and come back to the breath. Or, if you find yourself worrying about the future, label that "worry" and again, come back to the present moment, right here, right now, being with the breath. Perhaps there is judging … notice that, and then return to the present breath, bringing a quality of kindness and compassion to your experience.

Thoughts and feelings come and go in your mind and body. The breath remains in this moment. You are the observer of your experience and not what those thoughts and feelings say, no matter how persistent or intense they may be. You are the place and space for your experience. Make that space a kind space, a gentle space, a loving space, a welcome home.

As this time of formal mindful practice comes to an end, you may wish to commit to the intention of bringing this purposeful awareness of the present moment to the rest of your day. Then, when you're ready, gradually widen your attention to take in the sounds around you … and slowly open your eyes.

This exercise can be challenging to do at first. So remind yourself that you're learning a new skill. But don't let that challenge (a judgment) stand in the way of you doing the practice again and again over this week and the weeks to come. These judgments usually show up when you're trying to achieve a particular result—like calm, peace, or less anxiety, fear, or depression. If that result doesn't show up, it's easy to slip into thinking that the practice was a failure. This isn't so.

Remember, the goal is to experience what it is like to be right here, right now, not somewhere other than that. Many results are possible and all are okay. So, be kind with yourself as you do the practice.

It'll be helpful to track your experiences with this exercise over the next several weeks using the worksheet at the end of this chapter. This will give your practice some structure and give you a place to chart your progress over time. We've included an example of how to complete the worksheet. You'll also find the worksheet on the book website (http://www.newharbinger.com/33346) so you can print out as many extra copies as you need.

Of course, there are many areas of life where you can practice mindful awareness, and you don't need to close your eyes to practice it. In fact, the Mindful Walking exercise we introduced earlier is a great example of an activity you do regularly with eyes wide open. The skill is in learning how to come back to right where you are and to your life just as it is. Bringing mindful awareness to your experience will help you do just that. If you haven't done so already, give mindful walking another shot and look for routine activities in your daily life (e.g., doing the dishes) that you could approach more mindfully.

LIFE ENHANCEMENT EXERCISES

Centering exercises are a wonderful way to cultivate your observer mind. Here, we introduced one additional exercise: Acceptance of Thoughts and Feelings. This exercise is relatively simple to do. Focusing on the breath is a skill that you've already started developing with some of the centering exercises we covered early on. It will also be used in exercises in the chapters to come. The neat thing about this practice is that you can do it anytime and anywhere. Walking is something that most of us do anyway, and doing so mindfully will help you learn to move with presence.

The point is not to become overwhelmed by the material in this workbook, but rather to start doing something new in your life, however small that might be. Small changes will add up.

So, for this week, make a commitment to put the following activities on your to-do list:

- Practice the Acceptance of Thoughts and Feelings exercise daily.

- Practice mindful walking when you're going about your day.

- If you are willing, continue working with any of the exercises we covered so far. Focus on exercises that give you space and shift your perspective.

- Notice if you're resisting what we've covered so far. If you're resisting, pause, and look to see what you may be attached to—for instance, what would change in your life if you were no longer crippled by anxiety and fear? Some of these changes may be scary. You may have no clear sense of who you are and what you are capable of without the WAF label.

- Above all, be patient with yourself. The problems you are dealing with did not develop overnight. Working with the material in this workbook is an act of self-care and a journey on a new path and a new direction in your life.

THE TAKE-HOME MESSAGE

Everything you do happens in the present moment. Thinking happens here. Remembering happens here. Feelings unfold in the now, and so do urges. *Now* is where your life is lived. This is where you've experienced the costs too. The present moment is the only place where you can act to make a difference in your life.

But we must learn to be present. It is, as Elizabeth Lesser (2008) describes it, like learning "piano scales, basketball drills, ballroom dance class … With increasing practice, you become more skilled at the art form itself. You do not practice to become a great scale player or drill champion. You practice to become a musician or athlete. Likewise, one does not practice meditation to become a great meditator. We meditate to wake up and live, to become skilled at the art of living" (p. 97).

Developing any new skill takes practice and commitment. Mindful acceptance is no different. You must intend to be mindful. And you must be willing. And you have to do it over and over again to become skillful. That's why practice is important. But, as Elizabeth Lesser also teaches us, the practice is not the goal. Learning mindful acceptance is part of your journey out of suffering and back into your life. The more you do it, the better you'll become at it over time.

But be careful: using mindful acceptance like a new gold shovel to dig yourself out of your WAFs is just doing more of the same and will keep you stuck. There's no way to be mindful if you're holding on to the wish that things were different from how they are. You have to choose to let that thought go, and along with it your attachment to the pleasant moments in life, hoping that they will never change (because they will). You can also choose to let go of your attachment to the idea that unpleasant experiences in your life will always be this way (because they won't). You have to be open to everything that might show up—everything.

So ask yourself if there's enough room inside you to let all of you in—just as you are. If not, what's standing in the way of you experiencing yourself just as you are? And if there's something that shows up, see whether you can make space for *that*—not liking or condoning it, just acknowledging that it's there. By approaching WAF thoughts and feelings with mindful acceptance wrapped in compassion, you deprive them of the fuel they need to burn. You are no longer fighting. This will ultimately cool the flames feeding your WAFs and will free you to move in new and more vital life directions. You have control here.

Mindful Acceptance Can Pull Me Out of My WAFs and Into My Life

Points to Ponder: Acceptance is a vital and courageous activity. I can choose to acknowledge my WAFs without getting all tangled up in a struggle with them so that I can focus on what I really want to do with my life.

Question to Consider: Am I willing to approach my WAFs with more kindness and compassion?

ACCEPTANCE OF THOUGHTS AND FEELINGS:
Life Enhancement Exercise Practice Worksheet

In the first (leftmost) column, record whether you made a commitment to practice the Acceptance of Thoughts and Feelings exercise that day and include the date. In the second column, record whether you actually practiced, when you practiced, and for how long. In the third column, note if you did or didn't use the audio version of the exercise. In the fourth column, write down anything that comes up during your practice.

Acceptance of Thoughts and Feelings Life Enhancement Exercise Practice Form			
Commitment: yes/no Day: Date:	Practiced: yes/no When practiced? A.M./P.M. How long (minutes)?	Audio: yes/no	Comments
Commitment: (yes)/no Day: Saturday Date: 5/30/2014	Practiced: yes/(no) Time: A.M/(P.M.) Minutes: 20 minutes	yes	Was a bit difficult to keep my focus; easily distracted by negative thoughts; felt a bit scary to open up; am I doing this right? I will keep at it.
Commitment: yes/no Day: Date:	Practiced: yes/no Time: A.M./P.M. Minutes:		
Commitment: yes/no Day: Date:	Practiced: yes/no Time: A.M./P.M. Minutes:		
Commitment: yes/no Day: Date:	Practiced: yes/no Time: A.M./P.M. Minutes:		
Commitment: yes/no Day: Date:	Practiced: yes/no Time: A.M./P.M. Minutes:		

CHAPTER 11

Taking the Observer Perspective: You Are Much More than Your Problems

"I exist" is the only permanent self-evident experience of everyone. Nothing else is so self-evident as "I am." What people call self-evident, that is, the experience they get through the senses, is far from self-evident. The Self alone is that. So to do self-enquiry and be that "I am" is the only thing to do. "I am" is reality. I am this or that is unreal. "I am" is truth, another name for Self.

—Sri Ramana Maharshi

We've often found that people struggling with anxiety problems take on WAFs as their identity. Tonia, one of our patients with obsessive-compulsive fears, always talked about "my OCD" as if that was something she really owned. Or take Phil, who told us "his panic" was taking over at times and he was almost becoming it.

It's very easy to become so fused with and trapped by thoughts like "I am shy" or "I am depressed" that we don't even notice when it happens. Every time you say "I am ...," you become what comes after "I am"—in this case shyness or depression. You are literally "it." You become the very thing you most dread, and that is hurtful.

If you feel a bit queasy reading this, you should. But you should also congratulate yourself because it means that the healthy and helpful part of your mind is rebelling against being relegated to a psychiatric label or disorder.

YOU ARE MUCH MORE THAN YOUR WORRIES, ANXIETIES, AND FEARS

Recall that your thoughts and feelings—all of them—are a part of you. But they are not YOU. This is a very important distinction. But it's also a difficult one to understand with your rational mind. This is why we will rely on different exercises in this chapter so that your experience may come to guide your intuition.

Anxiety and fear are emotions you experience periodically. They may explode into your awareness, and after a while, they recede. You—the person who experiences and observes your life—are separate from feelings of anxiety, panic, or dread. Like every other thought or emotion, your anxiety has its moment on the stage, then slips into the wings. The only permanent, immutable thing is you—the audience—the observer of your life.

To get a sense of this, imagine the moment of your birth. Every person on this planet enters the world in the same way. We are born into the world, but have no experience of that world. No way to make sense of it. Yet, there are two eyes looking out onto the world. There is a you being born into the world—a you perceptive looking out on the world—without any experience of that world. In the beginning, we are much like an empty vessel.

And then quickly, we all start to collect experiences. We taste. We touch. We feel. We begin to speak, talk about our past, ourselves, our future. We collect experiences that are sweet, bitter, and mundane. Over time, from one moment to the next, we continue to collect experiences. Our vessel is no longer empty. Over time, it continues to fill and will continue that way for as long as we are alive.

You too have a vessel, containing everything you have lived through and experienced up to this moment in time. And, you might spend a lot of time with the stuff you have collected so far. Maybe you identify with it. Maybe you're trying to get rid of some of it, cover things up that you don't like very much, or rearrange things so that your load is easier to carry.

But here, we'd like to ask you: What's the one constant that's been with you throughout your life until now? Is it the experiences you collected? Or, is it that vessel—that pristine you? The you that was there at the moment you came into this world and before the hardship and pain, before the losses and joys, before the trauma, and before anxiety was a problem. That vessel is you—the holder and observer of your life—your safe refuge. It is there always, and with practice you can learn to sense it more clearly and let it help and guide you.

Rather than relying on more words to explain, let's look at some examples to let you experience what we mean by the impartial silent observer of your life—this presence within you that just witnesses everything happening inside of you.

Imagine listening to your favorite piece of music. As the music comes through the speakers or headphones, who is actually listening? It is true that your ears and brain are perceiving and processing the individual notes, but who connects the notes in a way that we call music? According to Deepak Chopra (2003), it is the silent observer within you who is always present and witnesses everything that is going on inside of you.

You can actually take on the silent observer perspective anytime with any of your experiences, especially those that often make you anxious. For instance, next time you notice your heart pounding, pay attention to who is noticing and who is listening to your heart: again, it is the silent observer—the still presence in you. It's still or silent because it's not commenting or passing judgment on your experiences. It just bears witness to them in an impartial manner.

Learning to look at your experiences from this observer perspective might help you take your WAFs a little less seriously. After all, they're just a moment in time—a wave on the sea of existence. You don't have to fight them. And you don't have to join them either. Your task is to notice your WAFs and disentangle your Self from them. Just let the WAF waves come and go. Watch them from the safety of the shore.

Here's another way to look at it: all your feelings and thoughts are projections. You are the movie screen on which they play. While the screen never changes, the images change constantly. Millions of scenes can play out in a lifetime. When unpleasant thoughts or feelings show up on the screen, wait. They will morph into something else soon enough. The screen doesn't fight or resist the projections. It merely provides the space for the movie to play out and waits for that movie to end. You are that screen upon which life manifests itself.

You might be thinking that we're asking you to become an automaton, a distant emotionless character like Spock from the popular TV series *Star Trek*. Perspective taking and mindful acceptance are not about becoming numb or detached from your experience. In fact, they'll help you more fully engage in your life, emotionally and mentally, as opposed to simply reacting to it with the same old habitual patterns of escape and avoidance. Being an observer gives you space to choose what to engage in, what to let go, and what to do with your time and energy.

So ask yourself if there's enough room inside you to let all of you in—just as you are. If not, what is standing in the way of you experiencing yourself? And if there's something that shows up, see whether you can make space for *that*—not liking or condoning it, just acknowledging that it's there with as much kindness as you can muster and without trying to fix it.

LEARNING TO TAKE AN IMPARTIAL OBSERVER PERSPECTIVE

If you want to really watch something, you have to plant yourself firmly in the present moment. The past and the future, where our thoughts so often dwell, must be abandoned in favor of the here and now. Remember: the present is the place where your life is lived out.

The first way you stay in the present is by listening to your body. You do that by noticing your breathing, your beating heart, your posture, and your areas of tension or hardness. You observe any significant sensations in your body—areas that hurt or that feel hot or heavy or shaky. This isn't an easy skill to learn, which is why we have exercises for you to practice every day. If you want to apply these skills in the heat of a WAF moment, it's best to practice them at other times first. The exercises help you do that.

The second way you stay in the present is to notice and track your conscious mind—your thoughts, emotions, and drives. During any WAF episode, you need to keep asking yourself some key questions. Here are a few:

- What am I feeling besides anxiety, panic, fear, or tension?

- What am I saying to myself? What "good" or "bad" or "right" or "wrong" thoughts am I experiencing?

- What am I driven to do now? Where's the urge to avoid discomfort trying to take me?

- What do I want to be about right now? What do I want my life to be about right now?

A useful strategy for staying in the present is to use a simple rhyme as a reminder of your role as observer. We like the one that children are taught when learning about school bus safety: *Watch, look, and listen, or you won't see what you're missing.* When you see negative evaluation and judgment, don't feed it. And if you find yourself judging, then simply observe that—without beating yourself up for the judging. Ultimately a judgment is just another thought. Don't allow it to hook you and suck you in. For the observer, there is no right or wrong—there's just noticing, experiencing, and learning.

What's It Like to Take the Observer Perspective?

Many of us find it hard to imagine what it's really like to look at life and our experience from an observer perspective. Although the silent observer is always there within us, we simply are not used to looking at life from that perspective. To help us get a feel for the observer self, our Australian colleague, Russ Harris (2008), came up with a simple weather metaphor.

Your observing self is like the sky. Your thoughts and feelings are like the weather. The weather changes all the time, but no matter how bad it gets, the weather cannot harm the sky. Not even the worst thunderstorm, wildest cyclone, or coldest snowstorm can hurt the sky. And no matter how bad the weather may get, the sky has sufficient space for it all. And if we are willing to stick around, sooner or later we will witness the weather getting better. Sometimes we forget that the sky is there because we can't see it through all those dark clouds. But if we go high enough, even the darkest, heaviest rain clouds cannot prevent us from eventually reaching the clear sky. That open sky space extends in all directions, without borders, and without beginning or end. Through meditation in particular, you can gradually learn to contact this part of you—an open safe space right inside of you, from which you can observe and make space for even the most difficult thoughts and feelings.

The Advantage of Taking an Impartial Observer Perspective

You may wonder why it's so important to be an observer and what it's actually like to look at your experience from that perspective. The great advantage of being an impartial observer is that you can watch what's going on (your experience) without having to take sides. It allows you to end the struggle with your judgments and drop the rope.

Until now you've probably felt as if anxious thoughts and feelings rule you because they're so strong and powerful. In the heat of the moment, it may seem like they're taking charge of you—so much so that you get lost in those thoughts and feelings. At moments like that, it's difficult for all of us to see that our thoughts, worries, or feelings are just a part of us. They're not us, and we don't own them. Like clouds in the sky, they come and go by themselves. We can't make them go away. We can't hold on to them either.

In a sense we're like a house. Just as a house provides the space (e.g., rooms with walls, floors, and ceilings) in which people live, we provide the space for our experiences. The house remains the same regardless of what goes on inside it. And for all we know, the house doesn't care about who lives in it, what people do in it, what they think or feel, or what furniture gets put inside. The house just provides a place for all that living to occur.

EXERCISE: WHAT CHESS CAN TEACH YOU ABOUT TAKING AN OBSERVER PERSPECTIVE

The impartial observer perspective can be illuminated by the game of chess (Hayes, et al., 2012). That game takes two players, each with a team of pieces. The players engage in all sorts of moves to win the game. When one player makes a move, the other player takes a piece and makes a counterstrike. Both players are working to outsmart each other.

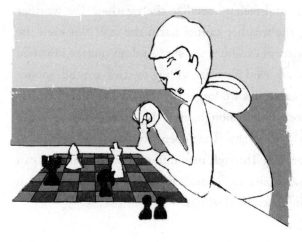

Now imagine you're a part of this game. The dark pieces are the team made up of your WAFs and everything that might trigger them. The other team represents your typical counterstrikes. So, when the dark knight attacks (e.g., "I'm about to lose it"), you get on the back of the white knight, ride into battle, and do something to knock the dark knight out: breathe … think of something else … reassure yourself that you can make it. Looking back at your experience and the work you've done in the previous chapters, you can once again ask yourself if this approach has worked. Or does the WAF team always manage to come back and make another move to get you?

There's a tricky problem in this chess game. Unlike a real chess game, it's not a game with different teams and players. In this special game, the two opposing teams are really one team: *you*. The thoughts, feelings, and actions on both sides of the board are your thoughts, feelings, and actions. They all belong to you—you are *both* teams.

So the game is rigged. Both sides know the others' moves. No matter which side wins, one part of you will always be a loser. How can you win when your own thoughts and feelings compete against each other? It's a war against yourself. This is why it's a war you cannot win. So the battle goes on, every day, for years. You feel hopeless. You sense that you can't win and yet can't stop fighting.

Let's step back for a moment and look at this situation from a different angle. What if we said that those chess pieces aren't you anyway? Can you see who else you might be?

How about this: let's suppose you're the board. This is an important role. Without the board, there's no game. As the board, you see all the pieces and you can just watch the action without taking sides. If you're a player, the outcome of the game is very important; you've got to beat those worries, anxieties, and fears as if your life depends on it.

But the board doesn't care about winners or losers. The board does not take sides or get involved in the battle. It just provides a space for the game and lets it happen. Can you imagine what a great relief it would be if you didn't need to be a player with a stake in the outcome? You simply provide a place for the game to play out. As the board, you can choose to be an impartial observer of your experiences.

If adopting a chessboard perspective to look at your experiences seems a bit hard for you, you may be able to relate more easily to a different sports-game metaphor—a game of volleyball. In volleyball, two teams (Team Anxiety and Team Struggle) strive to keep the ball in play, back and forth from one side of the court to the other, without letting the ball fall on their side of the net. Each time one team sends the ball across the net to the other side, an opposing team player in the front row jumps up to block it with her bare hands.

And so the game goes, on and on. As soon as Team Anxiety (A) serves up an unsettling thought, Team Struggle (S) responds to that thought by somehow arguing with it. This mental volleyball marathon of worries, intrusive thoughts, and feelings has replayed itself over and over in your head and without resolution. Yet there's another option.

Instead of choosing to be a member of Team A or Team S, you can choose to take the perspective of the volleyball court. As the court, you're an impartial observer, not a player with a stake in the outcome. Just like the chessboard, the court doesn't need to do anything. The court is merely there, watching and holding all of the players, the net, and the ball. In fact, the court doesn't care who wins or loses. The court doesn't worry about the outcome. The court will be around long after the game is over and as new players come and go.

We know from experience that thinking of yourself as a chessboard or volleyball court (or even as a vessel of your experiences) can be quite odd—at least at first. And yet over time, as you do these and the other exercises in this chapter, taking the perspective of the board or court will become easier *and* will provide relief. And this is no cheap, short-lasting relief that comes when you run away from your experiences by avoiding them. This relief is based on a deeper experience and understanding that, in a way, you really *are* the board, the court, and the vessel.

You see, your thoughts and feelings come and go. They are fleeting and ultimately don't really belong to you. They are only a part of you for a while, and then they leave—kind of like visitors. But the board and the court, they stay. They are always there—unchanged by anything that goes on around them. They really do nothing—they simply are (there).

This fusion of feelings, thoughts, actions, and self is an illusion that our mind creates. It's time now to pull each element apart so your observing self can watch—with mindful acceptance—your WAF experience as it really is.

EXERCISE: THE SILENT OBSERVER SELF

To get a clearer idea of how to separate the pieces of your experience from you as observer, let's look at Ellen's story. She's an office manager for a local ad agency. About six months ago, she was in a severe car accident. Ellen was fortunate to have walked away with minor physical injuries. Yet that event scarred her deeply.

Since then, she's felt unable to drive or be in a car, has suffered from nightmares and painful memories of the accident, and has struggled with panic attacks that seem to come out of nowhere. She's on temporary leave from her job and fears that she'll lose her position.

When first asked to explain the fears, Ellen saw no separation between herself and any of her thoughts, feelings, or actions. They were all crushed together in one upsetting experience. Here's how it looked in a diagram. Notice all the circles are overlapping.

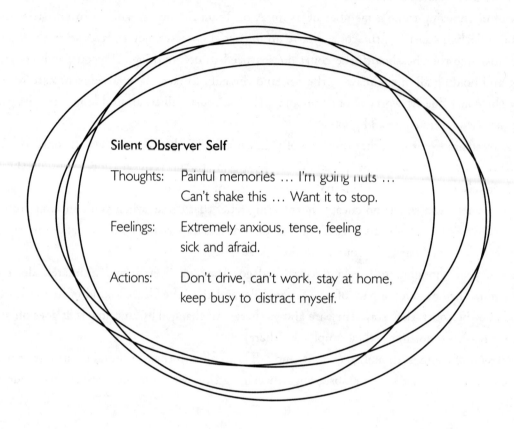

Silent Observer Self

Thoughts: Painful memories … I'm going nuts … Can't shake this … Want it to stop.

Feelings: Extremely anxious, tense, feeling sick and afraid.

Actions: Don't drive, can't work, stay at home, keep busy to distract myself.

Ellen's therapist asked her to do an exercise called Silent Observer Self. The therapist encouraged her to take a few moments to get centered, then drew a circle and wrote "Silent Observer Self" inside it. Below it he drew a row of three more circles. In the first he wrote, "Thoughts," in the second, "Feelings," and in the third, "Actions."

"Think of the chessboard exercise," he told Ellen, "and imagine being the board. This is the place we call Silent Observer Self—it's not so much a real place as it is a perspective that you can take to look *at* your experiences. It's where you can see yourself—watch what's really going on without having to comment or interfere. Now, from the perspective of that silent observing witness, fill in the other circles."

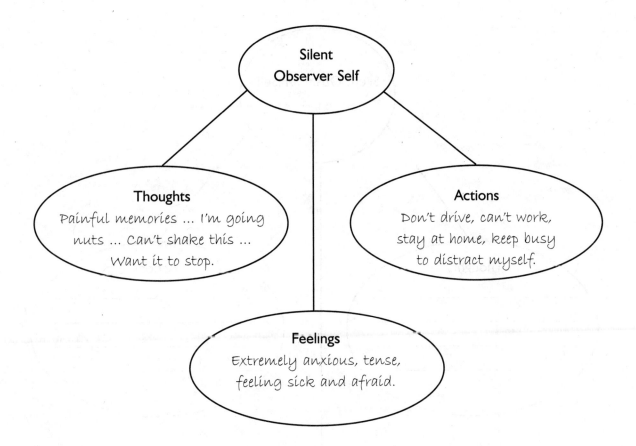

Here's what the exercise looked like when Ellen completed it. As you can see, the four circles aren't overlapping anymore. Thoughts, feelings, and actions are now separate and yet connected to and in touch with the observer self.

Right now, we'd like you to do the Silent Observer Self exercise using a recent WAF experience you've had. Pull out your LIFE worksheets from the past week and pick one that captures a situation that was difficult for you. Briefly review what you wrote down.

Then, when you're ready, take a few moments and bring your attention to the gentle rising and falling of your breath in your chest and belly. Just notice it. Wait a few moments until you feel centered. Now visualize that WAF episode from the LIFE Worksheet. From the perspective of your Silent Observer Self, observe each part of the experience. Separate your thoughts, feelings, and actions. Next, as Ellen did, write in the diagram below what you've observed.

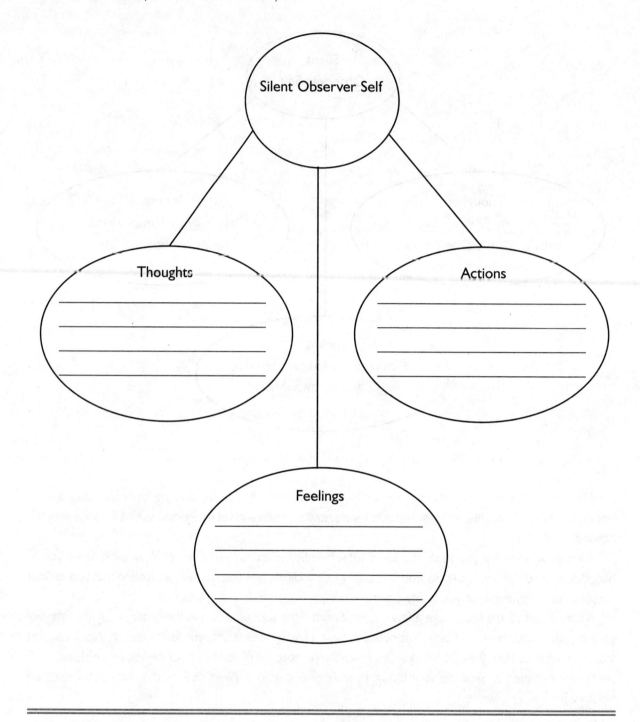

There's one more important insight that can be gleaned from the Silent Observer Self exercise. Your behavior is separate from your thoughts and feelings. You can be awash with anxious thoughts and feelings and still choose to act in ways that are potentially vital. Your thoughts and feelings do not create actions. You do!

The most important thing to keep in mind is this simple awareness: you can choose your actions. One set of actions is to act on your pain, to stuff or bury it. Another set of actions is to do what your history and mind tell you do to with your hurts.

Here's a third one: you can observe the discomfort arising from your mind and body and meet it with compassion, kindness, gentle curiosity, and openness. Just look at it from the silent observer perspective. When you do that, there's no need to take sides or judge. Instead, you'll have room to choose other vital life-expanding actions. Whenever you forget that your behavior is a choice, you're unlikely to exercise it. You'll let your old habitual history take over, where your thoughts and feelings drive what you do.

Developing your silent observer perspective puts all the activity happening inside of you in its proper place. And it'll help you learn the difference between *this activity*, *you* (the silent observer), and your *actions*. This softer approach will give you space to move and awaken your power to choose what you do. Remember: You can fight with your inner world or you can stay with and move with it. This choice is entirely up to you.

We'd like you to practice developing your silent observer skills with WAF experiences you've recorded using your LIFE worksheets over the past weeks. You may find it helpful to start with the least difficult episodes. The important thing is that you do the practice.

Pace yourself and commit to doing at least one Silent Observer Self practice a day. Get really good at simply noticing and watching your thoughts and feelings, and then place each in its own bubble with qualities of gentle kindness and compassion.

WHO AM "I"—REALLY?

Most people will be bewildered if you ask them, "Who are you?" They might say, "My name is ..." while pointing at their body. Or, you'll hear reference to a role in life such as mother, coach, doctor, construction worker, lawyer, receptionist, artist. But is this who we really are—our body? Our roles?

If we were our body, we would have to ask, "What model are you talking about, the 1960 model, the 1975 model, the 1989 model, the 2003 model, or the 2015 model?" Yes, we still have the same name that our parents gave us at birth, but we all know that our 2015 model looks nothing like the 1970 model. And modern science informs us that the majority of the cells in our body are replaced in less than a year—every year!

So if many of the cells in our body have been replaced many times over, we're clearly not the body we were born with. But does that mean we're not the same person we were born as? We all do have this uncanny sense of continuity. Deep down inside and in a very intuitive way, we sense that no matter what age we were, where we were, or what we were thinking, feeling, and doing, we have always been the same "I" that we are now. There is something about us that doesn't appear to change. We all know it and sense it, but none of us can really describe it and put it into words adequately. Remember the vessel was there before you had words to describe you!

If you persist with the "who are you?" question, people will start coming up with self-descriptions such as "I am an anxious woman," "I am a kind person," "I am not good at math," "I am someone who _____ [fill in the blank with your own descriptions]." Sometimes the answers are not just one-line statements, but they may involve long stories about why we have (or have not) become the person we are today. These are the stories we tell ourselves about ourselves. Telling yourself and others such stories is perfectly fine, *as long as we always keep in mind that they are only stories.* As plausible as they might seem, they are still stories made up by our minds. As in previous discussions, the real question is not whether the stories are right/correct or wrong/incorrect. The real question is: how helpful are such stories?

If you tell yourself in the morning that you've always been an anxious person, along with ten reasons why you have become such a person, and then end up staying at home because you felt panicky waking up, how helpful has believing that story been to you? These stories can turn from mind traps into utterly self-defeating life traps—they keep you literally stuck right where you are—if you really believe them *and* do as they say.

Throughout this book, we have encouraged you to become aware of any unhelpful stories and self-descriptions that pop into your mind without necessarily acting upon them. Taking the observer perspective greatly helps you to distance yourself from unhelpful stories and self-descriptions and look at them rather than continuing to act from them and on them.

At this point, many people have asked us this: "Well, if I'm not my body, or what I think, feel, do, or say about me, then who the heck am I?" This is an important question to ask. And, we're tempted to just give you an answer. But any answer we give you would just be another story for your mind to latch on to. So, we're not going to go there. Instead, we'd like to invite you to come up with a perspective on this question that goes way beyond your WAFs and the other self-descriptions you may be holding on to. To do so, it's helpful to first look at what your answers to the "who am I" question would be now.

EXERCISE: WHO AM I (BEYOND MY WAFS)?

As a result of years of struggling with your WAFs, you may have focused too much on what is seemingly wrong with you. So much so, in fact, that you've lost sight of other important aspects of yourself and your life. So in this exercise, we invite you to think about key aspects of yourself and your life that have nothing to do with your WAFs. How would you describe yourself? What are your likes and dislikes? You can go ahead and complete each line below right away, but if you find it hard to answer any of them, we suggest you close your eyes and think about a time when your WAFs were not yet a major problem in your life and then complete the item.

I am _____/_____/_____/_____/_____.

I am a person who _____.

I am not someone who _____.

I really like _____.

I do not like _____.

My most important relationship is _____.

How else would you describe yourself? _____

_____

_____

_____

If you had the time and inclination, you could go on with this exercise for quite some time. But the truth is that all of these descriptions—even the most detailed ones—are ultimately incomplete and inadequate. In fact, if you continued long enough, you would run out of words to describe who you are. And that's the point.

We will let you in on a little secret here. The problem is not that we don't have enough or the right words to describe ourselves, but that language can never capture ourselves fully. This is because there is an aspect of our selves—our core and essence—that goes beyond words. (Remember that vessel was there before you even had learned any words to describe you!) This aspect can be experienced as an unlimited and unbounded safe refuge. It is an experience beyond definitions, words, and content. The purpose of the exercises in this chapter is to help you experience this completely safe side of you.

ACT requires a lot from of us—it requires us to face aspects of ourselves that we'd rather not have at all or that we'd at least never want to experience for long. To move beyond fear and other emotional roadblocks, it would be very helpful for you to experience this place of safety that is just like an open space beyond any content. To contact this place, you need not go to a beautiful beach or climb up to a high mountaintop. This place is a space right inside of you—in the middle of your chest, just about where your heart is.

To help you experience this safe, whole, and pristine aspect of yourself that is beyond any stories and descriptions, let's start with an exercise, which is a variant of the self-identification exercise developed by Roberto Assagioli (1973) and modified by Hayes et al. (2012). In this exercise (with accompanying audio instructions, available for download at the book website), you use your imagination and try to experience that place where you are not your stories.

EXERCISE: THE CONSTANT OBSERVER

Close your eyes, get settled in your chair, and simply follow the instructions. If you ever find your mind wandering, just gently come back to the sound of the voice.

Before we start, take a couple of gentle breaths—in ... and out ... in ... and out. As you're doing so, notice the sound and feel of your own breath. Now turn your attention to being just where you are, here in this room sitting in a chair.

Now imagine you're watching yourself in a mirror. The eyes looking back at you now are the very same eyes that were also there on your first day of school. Can you still remember that day? What did you see with your eyes then? And what was happening inside of you that day? Do you notice any emotions you were having ... any thoughts? Now I want you to notice that, as you noticed these things, there was a part of you noticing them. A part of you noticed those sensations ... those sounds ... thoughts ... and feelings. And that part of you we will call the "observer you." There is a person in here, behind those eyes, who is aware of what I am saying right now. And it is the same person you've been all your life. In some deep sense, this observer you is that you, which you call "you."

Now I want you to remember the day you met your first girlfriend or boyfriend, or if your memory of that event is too faint, then remember the day you met your current partner ... The eyes looking back at you from the mirror are the very same eyes that were there with you then, noticing everything that was happening ... Remember all the things that were happening then ... Remember the sights ... the sounds ... the smells ... your feelings ... your thoughts ... and as you do, see if you can notice that you were there then, noticing what you were noticing. See if you can catch the person behind your eyes who saw, heard, smelled, felt, and had thoughts ... You were there then, and you are here now ... We're just asking you to notice the experience of being aware and to check and see if in some deep sense, the you who is here now, was also there then ... The person aware of what you are aware of now is here now, and that person was also there then.

Behind those eyes you see in the mirror now is the same you who was with you when you were a kid on vacation with your family, later in high school, in college, and still later on the job ... It's also the same you who is with you today when you leave the house in the morning, when you check your cell phone, go shopping, and when you're having dinner together with friends ...

What is important here is this: during all these moments you saw different things, had different thoughts, and experienced different feelings. Your looks have changed a lot over time as well. But one thing hasn't changed: it has always been the same pair of eyes that during all these different experiences looked *at* these experiences and watched everything. The observer behind your eyes was there then, and it is here now— and that observer was the same then as it is now ... Again, we're asking you not to believe this; just see if you notice this basic continuity—in some deep sense at the level of experience, not at the level of belief. This observer has always been the same. You have been you your whole life.

Your roles are constantly changing too. Sometimes you're a friend, a parent, a colleague, a business partner, a romantic partner. But no matter what role you happen to be playing at any given time, there is a you there behind your eyes who is not changing but simply observing how you move through life playing out all those different roles.

Now finally, let's look at your emotions. Notice how your emotions are constantly changing. Sometimes you feel joyful, sometimes you feel sad. At other times, you feel tense … and then comes boredom … excitement … relaxation. And yes, while these emotions come and go, notice that in some real sense the you who is registering all these changing emotions does not change … The same is true for your thoughts. They come and go, seemingly out of nowhere, and then go back there again … Sometimes you think about others, sometimes you think about yourself. Sometimes your thoughts make sense to you, and sometimes they don't.

So, as a matter of experience, not of belief, can you sense that you're not just your body … your roles … your emotions … your thoughts? All of these are the content of your life, while you are the arena … the place … the space in which they unfold … Notice that the worries, anxieties, and fears you've been struggling with and trying to change are not you, no matter how long this war goes, *you* will be there, unchanged and safe … See if you can take advantage of this connection to let go of your worries, anxieties, and fears just a little bit, secure in the knowledge that you have been you through it all, and that you need not be so invested in your emotional weather as a measure of your life … Instead, just notice the experiences in all the areas of your life that show up, and as you do, notice that *you* are still here, being aware of what you are aware of … *That* does not change.

Take a moment longer and just stay with this silent unchanging constant witness … Then when you're ready, picture yourself sitting on your chair in your room. And after a moment or two, come back to your room and open your eyes.

The Constant Observer is a powerful exercise because it not only lets you take on and experience the observer perspective in different aspects of your life, it also gives you a glimpse of a safe place inside of you that does not change and cannot be harmed, no matter what happens outside of you or inside of you. We suggest you listen to this exercise several times each week over the next few weeks to become well acquainted with you, the silent observer, your true self. Your mind may not always be your best friend, but your true self is.

I AM MANTRA MEDITATION—A SIMPLE ANSWER TO "WHO AM I?"

Becoming a good observer is important because it's such a helpful perspective and experience for anyone struggling with WAFs. To illustrate why this is so, take a look at the following list of statements. Notice what happens inside of you when you read the first four statements; then complete the last four statements with troubling descriptions of yourself that your mind offers up to you regularly:

- I am an anxious person.

- I am too shy.

- I am not good enough.

- ■ I am never going to make it.

- ■ I am _____.

- ■ I am _____.

- ■ I am _____.

- ■ I am not _____.

Did you notice how your mind almost immediately started to "work on" these statements, perhaps agreeing or disagreeing with them, rephrasing or qualifying them, making them stronger, toning them down, and so on? You're used to getting hooked by these *I am this* or *that* self-descriptions and end up spending much time and energy refuting them, struggling with them, and acting on them—the familiar tug-of-war situation. But as Ramana Maharshi reminds us in the chapter opener, our mind just makes up all these *I am this* or *that* statements, when the only truth and reality is that *I Am*—period!

This is not just some abstract philosophical idea but a very practical and helpful skill to learn. After they do the tug-of-war exercise, many people ask us, "How do I drop the rope in daily life? How do I drop the rope when my mind keeps throwing these evaluative *I am this or that* and *I'm-not-good-enough* statements at me?"

The answer is as simple as it is baffling: I am neither this nor that, but instead I Am—*I am that I am*. Answering the question *Who am I really?* with a simple, disarming *I Am* allows you to drop all those evaluative self-statements your mind constantly dishes out to you. It's the simplest and easiest way to drop the rope—once and for all, anytime. No more arguments, explanations, justifications and so on. I Am that I Am!

We have already started to introduce you to some defusion exercises to help you create some distance between those statements and your self. Learning the I Am mantra meditation below will help you leave all those unhelpful self-descriptions behind—or as Pema Chödrön (2001) so beautifully describes it: they will help you drop your story lines. Combining the I Am mantra meditation with a focus on your values is a powerful recipe for a good life.

I Am Mantra Meditation

Many mantras are Sanskrit words or short phrases (Sanskrit is an ancient language from India), but they can also be English words or phrases. Mantra literally means: "that which takes away the mind." Although mantras do not literally take your mind away, over time they do allow the mind to settle deeply inward—in a natural, effortless way. As you silently repeat a mantra, you automatically dive below the bubbling surface of the mind, which is always preoccupied with thoughts, memories, and desires, into a place of pure consciousness—a stillness that is deep within you and is waiting for you to contact it.

Mantras have been used for thousands of years, "Om" probably being the most famous one. They take you beyond your evaluative mind and give you glimpses of the experience of silence and pure awareness—your true Self. At first, you will only get brief glimpses of these experiences, but over time simply closing your eyes and gently thinking the mantra will settle your mind. With regular practice this meditation will become a very powerful and transforming habit.

The "I Am" mantra is not a clever philosophical or linguistic trick. I Am mantra meditations are mentioned in the Old Testament as well as in ancient Indian and other traditions (Dyer, 2012). "I Am" is simply an English translation of the Sanskrit phrases *aham* and *so hum*.

By now you can probably guess why this mantra is perfectly suited to the work you are doing: it literally makes you drop the story lines that typically follow your unhelpful *I am this* or *that* descriptions—what simpler and more elegant way could there be than to literally do just that?

By the way, we advise against using mantras such as peace, love, or compassion because they all have multitudes of meaning. The purpose of this meditation is to go beyond verbal meanings and leave your intellectual mind behind rather than engage it in thinking about such concepts, as uplifting and beautiful as they may be.

Many people turn to meditation techniques in the hope of quieting their mind. Yet no matter what type of meditation we practice, any attempt to quiet the mind using force and willpower doesn't work. Our everyday mind is full of thoughts, feelings, sensations, worries, daydreams, and fantasies. That is perfectly fine and normal even during meditation, with one important difference: during meditation we don't engage the mind in any of these mind games, and we don't direct it in any way.

So make no attempt to focus your mind on anything or to stop thinking. Instead, take it as it comes and make space for whatever your mind comes up with. Don't engage, struggle, or argue with it.

This meditation is relatively simple and there are only a handful of basic rules and directions to follow. We suggest you listen to the audio version in your first week of practice. Then you will be ready to do the exercise on your own. At that time, simply read the entire instructions that follow twice so you remember what to do. When you're done reading the instructions, close your eyes and begin the meditation. The audio version is fifteen minutes long and has a soft chime at the end to let you know when the time is up. When you practice on your own without the audio, you can extend your meditation time to twenty minutes if you like.

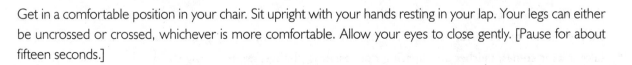

EXERCISE: I AM MANTRA MEDITATION

Get in a comfortable position in your chair. Sit upright with your hands resting in your lap. Your legs can either be uncrossed or crossed, whichever is more comfortable. Allow your eyes to close gently. [Pause for about fifteen seconds.]

- Let your breath flow naturally without attempting to influence it or breathe in any particular way. [Pause for about twenty seconds.]

- In a moment we'll ask you to start thinking the mantra *I Am* very gently and without any effort or strain. When we ask you to, start repeating the mantra silently to yourself without worrying about its tempo, rhythm, or sound. It's okay if the mantra becomes more faint and subtle and less distinct in the process. The mantra may also become faster, or slower, or completely disappear.

- After a while you'll notice thoughts or images or perhaps some bodily sensations. Let them all be. When you notice any of these, gently return to thinking the mantra in a very soft faint manner ... *I Am ... I Am ...* The most important thing is to take it all as it comes. So whenever you return to the mantra, do so ever so gently.

- Do not focus on anything and do not try to control your mind. Again, when you notice your mind thinking or any other diversions occurring, gently go back and think your mantra in a very faint and subtle way, ... *I Am ... I Am ... I Am ... I Am...*

- Now start thinking the mantra as instructed, and continue this process for the next fifteen minutes until you hear a soft chime ... *I Am ... I Am... I Am ... I Am...*

- Now stop thinking the mantra and take a little time to rest in the stillness and silence of your meditation. Continue to sit with your eyes gently closed for the next two to three minutes. After that time is up, open your eyes and resume your regular activities.

We suggest that you practice this I Am mantra meditation twice a day. Committing to a regular practice of daily meditation is one of the most important steps you can take toward healing and transformation. When you practice at home on your own, be sure to read the brief instructions again first before you start your meditation.

Remember, in this meditation you do not concentrate or focus on anything. This is not at all about thought or mind control. If a thought comes, do not try to push it out. Instead, just allow it to be there as in previous mindfulness exercises. When you become aware that you are not thinking the mantra, quietly and gently come back to it. Think the mantra very gently and faintly, and if at any moment you feel that it's slipping away, do not try to persist in repeating it.

There is also no need to think the mantra clearly—mental repetition is not a clear pronunciation. It is just a faint idea. The mantra may change in different ways, which is okay. It can get faster or slower, louder or softer, clearer or fainter. Its pronunciation and sound may change, lengthen, or shorten or even may appear to be distorted, or it may not appear to change at all. Don't try to make a rhythm of the mantra or align it with your breathing. Naturally, there will be times when you will simply forget thinking the mantra and thoughts will appear. That is normal and okay. When you notice thinking, simply return to repeating the mantra silently to yourself in a very gentle manner. In every case, just take it as it comes, neither anticipating nor resisting change, approaching the whole exercise with ease.

Am I Meditating Correctly?

In the beginning, people often wonder whether they're meditating correctly. *The simplest way to determine if you are meditating correctly is to ask yourself if you are meditating easily and effortlessly.* If you maintain an easy, open frame of mind as the mantra fades and you return to it, then you are indeed meditating correctly. Having many thoughts does not mean you're meditating incorrectly. In fact, your mind needs to wander off, get distracted, and lose focus in order for the awareness to move from the surface level of the mind to the deeper, expansive experience of consciousness. Let everything happen that wants to happen, without attempting to influence anything. Do not expect any particular effects, and never try to beat your thoughts down with the mantra to make them go away. Instead, always think the mantra gently and without strain.

Finally, the effects of meditation become apparent with regular practice over time in daily life during your regular activities, not during meditation. In fact, it really does not matter whether you feel particularly good or peaceful (or none of these) while you're meditating. So don't think you must be doing it wrong just because you don't feel relaxed or peaceful.

Remember, nothing in particular is supposed to happen—whatever happens, happens. Your task is simply to take everything as it comes and trust the process. Rely on the fact that over time, the grip that your mind seems to have on you will lessen as you become better at dropping the story line and just learn to be—I Am.

LIFE ENHANCEMENT EXERCISES

Below is a list of activities that we think will be helpful to you. Put them on a to-do list of ways to take care of yourself each day. You alone can decide to do them. Once you've made a decision, commit 100 percent to doing them. Be realistic and commit only to what you know you can reasonably achieve. For instance, if you know in advance that doing the I Am mantra meditation twice a day will be too much, then commit to doing it once a day. It's better to commit to less and follow through than to commit to too much and then break your commitments regularly. If you cannot commit to any of these exercises, then stop. Go back to the earlier material and ask yourself what is standing in your way. Perhaps you're taking things too fast. In that case, sticking with the earlier exercises a while longer might be helpful before going on.

Change can be scary, we know. Yet the prospect of doing the same old stuff that hasn't worked is even more frightening. If you want a different outcome in your life, you'll need to do something new, fresh, and different. Be patient. Do the work. It'll make a difference. Your experience will begin to tell you that.

- Practice the I Am mantra meditation at least once, preferably twice a day, for fifteen to twenty minutes. Be sure to read the instructions before you start your meditation.

- Practice being a mindful silent observer (the chessboard) during everyday activities at home and elsewhere—this can actually be very funny.

- Practice taking the perspective of the silent observer within you when something upsets or scares you.

- Practice being more mindful in your daily life.

- Take stock and notice what your experience is telling you. Even noticing your mind wandering off is a good sign—a sign that you are building your capacity to observe your experience and not buy in to everything your mind feeds you.

- Take stock of what you may still be giving up for anxiety this week.

THE TAKE-HOME MESSAGE

You can learn to stay with and bring patience to your WAFs and other forms of discomfort. This will free you to focus on the life you want to live. Learning to be a more accepting and compassionate observer of your experiences will make you more flexible—softer, kinder, and gentler with yourself, others, and the world in which you live. With that, you undermine and weaken everything your WAFs need in order to keep you stuck. You'll undermine the same old programming you've grown accustomed to.

Learning the Skill of Perspective Taking and Being a Silent Observer

Points to Ponder: Observing my thoughts, feelings, and behavior as separate from my true self is a vital and courageous step forward. I can learn to accept myself more easily by watching my WAFs from a safe silent observer perspective and be kinder with my WAFs on the road to living better.

Questions to Consider: Am I willing to observe all my flaws, weaknesses, and vulnerabilities from the perspective of a silent witness rather than a participant player? Am I willing to learn to separate my Self from my thoughts, feelings, and behavior by practicing regular mantra meditation as an important step to move on and reclaim my life?

PART 3

RECLAIMING YOUR LIFE AND LIVING IT

Take a stand against the habit of chaining yourself to your past and your mistakes. Take a stand against people who have purposefully hurt you time and again. Take a stand against thoughts and opinions seeking to diminish your worth. They shall not move forward with you. You will not allow them to deny you a new beginning. Make a commitment that their part in your life is over and done with, you are far too beautiful and far too strong to be a prisoner of things that do not really matter. Reclaim your life!

—Dodinsky

CHAPTER 12

Taking Control of Your Life

Life is a choice. Anxiety is not a choice. Either way you go, you will have problems and pain. So your choice here is not about whether or not to have anxiety. Your choice is whether or not to live a meaningful life.

—Steven C. Hayes

As Steven Hayes teaches us, nobody chooses to have anxiety. He's right! Every moment spent trying to control anxiety is a moment away from living your life in ways that are meaningful to you. This is why we talked a lot about what you cannot control early on in this book. You must decide if you're willing to drop the rope and let go of the struggle with anxiety so that you can gain the freedom to live your life. We asked you to look squarely at what WAF management and control has cost you in terms of energy, missed opportunities, and regret. These exercises were not intended to make you feel miserable. The intent was to position you to do something radically different from what you've done before—to give you space to exercise control in areas where you truly do have a choice.

In all of the previous chapters you took steps in that direction—taking control by choosing to simply watch your WAFs in different ways, more softly, less judgmentally, and with kindness. You can keep nurturing these skills from here on out. They're what will get you out from under your WAFs and free you to move with them as you do more of

> *By letting go of struggling with anxiety, I will gain freedom to grow.*

what matters to you. Keep this in mind as you read on and do the work: *By letting go of struggling with anxiety, I will gain freedom to grow.*

Earlier, we addressed an important area where you have control—your actions, or what you do with your precious time and energy. One set of actions has to do with your relationship with the world within you—your thoughts, memories, feelings, bodily sensations, and perhaps your sense of who you are and what you wish to become. This is important work and you've started on this already. But another set of actions is equally important. This has to do with what you want to be about in this life and what you do with your mouth, hands, and feet. Or, to put it boldly, what really matters to you?

In this chapter, you'll discover, or perhaps rediscover, what's important to you. This is a new moment to take stock. Look around the edges. Look deeply for places where your mind may be feeding you the same old false hope. Perhaps in the back of your mind you're still holding on to the idea that you can make the WAF monsters go away by attending to and appeasing them.

You may also think that if you trade in a little more flexibility in your life, eventually the anxiety monster will leave you alone. If you find yourself still stuck in this place, this waiting place, then spend some time with the following story before moving on.

Stop Feeding the Anxiety Tiger

Think of your WAFs as a hungry baby tiger. This baby tiger lives with you in your home as your pet. Although the tiger is just a baby, he's scary enough, and you think he might bite you. So you go to the fridge to get some meat for him, all the while hoping he won't eat you. And sure enough, throwing him some meat shuts him up while he's eating, and then he leaves you alone for a bit. But he also grows. And the next time he's hungry, he's just a little bigger and scarier, so you go to the fridge to get more meat to throw to him. Back and forth, over and over, the same drama plays itself out.

The problem is that the more you feed him, the bigger he gets, and, with that, the more frightened you feel. As this plays out over time, that little tiger isn't so little anymore. That tiger is now huge and he scares you more than ever. So you keep on going back to the fridge to get more meat, feeding and feeding him, in the hope that one day he'll leave you alone, and for good. Yet the tiger doesn't leave—he just gets louder and scarier and hungrier. And then one day you walk to the fridge, you open the door, and the fridge is empty. At this point, there's nothing left to feed to the tiger … nothing—except *you!*

Each time you actively struggle with your worries, anxieties, fears, panic, or just about any form of emotional hurt and pain, you feed the WAF tiger and it gets just a little bit bigger. Remember: hardness begets hardness. In the short term, it may not feel this way. But in the long run, that's what acting on your WAFs does—it feeds your anxiety and cripples your life.

Take another look at some of the LIFE worksheets you've completed as well as your earlier epitaphs, and ask yourself this (say it out loud or as a whisper): *Am I making choices based on what I deeply value and care about for my life? And am I doing things that really matter to me and make my life worthwhile? Or have my choices and actions been driven more by avoiding or minimizing my pain—my painful WAFs?* Pause for a moment before going on.

Now is the time to face some critical questions: Who's running your life? Who's in control here? Is it you or is it the tiger? You don't have to devote your life to feeding this tiger. You stop feeding it every time you practice using mindful acceptance and growing compassion for what you experience. This will keep the tiger from crowding out your life space. Then and only then will you be able to see that you do have the power to choose a different direction.

EXERCISE: LIFE WITHOUT ACTING ON MY WAFS

Have you ever wondered what your life would be like if you weren't always struggling with your WAFs? Think about the kinds of things you'd do with your time and energy if you weren't consumed with handling the people, places, and situations that hurt. How would you spend your day differently? And how might your relationships be different?

Go ahead, sit back, close your eyes, and take a moment or two to center yourself as you've done before. Then, when you're ready, imagine yourself feeding your life instead of the WAF tiger. Think—*This is my life as I'd like to live it.* In the space below, jot down what you were thinking about.

_____

_____

_____

We have a hunch that some of the images that came up in your mind had to do with important aspects of your life that you're missing out on, or may have given up on, because of your WAFs. We'd like you to reconnect with some of these important parts of your life—because we know that you can have them back. And you can have them without winning the WAF war! We call these important parts of your life values. Let's have a look.

WHAT ARE MY VALUES?

We understand that answering this question can be difficult. But before you get tangled up in the question, we want to be clear about what we mean by values. We're not asking you about your morals, beliefs, or philosophy—what you believe is right or wrong, just, or true. So, if that showed up, gently put those thoughts aside.

When we speak of values, we're talking about two things. First, what matters to you and only you! And second, what you do to express them in your life. The second piece is critical because your values find expression in your actions—in what you do.

So, you may believe that you should be a good parent, but without any actions, your belief is just that—a bunch of thoughts swirling around in your mind. If you want to move that belief into values, then you'll need to look at your actions in your role as a parent. You might even ask, *What do I do to express my value of being a good parent? What does that look like?* Likewise, if you're someone who believes in helping others, you need to act in ways that are helpful. If you don't act out your values, they're just empty beliefs. Beliefs or morality without action are dead ends.

So, to answer the question above, you need to allow yourself time to think about areas of your life that are deeply important to you and what you want to be about as a person. These are the things that make your life worth living, that you cherish and nurture, and that you'd act to defend when necessary. By completing the exercises in this chapter and the next, you'll get a very clear sense of what *you* value.

Values Are Like a Beacon in the WAF Storm

You can think of values as the shining lighthouse in the stormy sea of life. Like a lighthouse, values orient you in a direction, pointing the way toward what's important in your life. Without values, you'll end up like the person in the image to your right.

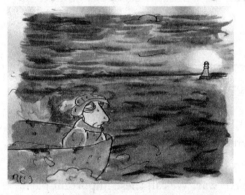

That person is stuck, being tossed about in the relentless churning seas, wind, and dense fog of the WAF storm. She's lost her bearings and any sense of direction. The storm has become the main concern, not the shining light in the distance.

You may feel that way too—directionless, pulled and pushed around in a sea of worry, anxiety, and doom and gloom. There seems to be no hope, no way out, and no place to go. That is, unless you turn your attention to the light coming from the lighthouse.

That light, that wondrous and wonderful light, is waiting for you—calling out to you: "This is the way toward the things that matter in your life!" You need to look for it to see it. You need to focus on ways that you might move toward that light instead of bobbing in place, wallowing, and waiting for the storm to pass. Ask yourself: How well has waiting in that boat worked for you so far? Do you feel stuck in there?

Values are the lighthouse that can help guide you out of the storm and into your life. You don't need to wait for the storm to pass. You can move yourself, storm or not, in directions that are important to you. You know that your WAFs come and go just like the weather—sometimes strong, sometimes weak, sometimes surprising, and at other times entirely predictable. Other thoughts and feelings do this too. Yet your values tend not to change the way your mental and emotional weather does. The trick is to start looking for those values and nurturing them.

When you do that, you'll probably want to do more of it, WAF storm or not. Once those value-guided directions are clearer to you, you can begin to focus your efforts on moving in those directions. This is how you create a life.

Values Help You Stay Focused

Focusing on living well instead of thinking and feeling less anxious is a radical step, and it is a vital step! Keeping your sights set on your values and life will help motivate you to keep up with the exercises in this book. Doing the exercises, in turn, will give you the space to live your life. We know that this isn't easy and requires commitment. We also know that few things worthwhile in life are easy.

As you start spending more of your time living consciously and consistently with what you value, and do so mindfully and with compassion, your life and everything you want to be about will come into focus. Valued living plus mindful acceptance is *compassion in action*!

Life is energy—and this energy is a precious gift. Right now, you are beginning to nurture that energy by developing mindful acceptance and observation skills. These skills will help shift your attention and energy from WAF struggles and utter exhaustion to a place where you have energy to focus on and engage in other more meaningful life activities. Remember this: you can choose how you expend your energy.

In fact, you can think of your energy as being like a hammer. You can use a hammer to build or destroy. You can also spend your energy constructively or destructively. It's up to you. You can choose to waste your energy struggling against WAFs, or you can decide to focus that energy on being a loving partner, a good friend, an athlete, or whatever else is important to you. As you explore your values, keep this question in mind: *How can I use my time and energy wisely?*

Values Are a Wise and Vital Alternative to WAF Struggle and Control

Values serve as a benchmark for deciding which actions are useful and which aren't. This is especially important when you feel anxious, worried, or panicky and wonder what to do. At those times, you know from your experience that your mind will put you in overdrive, feeding you all kinds of "solutions" that haven't really worked. Even now, you may still feel the pull of your old history, *Listen to us … Give us one more go … Maybe it'll work this time.* In those moments, it's critical to focus on your values because they'll guide you toward the actions that you want your life to be about.

> *The value question: Does this action I want to take move me toward or away from my values?*

When you're in the grip of your WAFs, you will know what to do and what not to do by answering one very important question: *Does this action I want to take move me toward or away from my values?* Our experience tells us that in most instances, it won't be difficult for you to come up with the right answer. Thinking about this question and answering it will help you move forward rather than resorting to old strategies that haven't worked. To help you remember the value question in those critical moments, we put it in a special box for you, on the right.

You may worry that your values will act as a clever distraction from your WAFs. In truth, you could use anything you do as a clever distraction from pain and difficulty. But what really matters here is your intention and purpose. Someone who values working may pour long hours into her job because it brings her a sense of purpose, and allows her to create, share, stretch her limits, express her talents, support herself and her family. This person still may have significant obstacles, problems, and pain too, but work is not being used as a distraction from that. Instead it serves to help the person live more in accord with what is important to her. Another person may pour himself into work as a clever escape from life's demands, worries, and other forms of pain and difficulty. So here we have two people engaging fully in work, but only one of them is doing so as a choice and not as a distraction from WAFs and other life challenges.

The key message here is this—values don't act as a distraction from WAFs. Instead, they give you direction and traction in your life. They will help you decide what matters and where you are putting your energy: winning the battle with WAFs (or at least keeping them at bay) or living well.

As you become aware of your values, situations will arise that require a choice from you. There are really only two options here. One choice is to continue spending your life managing anxiety. This choice, as you have learned yourself, is an away-move from what matters to you.

Another choice is to take your anxiety with you as you move in directions you want your life to take. This is a toward-your-values move, and all of the new skills you are learning in this book are for the sole purpose of keeping you moving toward your values even when anxiety shows up.

PROBLEMS WITH FINDING VALUES

We've found that some people struggling with anxiety have problems identifying their values. At times, they also confuse goals with values and have a hard time separating values from feelings. If left unchecked, these and other concerns can keep you stuck. To help you avoid that, we'll briefly discuss them.

I Don't Have Any Values!

Sometimes we hear people say they don't really have any values. When we ask more questions, it turns out that most of those people do have values but feel too helpless and afraid to move in valued directions. They're simply overwhelmed by their WAF barriers.

Doug is one of many people who struggled with this problem. For much of his life, he suffered from obsessive-compulsive problems and excessive worrying. He told us, "I don't really care anymore about friends and intimate relationships. Every time I try to get closer to people I like, they just seem to push me away. And after going on a date with a new potential partner, I find she's usually not interested in seeing me again—probably because she noticed some of my peculiar habits."

On the surface, it sounds like Doug doesn't care about his social life and intimate relationships. Yet if you look more closely, you'll see that his values were lurking inside his pain. In fact, the pain he shared says that he does care about having meaningful social bonds. Otherwise, there'd be no reason for him to feel pain about missing social connectedness in his life.

This may be true of you too. Perhaps the pain you experience in areas of your life is a reminder that you also care, and care enough to feel strongly about something that has been missing, diminished, or put off in your life. To help Doug out of this apparent dilemma, we asked him to reframe the way he identified his values. Instead of asking, *Can I* achieve *this?* we recommended he ask himself, *Do I* care about *this?* You can ask yourself this question too.

Doug was thinking about his values in terms of goals and achievements. He was disappointed that he hadn't reached his goal of having a number of close friends and an intimate relationship with a woman he cared about. However, he certainly cared about having meaningful personal relationships. So we brainstormed things he might do to support his social values. And we acknowledged that forming loving and deep social bonds takes time.

Focus on the Process of Living Your Values and Less on Outcomes

Doug got stuck thinking that values are about achieving some future outcome or result: *If I do this or that now, then I will get this or that in the future.* This is a trap.

In truth, there is no way to know if the steps you take to live your values now will get you exactly what you want later on. You simply don't know. But it's so easy to get stuck on achieving results. In a way we're always looking into the future and miss the moment-to-moment process and sweetness of engaging our values right here, right now.

Value-focused living, like life in general, is more like a journey, not a destination. Destinations are the steps along the way of creating a life, but the outcomes—good, bad, and sometimes ugly—of reaching certain destinations will not be known to you until you reach them. And even then, they need not diminish the value that guided you in taking the journey in directions you care about. The point of valuing is that you do your part and you do what's most important to you in life. And you do it in the here and now. You do it because that doing so matters. It's not about outcomes.

Consider parenting as a value. Most parents wish the best for their children and do what they can to help make that outcome more likely. Yet engaging the value of parenting is absolutely no guarantee that your children will be healthy, safe, and grow up to be good citizens or functional adults. Not knowing the outcome for their children doesn't stand in the way of parents, who value parenting, doing what they can as parents. The same is true of other values that involve actions that might be risky or outcomes that are largely uncertain—for example, with career and financial stability, health, love and friendship, or recreation.

The point here is that values focus your attention on the here and now—the process of living your life. If you choose values solely on the basis of results and outcomes, you'll be waiting a very long time to see them. And you'll likely be disappointed if things don't turn out a given way.

When you persist, trust that you will eventually progress so long as each step you take is guided by something that matters to you. Think of it this way: Each day you're given 86,400 seconds to use wisely or to squander. Time is a nonrenewable resource. It can't be saved and stored for tomorrow. If you don't use it, you'll lose it. So spend your time wisely each day. Use all of it as well as you possibly can. When you do that, you'll position yourself to be able to say at the end of the day, "There were 86,400 seconds lived well." And you may find that the results and outcomes will be more or less what you are looking for.

Connect with Your Heart and Choose Values That Are Important to You

When thinking about values and goals, listen to your heart and don't just blindly follow your mind. When we ask people about what's important to them, we sometimes hear them say, "It's important for me to contribute to my community" (a value) or "I want to be a good parent" (a value) or "I want to spend at least two nights a week reading to my children" (a goal). And yet they don't sound very enthusiastic when talking about any of their values and goals. As you come up with values and goals, always ask yourself, *Is this* really *important to me, or am I doing it because I'm supposed to?*

We find that some people don't freely choose values. They choose a value because it sounds socially appropriate, makes them look good, or meets others' expectations of them. What's important here is that you listen to your heart, not outside pressures to conform to valuing this or pursuing that. So be absolutely sure that your values are *your* values, not values that society, friends, or family impose on you. Ask yourself: *Why am I doing this? Am I doing this for me or for someone else, or to avoid someone else being hurt or disappointed by my choices?* Remember that the pursuit of values is about discovering or rediscovering what's truly important in your own life—what *you* want your life to stand for, not what other people want from you or for you.

Vitality and a Sense of Aliveness Are Your Benchmarks

Goals can help you physically move in your valued directions, but in order to regain your quality of life, you need to judge the quality and vitality of each activity against your values. This sound advice was shared with us by two of our colleagues—JoAnne Dahl and Tobias Lundgren. We think it's right on the mark.

Vitality is your benchmark. Moving toward important values makes you feel energized and alive. Sometimes you'll experience that vitality as you take a step, but other times you won't. Some steps might not come with a "good feeling." Here, just think of something you care about in life and important things you've done in the service of that important value. You've probably had many "not feeling great at the time" steps along the way. And still, you may be able to connect with a greater sense of purpose or an inner knowing that you are doing something good for you and your life.

In fact, reading this book and doing the hard work of changing your life for the better (a value of health and wellness) isn't all roses. Yet you persist, because when you look back at your steps against the backdrop of your values, you can say, "Yes, my actions are part of something bigger ... They leave me feeling more vital and alive at the end of the day." When you can say that, you've found a value and a goal that really strikes a chord in you.

If you find that what seemed like a worthy goal doesn't advance your sense of vitality, then reexamine that goal and adjust your course. This is a smart thing to do. Adjustments are normal steps on your valued path, and if you keep your values in sight, they'll steer you in the right direction.

Without identifying the direction you want to move in, and without a plan on how to move in that direction, you're unlikely to go anywhere. This is why goals are so important. Setting goals allows you to establish a game plan for the way you want to express your values in your life. In chapter 19, we'll help you set goals based on your values. For now, it's enough that you understand the difference between goals and values, and that you choose values that are truly your own.

Is It a Goal or a Value?

It's easy to confuse goals with values. Here's how to think about the difference. Goals are stepping stones that lead you down the path of a valued life. Goals involve actions you can put on a list, complete, and then tick off. Once you reach a goal, the work is done, and you're finished.

Taking out the garbage is a good example. If you set that as a goal, you could put it on a list and tick it off when you're done. Other goals might include losing ten pounds, taking a vacation, getting a degree, or mowing the lawn. Even the act of getting married fits our definition of a goal. Once that ring is on your finger, your goal is achieved. So you can tell if something is a goal by whether you can do it and then tick it off your list.

Unlike goals, values are lifelong journeys. You can't answer the question "Am I done yet?" about values. Values have no end point. Instead, they direct us throughout life. If values are the map or compass that shows you the direction you want to move in, then goals are the waypoints on the map, places you plan to visit as you move in the direction of your values.

For example, reaching a particular goal (getting married) is just one of many steps in a valued direction (being a loving partner). The value of being a loving, devoted partner isn't done the moment you say, "I do." Being a loving, devoted partner is something you must keep working toward—there's always room for growth. You'll get a better sense of that in a bit when we share Danny's experience.

The same can be said of parenting as a value. Reaching your goal of spending two hours of quality time with your child every weekend doesn't complete the value of being a good parent. Values such as being a loving person or a good parent are ongoing commitments that manifest in moment-to-moment actions. You cannot ever "finish" a value.

Although values and goals aren't the same, they're related. Just think of one or two goals you have set for yourself. Be open to the seemingly mundane here too—things like taking out the garbage. To determine the value that underlies the goal, you can simply ask yourself, *Why am I doing this? What am I trying to accomplish in my life with this goal?* and *Where am I heading with this?*

Answers to these questions will point you in the direction of your values. And they'll change the way you look at things too. You may find that the simple act of taking out the garbage reflects a value of helping, taking care of the environment, creating a clean healthy home, and/or being a supportive spouse. It's no longer a stinky "I have to do it" task. Taking out the garbage with an eye on your values changes the act of taking out the garbage. See if you notice the difference the next time you take out your trash.

> *You cannot ever finish a value.*

Valuing Involves Action, Not Feeling

Many people assume that valuing is about how they *feel* about a particular area in their lives. This is another trap. Here's why. You do lots of things in life regardless of how you may feel at the time. Breathing is one of them. If you waited to feel good or happy before taking your next breath, you'd be in serious trouble. Many other actions are like this too. We do many things despite how we think or feel at the time.

You probably go to work in the morning regardless of whether you feel anxious, sad, irritated, worried, or happy. Or you may have paid a visit to Aunt Edith even if you don't like her very much. Let's take this a step further.

Suppose you value social interactions and feel anxious about talking to a group of strangers. Not waiting to feel less anxious in this situation means that you can still talk to them regardless of how you may feel inside. Or if you're feeling panicky while attending a ball game with your son, you can stay in the stadium even though you feel like heading for the closest exit.

Put simply, values are the cumulative effect of what you spend your time doing, not what you think and feel about what you're doing. Many research studies have shown that if you focus on your actions, your feelings will eventually follow and take care of themselves.

This is why we stress that valuing is all about doing things. You actually value with your hands, feet, and mouth (that is, by what you say). So valuing your career means that you're acting on that: working to build your career. If you don't work to build your career, then you don't value it, regardless of how you *feel* about it. Values are expressed in action—period.

Emotional Outcomes and Traits Are Not Values

When we ask people what's important to them, they often make statements such as:

- "I want to be calmer, more at peace."

- "It's important for me to be happy."

- "I want to feel more confident."

- "I need more motivation."

- "I want to be less anxious and more easygoing."

- "I want people to like me."

- "I need more self-esteem."

- "I want people to accept me so I can accept myself."

All these statements sound like values, but they're really goals masquerading as values. In fact, they're emotional goals—different types of feelings and traits. Being calmer and happier are emotional outcomes too. You could even tick them off when they show up. They are states that may or may not happen *after* you start moving toward your values. Remember that you can't really control what you think or feel or how others think or feel about you. You can only control what you do.

You set yourself up for disappointments if you make feeling better, happier, more confident, or more accepted the reasons for your actions. Chances are good that you'll *sometimes* feel better about yourself and generally more contented once you start moving in the direction of your values. But when you do things just to feel better, you're walking on thin ice, because no matter what you do, you won't always feel good, calm, confident, motivated, or accepted. Feelings are fickle. They come and go. That's why they cannot serve as a solid foundation for your actions.

Values are like stars in the sky.

If you look deeply inside yourself, you can connect with aspects of your life that are precious—for whatever reason. Those precious things are that way just because they are. You don't need to justify them. They're present despite your emotional weather, much like the stars are forever present, even on an overcast evening. You know the stars are there even when you sometimes can't see them. And you know they'll be back in view. Even the clouds don't stick around forever, but the stars surely will. Your values are like the stars in a way. They don't change overnight, nor do they go away. This is why values provide a more solid foundation for your actions than fleeting feelings ever could.

YOU'RE AT A CROSSROAD

Right now, you're at a critical crossroad in your life. You can choose to live your life in a way that upholds your deepest and most cherished desires, or you can choose to live the same old way, constantly avoiding or struggling against WAFs. It's up to you.

Take a look at how Danny handled this important choice in his life.

■ *Danny's Story*

Danny came to us suffering from panic disorder. His panic was taking a huge toll on his life, snuffing out just about everything that mattered to him. One of Danny's values was being a loving husband. Danny was faced with a tough choice—his panic or his relationship.

Danny and his wife enjoyed classical music. Yet they hadn't been to a live performance in years because to do that meant that Danny would need to sit in a concert hall for two hours amidst hundreds of people. Then, the unexpected happened.

Danny's wife approached him with some exciting news. Her friend had offered her two tickets to the symphony at a bargain price. That news sent Danny's mind into a tailspin and headed straight into a pit filled with the usual worries and scenarios: What if you have a panic attack? It'll be difficult to leave. Everyone will stare at you as you try to make it to the exit in the middle of the show.

In the past, Danny's default response was a flat out "No!" And he knew that opting out made him feel safe and then sad. His wife would feel unhappy too. That's how it went when his choices were about panic management. This time though, things were a bit different.

He asked his wife for a bit of time to think about it. He knew how much his wife would love to go with him, all dressed up by his side. And he was well aware of his deep love for her (and for the music). So he took time to think about it and make a choice. This wasn't easy. He wanted to go and tell her, "Yes, let's go." Yet his mind was feeding him doom and gloom—cycling through an endless stream of frightening scenarios of what might happen at the concert. His old history was at work here, and it was pointing him to same tiresome conclusion: don't go—stay home.

He was torn and didn't know what to do. It was at this point that Danny remembered the value question we had talked about. And focusing on this question helped him resolve his dilemma. He saw that listening to his mind and staying at home wouldn't move him any closer to his value of being a loving husband. And with that, he made a courageous choice to go to the concert with his wife.

Like Danny, you have an important choice to make: Are you going to start living the life you want to live or are you going to keep on struggling with or trying to avoid your WAFs?

You can think of these choices in this way. Imagine life as a walk down a long corridor with many doors on either side. You have the power to choose which doors to open and enter. One of those doors is labeled "no more anxiety." You've chosen the no-more-anxiety door for so long that you may have lost sight of other doors available to you. Now's the time to venture out and open up other doors. You can do this!

What choice do you want to make? Going back to the no-more-anxiety door sure sounds tempting. Now consult your experience: has this action moved you closer to your values or further away from them? By now, you know the answer. If not, just go back to the Costs of Anxiety Management exercise in chapter 6.

Now is the time to muster the courage to explore other doors in your life corridor. Think about your life. Besides the no-more-anxiety door, what other doors would you like to open? Maybe there's a door labeled "love" and another sporting a sign that says "physical fitness." There's a door to professional satisfaction and another that leads to political activism. Yet another is marked "inner peace." It's a long corridor with many, many doors.

LIFE ENHANCEMENT EXERCISES

In chapter 11, you created a to-do list of ways to take care of yourself each day. Continue to practice the exercises, listed below, from that chapter. Remember that you're learning new skills, and be patient with yourself. Make your practice an important part of your daily routine.

- Practice the I Am mantra meditation once a day and work on "taking an observer perspective" with thoughts, feelings, sensations, and the world around you. Get curious and notice. Develop your observer skills by practicing the silent observer perspective (the chessboard) during everyday activities at home and elsewhere—and have fun with it.

- Pause throughout the day and ask yourself this: *Is what I am doing right now a move toward or away from what I care about?*

- Take stock of what you may still be giving up for anxiety this week.

THE TAKE-HOME MESSAGE

You can take charge of your life by focusing on what you can control: what you do with your hands, feet, and mouth. Instead of struggling with WAFs, you can identify what truly matters in your life and then focus your energy on pursuing goals that will move you in those directions.

The values you choose are the road map for guiding you in the process of reclaiming your life from anxiety. They help you stay focused on what matters. When the WAFs are yelling at you and demanding your attention, you can stop, observe your thoughts and feelings, and then listen to your values and do as your values say. They'll help you choose a course of action that moves you closer to your dreams.

Focusing on My Values

Points to Ponder: My values are the beacon guiding my actions. My actions create my life. My actions are what others see about me.

Questions to Consider: Am I willing to let my actions be guided by my values rather than my WAFs? Am I willing to make valued living my No. 1 priority?

CHAPTER 13

Finding Your Values

Follow your bliss!
If you do follow your bliss,
you put yourself on a kind of track that has been there all the while waiting for you,
and the life you ought to be living is the one you are living.
When you can see that, you begin to meet people who are in the field of your bliss,
and they open the doors to you. I say, follow your bliss and don't be afraid,
and doors will open where you didn't know they were going to be.

—Joseph Campbell

So many of us have chased happiness now and then, but like a butterfly it eludes us. It is not something we can grasp and hold on to. When you feel happy, the feeling comes after or alongside something you were doing in the moment. It does not float around "out there" waiting for you to discover it.

As Joseph Campbell teaches us, happiness flows from listening to your heart and then doing things that matter. Like a river, true happiness—and by this we mean an enduring sense of contentment in life—flows like water from a source. That source is having a clear purpose in life and acting in ways to uphold that. We want nothing more than to help you get in touch with that clear purpose that resides in your heart and then follow its calling—follow your bliss.

To create the conditions for genuine happiness in your life, you'll first need to know what matters to you (what your bliss or passion is) and then find ways to do what matters in your daily life. There are enormous benefits to this too, apart from reaping the rewards that come from spending your life doing what you care about. One recent study by Hill and Turiano (2014) showed that people who cultivate a sense of value-guided purpose actually live longer than those who have no sense of purpose. So, by getting clear about your values, you may create the conditions not only for a more meaningful, blissful life, but also for a longer one.

Having a purpose in life really boils down to knowing what matters to you. In this chapter, we're going to help you do just that. Identifying your own values is the most important first step on the road to living the life you want to lead. It may also seem like quite a daunting task. And you may even think that you have no values. Asking yourself a few simple questions will always point you in the right direction:

- What do I want my life to be about?

- What really matters to me?

The epitaphs you completed in chapter 7 have already primed you to get to a place where you're able to consider such questions.

WHAT ARE MY IMPORTANT VALUES?

In this section, we're going to guide you in exploring your own values more deeply. We've structured this process with an exercise using the Valued Directions Worksheet. This worksheet will help you identify areas of your life that are most important to you right now.

You'll see that the worksheet covers ten common life domains that many people engage in to varying degrees: work/career, intimate relationships, parenting, personal growth/education/learning, friends/social life, health/physical self-care, family of origin, spirituality, community life/environment/nature, and recreation/leisure. You may find that many of these life domains are important to your life right now, or just a few. Either way is fine.

Each area you consider important makes up the fabric of your current life—the areas you engage in now because, in some sense, they matter to you. It is natural though that where you spend your time and energy may change over time. Work and career may give way to retirement and more time and energy spent with leisure pursuits. Or, if you have kids, you know that they will eventually grow up and move away. So, you may shift your energies from what was once the important area of parenting to personal growth or volunteer work. And so it goes.

Our point is that the worksheet covers life areas where you can express your values. But the ten areas covered in the worksheet are not values themselves. They are life domains where you express and live out your values. As you go through the exercise, you may also find that some domains are missing from your life. You want to engage in them, but for whatever reason it has been difficult for you to do so. That's okay too. A bit later, we'll look at what is getting in your way.

For now, the first step is for you to identify areas of your life that are important to you—life domains where you would like to express your values. Be mindful that you may not deem many or all of them as important to your overall life right now. Be aware too that areas of life that you consider important may not be exactly what others consider important. This is exactly how it should be.

Once you identify those important areas of your life, you'll move on to consider your values—what truly matters to you in each of your important life domains. To help you along, we've created *The Common Core Values Guide*, which is nothing more than a list of words that embody common values. We adapted this list from the Life Compass Cards exercise created by Joanne Steinwachs. The list itself is simply a starting point for deeper reflection. If you don't see one of your important values on the list, that's okay. Feel free to come up with your own words that capture the essence of what you care about and wish to be known for.

But knowing the domains of life that are important to you, and identifying words that capture your values, is not enough. What you need to do next is consider your valued intentions.

Your valued intentions reflect your actions, or how you wish to express your important values in each domain of your life. Intentions are really all about behavior, or what you would like to do or do more of. So, if you value integrity in your work and career, you'll need to ask yourself these important questions: How do I show or express this value of integrity by my actions? What do I do to uphold the value of integrity? How would others know that I value integrity? What would they see me doing with my mouth, hands, and feet? The answers you come up with will capture your valued intentions. We emphasize intentions because without a clear intention, you won't know what to do. Intentions make your values concrete, personal, and doable.

And, as you move on with this workbook, making an intention to act on your values can go a very long way in helping you make them a habit and priority in your life. So, with valued intentions we are asking you, in each life domain, "How do you want to express your values?" We all have different valued intentions. How you express integrity will be different than how someone else shows integrity. There is no right or wrong in any of this.

Be forewarned—this exercise will take a while to complete, and it should. It's one of the most important exercises in this book and in your life. We'll guide you along. You'll see it's time well spent. Here's how you do it.

EXERCISE: THE VALUED DIRECTIONS WORKSHEET

Follow each of the four steps in order as you complete the worksheet.

Step 1: Make Your Importance and Satisfaction Ratings

Start by considering your life right now. And from that place, rate the importance of each area by circling either "Yes" or "No" on the Importance Scale according to *your own personal sense of its importance.* It doesn't matter how many areas you rate as important to you. What matters here is that you look inside yourself and make an honest rating of what's important to you personally when you consider your life right now, with the understanding that areas you consider important now may shift and change over time.

If you rated an area as "No," or unimportant, then move on and rate the next area. Continue until you've rated the importance of all life domains.

Now, go back and rate how satisfied you are with each life area that you rated as important. When you make your satisfaction ratings, listen to your gut. A low sense of satisfaction may be a clue that something is amiss—that something is getting in the way of you engaging your values in important areas of your life right now. Becoming aware of areas in your life where you are less than satisfied can help you later when you move on to identify barriers between you and your values using the Life Compass.

The following steps apply only to those life domains that you rated as important.

Step 2: Identify Your Values

The next important step is to consider your values for those life domains that you rated as important. For each of those life domains, you'll see space where you can list up to three values that you care deeply about.

This is a time to slow things down and reflect deeply on what matters to you and what you wish to be about as a person. If you find yourself stuck here, then feel free to refer to *The Common Core Values Guide* at the end of this worksheet. And then, with each area you rated as important, list the words in the spaces that truly reflect your core values in that important area. As you do this important work, be mindful that values are not goals.

You'll notice that we limited the number of values you can list to three for each life domain. That was intentional to help you focus on what's most important to you. You may come up with three values for each important life area, or you may have just one or two. That is fine for now. Just do the best you can. If you come up with other words that better capture what matters to you, then please use them. For now, it's best if you can embody your values in a word or two.

Try not to select a value that is almost identical to the name of a life domain (e.g., don't select family as a value under the life domain "family of origin"). If you find yourself doing that, think more deeply about what it is about family of origin that is important to you. From there, you'll likely find other words to capture the essence of what matters to you (e.g., love, support, connection, sharing). You might even find that family shows up as a value under work/career, where you consider the contribution to your family's support and care by working. Stick to no more than three different words for each important area of your life.

You may also find yourself using the same words to reflect your values in different life domains. This is important to notice, for these common words are like golden threads that capture the real essence of what matters to you, regardless of where you find yourself.

Step 3: Write Your Intentions

To complete the worksheet, go back to each life domain that you rated as important and look at the values you wrote down. For each value, come up with a valued intention—a statement that makes your values personal and meaningful. They should reflect what you wish to stand for, or be about, with each of your values within a specific important life domain. You can think of your intentions as capturing how you'd like to live your life. They should bring to light what's most important to you for each value in each life area.

These statements should be real in the sense that they genuinely reflect your wishes. And, they should be real in the sense that they reflect how you express your values—the kind of person you wish to be, or what you want to show the world. So listen to and follow your heart and bliss. Really make an effort to come up with statements rooted in your experience. This will give your values greater pull over your actions when your WAFs are in danger of pulling you away from where you want to go.

Now go ahead and write your valued intentions next to each value on the lines provided. Do this for all areas you rated 1 or 2 in terms of importance.

VALUED DIRECTIONS WORKSHEET

1. Work/career

Is this life domain important in my life NOW (circle one):

YES = It's important to me   **NO** = It's not important to me

How satisfied are you with this life domain right NOW (circle one):

0 = Not at all satisfied   1 = Moderately satisfied   2= Very satisfied

Reflect on your values and intentions

Work may involve a paid job, unpaid volunteer work, or homemaking. What's important to you about your work, and what qualities does having a job provide for you? For some people it means financial security, independence, or prestige; for others it involves intellectual challenge or interacting with or helping others.

Have you put a valued career or volunteer job on hold because of emotional or cognitive barriers? Maybe it's a fear of failure or sense of unease as you consider a career that may mean giving up some of the comforts or luxuries of your current lifestyle. Or maybe you think it would be irresponsible to pursue your dream job.

Don't let those thoughts and emotions stop you from exploring this area. After all, most of us spend a major chunk of our waking hours involved in work. There are many ways to make whatever you do personally rewarding. Keep that in mind as you envision your dream job or how you'd like to use your energy, talents, and skills productively. What would that look like? What would you do if you could be doing anything? Describe the qualities of a job or endeavor that you believe would be perfect for you.

What do you want your work or career to be about or stand for? What is important to you about your work (for example, financial security, intellectual challenge, independence, prestige, interacting with or helping people)?

My Core Values in This Domain	*My Valued Intentions for Each Value*
1. _____	1. _____
2. _____	2. _____
3. _____	3. _____

2. Intimate relationships (e.g., marriage, couples, partnership)

Is this life domain important in my life NOW (circle one):

YES = It's important to me   **NO** = It's not important to me

How satisfied are you with this life domain right NOW (circle one):

0 = Not at all satisfied   1 = Moderately satisfied   2= Very satisfied

Reflect on your values and intentions

This area focuses on intimate relationships with a partner or spouse. Here, we're asking you to look and see what you'd like to bring to those kinds of relationships. What kind of partner would you most like to be within an intimate relationship? What values do you want to express here in your role—what would you like to bring to such a relationship (not what others may give you in return)? What would you be doing to show greater intimacy with a close partner or spouse? What type of marital or couple relationship would you like to have? How do you want to treat your partner, or a person that you share a special commitment and bond with?

My Core Values in This Domain	*My Valued Intentions for Each Value*
1. _____	1. _____
2. _____	2. _____
3. _____	3. _____

3. Parenting

Is this life domain important in my life NOW (circle one):

YES = It's important to me   **NO** = It's not important to me

How satisfied are you with this life domain right NOW (circle one):

0 = Not at all satisfied   1 = Moderately satisfied   2= Very satisfied

Reflect on your values and intentions

You may be a father, mother, or caretaker for a child. Or, you may have plans to someday be a parent. Here, look to see what you want to be about in this area. What type of parent do you want to be? How do you want to act to support your role as a parent? How do you want to interact with your children? What would your child see you doing to support your values here? What would others see you doing? What is it about being a parent that is important to you?

My Core Values in This Domain   *My Valued Intentions for Each Value*

1. _____   1. _____

2. _____   2. _____

3. _____   3. _____

4. Personal growth/education/learning

Is this life domain important in my life NOW (circle one):

YES = It's important to me   **NO** = It's not important to me

How satisfied are you with this life domain right NOW (circle one):

0 = Not at all satisfied   1 = Moderately satisfied   2= Very satisfied

Reflect on your values and intentions

You nurture your personal growth when you explore yourself and develop as a human being—emotionally, intellectually, physically, spiritually, behaviorally. This often means gaining a deeper sense of who you are. In fact, many of the domains you've already read about have everything to do with your personal growth as a human being.

Personal growth is often related to learning. Traditional schooling certainly counts, but growth and learning can happen just about anywhere. You don't need a classroom for that. For example, amateur athletes may experience health or social benefits from participating in a sport, but these activities can also offer a sense of being challenged and the pleasure of learning or refining a skill.

So look within yourself and see if you can find anything about personal growth and learning that's important to you. Would you like to sharpen skills you already have, or develop new ones? Are there areas of competence you'd like to explore? Do you enjoy learning new things? Do you enjoy sharing what you've learned with others? Why is learning important to you? What skills, training, or areas of competence would you like to acquire? What would you really like to learn more about?

My Core Values in This Domain   *My Valued Intentions for Each Value*

1. _____   1. _____

2. _____   2. _____

3. _____   3. _____

5. Friends/social life

Is this life domain important in my life NOW (circle one):

YES = It's important to me   **NO** = It's not important to me

How satisfied are you with this life domain right NOW (circle one):

0 = Not at all satisfied   1 = Moderately satisfied   2= Very satisfied

Reflect on your values and intentions

While we're all social creatures, there's a lot of variation in what we value in the realm of social relationships and their depth and scope. Some people value knowing many people, even if they don't know any of them particularly well. Others place a premium on having a few close friendships. Still others prefer a mix of friendships, some with depth and others relatively shallow. And then there are people who prefer to be alone.

Depth relates to degree of intimacy, whether emotional, spiritual, or intellectual. So think about the importance and quality of your social life. Are social bonds important to you? What kind of relationships would you like to have? What personal qualities would you like to develop in and through your relationships? How would you interact with your friends if you were the "ideal you" with them?

Give some thought to your talents and passions, and to what might currently be missing in this area. What is unique about you as a person? What can you bring to any friendship? What kind of friend do you want to be? What does it mean to be a good friend? How do you behave toward your best friend? Why is friendship important to you?

My Core Values in This Domain   *My Valued Intentions for Each Value*

1. _____   1. _____

2. _____   2. _____

3. _____   3. _____

6. Health/physical self-care

Is this life domain important in my life NOW (circle one):

YES = It's important to me   **NO** = It's not important to me

How satisfied are you with this life domain right NOW (circle one):

0 = Not at all satisfied   1 = Moderately satisfied   2= Very satisfied

Reflect on your values and intentions

How and why do I take care of myself? Why do I want to take care of my body and my health through what I eat, by exercising, or by being physically fit? How important is physical health to me? What roles do exercise and healthy eating play in my life?

People have a variety of motivations for trying to stay healthy. Some do it out of sheer enjoyment; others do it in order to be successful in a physically demanding job. Still others see a healthy lifestyle as a way of taking care of themselves, perhaps so that they stand a better chance of living to a ripe old age and being around for those they love.

Many of us also have old wounds from losses or unfair treatment by others, and, sadly, some have suffered abuse and trauma. These experiences can change us for good or for ill. So often the darkness is all we can see, and this makes us harden up. We blame ourselves or others and retreat from the world and all it has to offer. This ultimately hurts us in the end.

The antidote is to practice acts of kindness and loving care—starting with yourself and then expanding out to other people in your life. This can help you stop being at war with yourself and will also take the sting out of the psychological pain and unhappiness you've lived through and may continue to experience now. And even if you don't have much pain in your life, you still might value kindness and compassion.

How important is it to you to learn to be kinder to yourself? How would your life be different if you were to practice more acceptance and compassion toward your feelings, memories, and wounds? Do you look for ways to practice acts of kindness toward yourself, and if so how does that look? What do you do? If you don't do this currently, what form might it take? Even if self-compassion seems difficult, does it seem important for you to start moving in that direction?

Think about what motivates you to stay healthy—mind and body. There are many possible reasons for actively pursuing good health, and all are valid. What is it about caring for your physical and mental well-being that's appealing to you, and how important is it to you to act in accordance with this value?

My Core Values in This Domain

1. _____

2. _____

3. _____

My Valued Intentions for Each Value

1. _____

2. _____

3. _____

7. Family of origin (parents/caretakers/siblings you grew up with)

Is this life domain important in my life NOW (circle one):

YES = It's important to me   **NO** = It's not important to me

How satisfied are you with this life domain right NOW (circle one):

0 = Not at all satisfied   1 = Moderately satisfied   2= Very satisfied

Reflect on your values and intentions

Take a moment now to consider your relationships with members of the family in which you were raised. This may include your stepfamily members too. Are your family bonds important to you? Do they give you a sense of meaning and purpose? What kind of relationship do you want to have with your parents, caretakers, or siblings? Are these roles and relationships important to you, and if so, how?

Be mindful of your passions and talents in this area too. What do you bring to this domain and what do you feel strongly about in this area? Also think about whether there's anything missing from your life in this area. How do you want to interact with your family members? If you have siblings or stepsiblings, what type of stepsister or stepbrother do you want to be? If your parent(s) is/are alive, what type of son or daughter do you want to be?

My Core Values in This Domain

1. _____

2. _____

3. _____

My Valued Intentions for Each Value

1. _____

2. _____

3. _____

8. Spirituality

Is this life domain important in my life NOW (circle one):

YES = It's important to me   **NO** = It's not important to me

How satisfied are you with this life domain right NOW (circle one):

0 = Not at all satisfied   1 = Moderately satisfied   2= Very satisfied

Reflect on your values and intentions

We are all spiritual beings in a sense. This is true whether you practice a faith, pray, meditate, ponder life's questions, or seek out ways to grow in awareness of yourself and your connections with other human beings and the world around you. So participating in an organized religion counts here, but for many people spirituality transcends the boundaries of a religion, place of worship, or belief in a higher power.

Take a moment to reflect on your spirituality. Do it broadly and on your own terms, and don't limit yourself to cultural or social expectations. What seems most appropriate and suitable for you? Are there things larger than your own life that inspire you? What are the mysteries of life before which you stand in awe? In what (if anything) do you have faith? Describe the role you'd like to see spirituality play in your life and how that would manifest. If you had this in your life, what kind of qualities would it provide for you?

My Core Values in This Domain

1. _____

My Valued Intentions for Each Value

1. _____

2. _____   2. _____

3. _____   3. _____

9. Community life/environment/nature

Is this life domain important in my life NOW (circle one):

YES = It's important to me   **NO** = It's not important to me

How satisfied are you with this life domain right NOW (circle one):

0 = Not at all satisfied   1 = Moderately satisfied   2= Very satisfied

Reflect on your values and intentions

We all belong to a community of some sort. You can think of this area broadly or narrowly, from being a citizen of a country or state to being involved in your town or neighborhood to the particular role you play in a social group, your workplace, a religious or secular group, or an organization. You may feel a connection with community on one or many of these levels. And it's also likely that you place varying degrees of importance on giving back in terms of your time, talents, and resources.

With all of this in mind, is being part of a community—something larger than yourself—important to you? Do you care about giving back or making a difference in the lives of others in your community? What kind of person do you want to be at whatever level of involvement you find yourself? How would you like to share your talents and passions in your community? What pulls at your heart here?

Taking care of the environment is on the minds of many, and there are many ways to do that. But you can also think of environment more broadly, as anywhere you might be: school, work, home, shopping, and so on. So, as you think about environment and nature on your own terms, consider some of these questions.

Is serving the planet important to you? For instance, do you enjoy taking care of your surroundings? Beyond things like recycling or conserving energy or water, this could include landscaping, planting a tree, or caring for a garden, or it might mean attending to your home or work space. Enjoyment of the natural world can take many forms: hiking, camping, hunting, fishing, rock climbing, sailing, relaxing on the beach—the list goes on and on. Maybe you simply like to commune with nature in a contemplative way.

Look to see if sharing, helping, or reaching out is important to you, and if so, how you might express that. Also consider if you feel that anything is currently missing in this area of your life. What can you do to make the world a better place? Why are community activities (such as volunteering, voting, recycling) important to you? What do you care about when you consider the environment or nature?

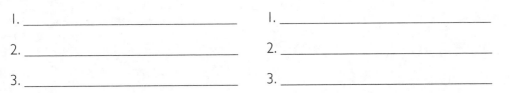

My Core Values in This Domain   *My Valued Intentions for Each Value*

1. _____   1. _____

2. _____   2. _____

3. _____   3. _____

10. Recreation/leisure

Is this life domain important in my life NOW (circle one):

YES = It's important to me   **NO** = It's not important to me

How satisfied are you with this life domain right NOW (circle one):

0 = Not at all satisfied   1 = Moderately satisfied   2= Very satisfied

Reflect on your values and intentions

The way you spend your leisure time can profoundly affect your quality of life, so it's important to consider it carefully. This domain can include just about anything. You can have a spirit of play outside of work, and at work too.

When children are playing for fun, they're doing much more than just having fun. Children love playing because it allows them to fully absorb themselves in activities that often call on all of their senses. Children also use play to express themselves—their feelings, moods, and dreams. But play isn't just for children! Adults can and often want to play for the same reasons that children do: to be fully absorbed in an activity that's fun and that allows them to express the playful and creative part of themselves.

In this domain, look for the value you place on expressing that playful spirit. Do you cherish having time to unwind, have fun, be a kid again, challenge yourself, or develop new interests or skills like playing a musical instrument? Any activity that has a playful quality to it counts here.

So how would you describe the quality of this part of your life if it were exactly the way you would like it to be? And with that in mind, what activities, interests, or hobbies would you love to cultivate and explore if you could? How do you feed yourself through hobbies, sports, or play? Why do you enjoy these things?

My Core Values in This Domain	*My Valued Intentions for Each Value?*
1. _____	1. _____
2. _____	2. _____
3. _____	3. _____

The Common Core Values Guide

Listed here are common values people find important to them. This list is by no means exhaustive, so feel free to add your own values. This list is a guide to help you identify and clarify what is truly important to you.

Empathy	Quiet	Kindness	Risk-taking	Appreciation
Parenting	Admiration	Surrender	Action	Excellence
Inspiration	Beauty	Peace	Control	Challenge
Belief	Nurture	Hope	Gratitude	Self-Expression
Sacredness	Calm	Change	Learning	Accomplishment
Nature	Community	Fairness	Partnership	Faithfulness
Adventure	Contribution	Truth	Pleasure	Security
Service	Happiness	Power	Serenity	Enlightenment
Play	Relationship	Inner Strength	Invention	Encouragement
Fun	Equanimity	Reliability	Honor	Work
Order	Connection	Structure	Strength	Intellect
Spirituality	Passion	Self-Respect	Imagination	Planning
Humor	Patience	Friendship	Joy	Honesty
Wholeness	Thoughtfulness	Intuition	Rules	Dignity
Family	Love	Home	Leadership	Dependability
Consistency	Grace	Mastery	Laughter	Integrity
Support	Winning	Growth	Creativity	Loyalty
Health	Tradition	Compassion	Sexuality	Respect
Safety	Attention	Spontaneity	Courage	Understanding
Pride	Rituals	Wealth	Sensuality	Justice
Trust	Discovery	Vitality	Feelings	Self-Control
Freedom	Generosity	Independence	Openness	Curiosity

Use the spaces below to add your own words:

_____ _____ _____ _____

_____ _____ _____ _____

CREATING YOUR LIFE COMPASS

The Valued Directions Worksheet is the foundation for creating a "life compass" (adapted from Dahl & Lundgren, 2006). We call it the Life Compass because it gives your life direction—with it, you'll know where to go from here. The next exercise will help you create it.

EXERCISE: BUILDING YOUR LIFE COMPASS

We've broken this exercise up into four easy steps. Referring back to your Valued Directions Worksheet will make building your Life Compass easy. The Life Compass appears at the end of the exercise.

Step 1: Focus on Life Domains You Find Important

You'll notice that there are two small, blank boxes attached to each life domain in the Life Compass below. These boxes are for rating each area in two different ways: how important the life domain is to you right now ("i" is for "importance") and how often you have actually acted on your values and intentions in that area over the past two weeks ("a" is for "action").

Let's start with the importance rating. Go back to the Valued Directions Worksheet. Identify each life domain that you rated as "yes," this is important. Then switch to the Life Compass and put an "X" in each "i" box connected to life domains that you see as important to you.

Step 2: What Are Your Intentions?

Write a brief intention statement in those value boxes you rated as important. You can start by going to the intention statements on the Valued Directions Worksheet. We suggest that you boil these down to a shorter statement that will fit into the box of the Life Compass so that you'll be able to remember the intentions more easily when you're in the grip of WAFs. Do this for all domains you rated as important in your life now. Remember, intentions are statements that reflect your core values and should capture the essence of how you would like to live your life in that area—what is most important to you. Now go ahead and write your intentions in each box.

Step 3: Are You Doing What Matters to You?

After you've finished writing down your intentions, please think about your activities in the past two weeks. Are your actions consistent with your valued intentions in each area? We call these activities "your feet."

So, were you doing things consistent with the intentions you just wrote down? For each intention, rate how much action you've been taking on your important values during the past two weeks.

Use the following scale for your action ratings:

Y = Yes. A "Y" here means that nothing gets in the way of you living out your valued intentions in this area.

S = Sometimes. An "S" means that there are times when you can express your values, but other times you can't. You sense an inconsistency, perhaps due to competing demands, priorities, life challenges, or because of your emotional weather.

N = No. When you reflect and come up with a "N" rating, you are sensing that you are stuck, stalled, and taking no action to live out your values in an important life domain of yours. You may even feel like you are moving in fits and jerks, or white knuckling your life. It means that you're not living your valued intentions in this area. Something is getting in your way.

Write your ratings (Y, S, or N) in the "a" (actions) box next to the "i" (importance) box that's connected to each valued intention within each important life domain. Be mindful too that we're not asking about your ideal life in each area or about what others may think of you. Just rate how actively you've been living out your intentions over the past two weeks.

Now go back and look at your intentions and actions. How well do they match up for each value domain you rated as important to you? Take stock here. Look for areas where the "i" box has an "X" and the "a" box has either an "S" or an "N." What this mismatch tells you is that you clearly have an important area of your life, but you're not living out your values (an "N"), of if you are, then you're not able to do so freely and regularly (an "S"). These inconsistencies are what you want to focus on because they mean that you're not living your life as you want to live it.

For instance, if you consider family important (say, "i" has an "X") and your action rating is low ("S") or nonexistent ("N"), you're living a life that is quite different from the one you want. If you're like most people with anxiety problems, you might find discrepancies between your importance and action ratings.

Step 4: What Stands in Your Way?

Discrepancies between your intentions and actions in valued areas are often related to internal barriers. A barrier is anything that stands in the way of you living out your values. Go back to each value area that's important to you and examine what exactly stands in the way.

Here, it can be helpful to break the barriers down into the following categories:

Thoughts and images—What thoughts or images show up that get in the way of you living out your valued intentions?

Feelings—What emotions get in the way of you taking action for your valued intentions?

Physical sensations—What are the physical sensations in your body that seem to stand between you and what matters to you?

Urges and impulses—What urges or impulses (e.g., shutting down, turning away, responding in anger, or using and abusing alcohol or other substances) get in your way?

THE LIFE COMPASS

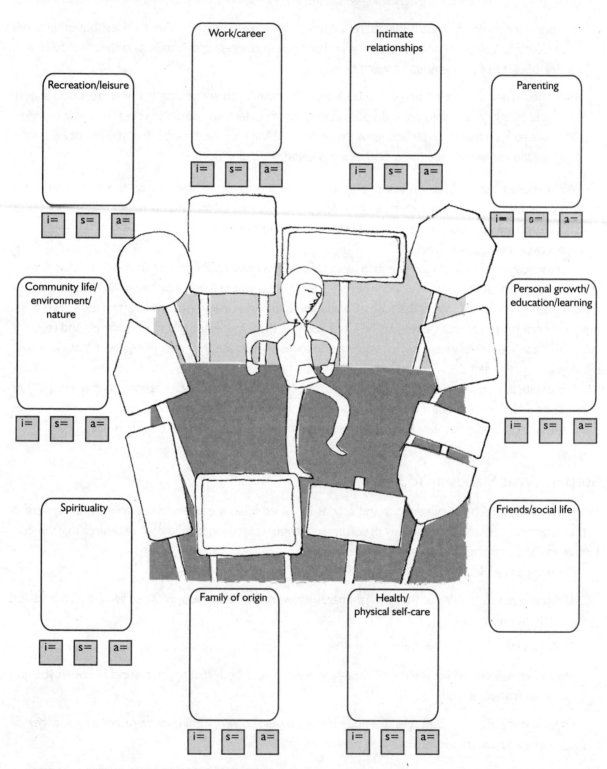

Recreation/leisure

i=   s=   a=

Work/career

i=   s=   a=

Intimate
relationships

i=   s=   a=

Parenting

i=   s=   a=

Community life/
environment/
nature

i=   s=   a=

Personal growth/
education/learning

i=   s=   a=

Spirituality

i=   s=   a=

Family of origin

i=   s=   a=

Health/
physical self-care

i=   s=   a=

Friends/social life

Now stop and review your Life Compass. If you look carefully, you'll see that many of your barriers have to do with your WAFs—thoughts, negative evaluations, judgments, feelings, and bodily sensations you don't like. The barriers are happening inside you.

Worries about anxiety and what might go wrong can definitely sidetrack you from seeing your valued intentions and following through with them. This isn't something to beat yourself up over—many people with anxiety problems are in the same boat that you are in.

Here's what you can do: you can choose to take what you've learned during this exploration of your values and use it as inspiration to stick with this workbook and to learn how to follow your bliss by bringing your life into alignment with your core values. If you find that WAFs have steered you away from the life you value, the next chapters will show you a way out of the avoidance detour and back on the road toward your value mountains. This is the opportunity that this book offers you: learning to live the life you want without being held back by your struggles with WAF barriers.

You may have a clear sense of your internal barriers. If so, that's wonderful. But if you're struggling here, then the exercise below will help you get more clarity about the barriers that stand between you and the life you wish to lead. You can read the exercise if that works for you, but it can be more powerful if you listen to the audio and follow along by downloading it at http://www.newharbinger .com/33346. The exercise should take about ten minutes and will leave you with a better sense of your barriers.

EXERCISE: IDENTIFYING INTERNAL BARRIERS

Take a moment to close your eyes and get yourself centered right where you are. Then, when you're ready, imagine that you're sitting in front of a window, trying to look outside to your life. But you notice that the window is fogged up, and your view is fuzzy. You know there is something precious out there beyond you, but you can't quite see it yet.

In your mind's eye, imagine that with each breath the window on your life is becoming clearer and clearer. Do it slowly and notice that with each breath, the fog is lifting as your valued intentions come into view. Sink into the sweetness and goodness of this moment as you look out the window on the life you wish to lead. If that's hard to do, come back again to your breath, noticing the fog lifting as you simply gaze out the window on the person you wish to be about and the life you so desperately want to have.

As you continue to gaze out, imagine that you're watching yourself living out your intentions. Focus on the very first step or two just as you decide to act on your intentions. Notice where you are. Notice what you're saying. Notice what you're doing with your hands and feet. And, if other people are involved, watch how they might be responding to you. And now, take an inventory of what's showing up inside of you. If the window on your life starts to get foggy again, just breathe the fog away.

Observe what your mind is telling you. Is there judgment of you, or the situation, or other people? Do you notice blocking thoughts, like *I can't do this … it's too much*? Or, discouraging thoughts, like *nothing matters … so don't bother*? Or, maybe your mind is conjuring up images of catastrophe, old wounds, doom and gloom, or maybe it's telling you something else like *I don't have enough time*. Just notice what's there and take stock.

Now move on to what's going on in your body. What are you feeling? And, if that's still difficult for you, see if you can notice any sense of hardening, closing down, or pulling back. As you observe, notice what's showing up just as it is, like *I'm noticing hardening* (or *tensing*, *fear*, or *shutting down*).

And, as best you can, see if you can detect any physical sensations in your body like tension, heat, energy, your heart pounding, or maybe holding your breath or breathing really fast. Just take stock of that too and observe it as the chessboard would.

Now look and see if your mind is commanding you to do something. Is it telling you to cut and run, turn away, lash out, or give up? Just notice these urges and impulses and ride the wave.

And, if we've left anything out, just notice what that may be in your experience—it could be thoughts, emotions, sensations, or urges to act or react … Look to the barriers you've been working on to guide you here.

And now, let's come back to where you are right now, sitting at the window looking out on your life. Bring your awareness back to where you are sitting and allow yourself one or two rich breaths in and out. And then, slowly open your eyes with a clearer sense of what matters to you and the barriers that get in your way.

Use what you learned from the imagery exercise you just did to get clear about your barriers. You can also look to past experiences of when you tried to take steps toward what matters to clarify what gets in your way.

Perhaps it is a fear of a panic attack or other intense feelings; thoughts about being overwhelmed, embarrassed, or exposed; intrusive unwanted thoughts that seem to show up out of thin air and invade your mind; painful images or memories; specific worries about what will happen if you move in that direction; thoughts about failure, incompetence, or inadequacy; or other worries and doubts.

We strongly encourage you to take your time with this part. It makes no sense to move forward unless you are clear about what is getting in the way of you living your life in ways that truly uphold your values.

Whatever the barriers may be, just write them down (in a word or two) in the signposts on your Life Compass. Be as specific as you can. These are the barriers between you and your values.

LIFE ENHANCEMENT EXERCISES

Below is a list of activities that we think will be helpful to you. We've added a new activity about your values. Add them to your daily to-do list and commit to doing them as best as you can.

- Practice the Acceptance of Thoughts and Feelings exercise (chapter 10) once a day.

- Practice developing your skills as an observer (the chessboard, Silent Observer Self, and the I Am mantra exercises from chapter 11) anytime, anywhere.

- Continue with any of the earlier exercises that worked well for you, and commit to cultivating a sense of compassion and kindness within you.

- Really spend time with your values and what stands in your way. Work with the Valued Directions Worksheet and Life Compass to help you along.

- Start doing something in line with your most important value(s) at least every other day. A tiny step or two is fine here too!

- If you commit to taking a step to support an important value of yours, remember to bring along the skills you've been learning to help you be present, get some perspective, and focus on what matters.

Doing the exercises won't always go smoothly. And you won't always get the result you may be hoping for. That's okay. Be patient and trust that doing the work will make a difference. We've seen the exercises make a difference with many people who have worked with this program.

THE TAKE-HOME MESSAGE

The values you choose are the road map for getting the most out of your life. They help you stay focused on what's important. When WAFs are demanding your attention, you can stop, observe your thoughts and feelings, and then listen to your values and do as your values say. A life lived well is a product of many small, valued actions. You write your own eulogy and epitaph through the choices you make and the actions you take every day. Each day provides you with opportunities to move in valued directions *and* to take your anxious thoughts and feelings with you.

Identifying and Thinking About My Values

Points to Ponder: Life is short. My values are lived out by my actions and make my life worthwhile. Anxiety management is not a vital value and no way to live. I want to follow my bliss!

Questions to Consider: What do I want to be about in this life? Am I living my values? Am I letting my WAFs get in the way of my values? Am I willing to make valued living a priority? Am I willing to do what I care about?

CHAPTER 14

Breaking Free from Anxiety with Mindful Acceptance

*And then the day came
when the risk to remain
tight in a bud was
more painful than the
risk it took to bloom.*

—attributed to Anaïs Nin

Resisting the natural flow of your experience keeps you small. There may even be some comfort in remaining tight as a bud with your anxieties and fears. After all, this is what's familiar to you. But you'll never flower that way. To flower, you need to stop resisting the flow of your inner life. You need to decide, as the opening quote teaches us, that the pain of remaining tight as a bud is more painful than the risk to bloom.

You decide that you no longer wish to remain small, stuck in the anxiety management and control trap. Instead of remaining tight, you choose to grow and expand. You decide that your life is worth the investment of your time. No more fighting or struggling. No more coping with your WAFs just to get by. No more waiting for your life to begin. It's time to let go of all the needless struggle and resistance once and for all to make room for the life you wish to have. This much you know and can control.

This moment of flowering is the expression of who you are and what you care about. With each unfolding moment, you manifest your heart in the world and stand to reap the rewards of doing what matters to you. When one of our readers shared what led him to open up, he said, "The pain of avoidance and struggle with my anxiety became greater than the pain of allowing anxiety to happen and be there." His willingness to open was risky, but he used the tools in this workbook to guide him along the way. You can do that too.

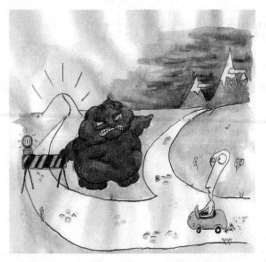

The epitaph and other values exercises in previous chapters have shown you that you don't want your life to be about an endless struggle with WAFs either. The exercises also provided you with an opportunity to discover what things you care about. Now it's time to start taking the first steps in directions that you really want to be headed.

You may ask, "But what about my anxiety? If I start doing all those things I want to do, my WAFs are going to stand right in the way and keep me from going forward."

You may feel that your situation is like the one depicted in the drawing you see to the right. Notice that the anxiety monster is blocking the way to Value Mountain—the direction you want to go with your life. The anxiety barriers are still there, hurting you. Your experience has shown you that listening to and doing what your WAFs ask you to do has only made the space they occupy larger while your life space has become smaller and smaller.

YOU'RE IN CHARGE

You already know what it's like when you turn your life over to fear and anxiety. You don't get to live it. But here's the deal. You are the master and creator of your life. It is you who has the power to choose how you respond to the fear, the dark images from your past, or the sense of foreboding about an uncertain future. It is you who can decide to fight the war with anxiety or to make peace with it.

Everything from this point forward will focus on developing skills to help you take back control over your life. Many of these skills build upon those you've started practicing already—a more gentle and friendlier approach to your anxiety, panic, thoughts, and bodily sensations. By continuing to practice and apply mindful acceptance and observer skills, you'll come to see your anxiety for what it is rather than what your mind screams that it is. We'll also teach you new skills to make more space for what your judgmental mind comes up with and to handle all the hooks and snares that pull you out of your life.

The foundation for all this work is your values. You've already created a compass to guide you. Keep your eyes and heart focused on following your bliss as you move through the rest of this book. For in your values, you will find your north star, your guiding light and inspiration. They will motivate you to go forward and take steps in a more vital, meaningful direction—one where you, and not your WAFs, are in charge. It is from this place that you create a life that's truly in alignment with your core.

WHAT TO DO WHEN YOU'RE ANXIOUS OR AFRAID

As you're getting ready to face your WAFs in a new way, one nagging question may be on your mind: what do I do when I'm getting anxious or afraid?

This is a natural question with a simple and challenging answer. Don't do what you've always done. Instead, do something radically different from what you've done before! That's it. But notice that your mind might follow with this thought: *Well, how do I do that?*

Here, it's important to be mindful that you're already doing something radically new with your WAFs. If you've gotten this far in this book, and have honestly and wholeheartedly practiced some of the exercises we've covered so far, then you're moving in a new direction. You're becoming more skillful. The exercises that come later in this chapter simply build upon the skills you've been learning about and practicing. Give yourself time with them.

For now, here are a few bits of advice for when you find yourself right in the middle of your WAFs.

Choose What You Do and Attend To

This is probably the most important choice you will make when you notice your WAFs coming on. You can choose to attend to and listen to what your WAFs are telling you and do as they say. Or you can choose to watch all the activity from an observer perspective, without buying in to it, and move with your hands and feet, guided by your values.

Acknowledge What's Happening Anyway

Anxiety happens. Remember that it's not a choice whether it comes or not. But it's your choice what you do with it. You can choose to fight it or you can choose to get curious about it, open up to it, and let it be. Like waves on the ocean, it will pass.

Do the Opposite of What Your Anxiety Compels You to Do

When your WAFs tell you to stay put sitting on your hands, you get up. When you are compelled to turn away, you get curious and lean in. When you are inclined to freeze, you move. When you feel like you're losing touch or you find yourself lost in the past or future, you take a rich grounding breath and bring your awareness back to where you are right now. When you find yourself agitated, you allow yourself to sit still with the energy inside. Doing the opposite of what your WAFs command is a powerful way to take back control of your life.

Be Kind and Gentle with Yourself

Above all, practice being gentle with yourself. This is not the time to go to war with your anxiety again. In a way, being gentle and kind is the exact opposite of warfare. This is why it can be so powerful. Just don't use it as a clever way to make the anxiety go away. If you do that, you'll likely just find yourself right back where you started and in another war, except using a new set of weapons. We've given you a few kindness exercises already to help you develop a new relationship with your mind, body, and experience. There will be more of them as you read along.

MOVING WITH BARRIERS

As you embark on your journey, you'll find the road to be full of barriers. Some barriers are external, such as lack of money; competing life demands that pull for your time and resources; opportunity; physical space; geographical constraints; or even foul weather. You can work through some of these barriers by brainstorming alternatives or by talking with a good friend to get some perspective and fresh ideas. Yet by far the most frequent and tricky barriers that you'll face are those nagging, pesky WAF-related thoughts, feelings, bodily sensations, or impulses that have slowed you down in the past.

In this chapter, we want to help you get ready for the moments when WAF barriers show up. These are the moments to employ some of the observer, mindfulness, and acceptance strategies you've been learning about in this book. These are also the moments of choice where you can determine the direction that you're headed by controlling what you do with your hands and feet.

Remember that we're brought up and socialized to believe that when a barrier comes up, we should just get rid of it—overcome it. The problem with this strategy is that getting rid of and overcoming a barrier awakens our natural inclination to struggle. You know by now that struggling with your WAFs doesn't work well. So when a barrier comes up, you need to listen to and trust your experience, not your mind!

You don't need to get rid of WAF barriers on your road to living your values. The key is to accept and move *with* the barriers—take them along for the ride! You can deal with any WAF-like obstacle in the same way that you deal with other thoughts and feelings. You don't push them aside; instead, you make room for all the unwanted stuff that has been stopping you from doing what's best for you. You acknowledge that stuff and watch it from your observer perspective. Above all, you let it be without getting involved with it *and* keep on moving in the direction you want to go—all at the same time, just like the person in the cartoon to the right.

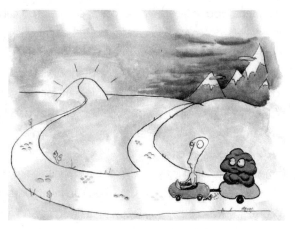

EXERCISE: DRIVING YOUR LIFE BUS

You can think of yourself as the driver of a bus called "My Life." You're headed north toward your Value Mountain, _____ [insert one of your important values here].

Along the way, you pick up some unruly passengers, like frightening thoughts and images that your mind comes up with. Other passengers on the bus traveling with you are feelings of panic, apprehension, and tension. These passengers are loud and persistent. They frighten and try to bully you as you drive along your chosen route, "Don't go there! It's too dangerous. You'll make a fool of yourself. You'll never be happy. STOOOPPPPP!"

After a while, you realize that while you were busy trying to come up with arguments and strategies to quiet them, you missed a road sign and took a wrong turn. Now you're an hour out of your way, headed south. You are, in a very real sense, lost. So you stop the bus and focus on getting your passengers in line. This time you turn around, face them, and let them have it: "Why can't you leave me alone? I'm sick of you. Just give me a few moments to relax."

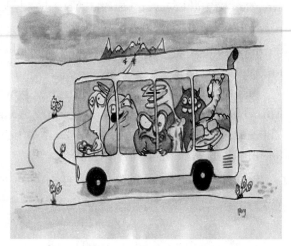

Look at what happened here: You've stopped the bus, let go of the steering wheel, turned yourself around, and your eyes are looking at the back of the bus instead of staying focused on the road ahead and your real destination. You're not moving. Instead, you're paying attention to the stuff that has nothing to do with your values.

Here, you're faced with another choice. You can stay tangled up in arguments and strategies to calm the passengers down or you can let them be, get back in the driver's seat, turn on the engine, grab the steering wheel, and find your way back onto the road toward your Value Mountain.

If moving toward what you care about is important to you, then you need to stay in the driver's seat of your Life Bus at all times. The unpleasant passengers will still be on the bus with you. You can't kick them off. While you're driving your Life Bus on the road to your Value Mountain, every now and then they creep forward and scream, "Pay attention to us! Turn around! Go back! Take this detour—it's safer, easier—and it'll make you feel better."

Here, life is asking you to make a choice again: what will you do? Stopping won't get you to the mountain and neither will the detour. Only you can take yourself to where you want to go—and you have no choice but to take the whole crowd with you. Thoughts and feelings cannot prevent you from turning your bus around and heading north again toward the mountain. That is, unless you give them that power.

The passengers on your Life Bus are not all dark and menacing. In fact, if you listen closely you may notice the voices of other passengers on your Life Bus who are desperately trying to be heard. These are the voices of your values. They've been drowned out and ignored until now, but if you stay in your driver's seat and listen, you will hear them. They will remind you of the good that you're doing for your life each time you stay in the driver's seat and move your bus in directions that matter to you!

Remember, your WAF passengers will grab every opportunity to steer you off course. They'll try to convince you that you don't feel like doing this anymore, that it's all too much, too difficult, not worth it … *and* you can still choose to keep on moving north. You can't control what kinds of feelings, thoughts, or fears will ride along with you. What you can control is where your Life Bus is going—you control the steering wheel with your hands and the accelerator with your feet.

Tuning In to Just So Radio Instead of Anxiety News Radio

To gain freedom from anxiety and fear it is important to learn that you can choose what you pay attention to and how you respond. You already know what this is like if you listen to the radio. If you have a few favorite stations, you probably choose to tune in to one of them. You may even surf stations during commercials, or change stations altogether when you're tired of listening to the same old news, messages, or songs.

Just like a radio dial, you also have the power to tune in or tune out to your WAFs or your life. This choice is humorously illustrated in the Anxiety News Radio metaphor from our colleague, Peter Thorne, a clinical psychologist in England. When we met him, he shared an interesting comment from one of his clients. We'll call her Amy.

Long before Amy came into therapy, she'd been an avid radio listener. The station she tuned in to most often was WANR—Anxiety News Radio—and she was sick of it. This wasn't the kind of radio most of us think of, nor was it something that Amy wanted to listen to. This radio was broadcasting from her head, and she couldn't tune it out or turn it off. This brought Amy to Peter.

Over time, she learned that she didn't have to stay tuned in to WANR around the clock, slavishly listening to and believing all the broadcasts inside her mind. The idea that she could tune in to more helpful sources of information was a revelation and the beginning of a new direction for her. Perhaps it will be for you too.

Read the next exercise to find out, or better yet, go to http://www.newharbinger.com/33346 and listen to the audio with your eyes closed. If you decide to listen, notice the different style and tone of voice of the two messages.

EXERCISE: CHANGING RADIO STATIONS

Anxiety News Radio (WANR)

Here's the message you've been getting:

Welcome to Anxiety News Radio, WANR, broadcasting inside your head twenty-four hours a day, seven days a week. We're the news station you've grown up with and we're the station that never sleeps. Anxiety News Radio is known for its cutting-edge coverage of all of your deep-seated fears, worries, and all that is wrong with you. We'll offer you round-the-clock compelling listening of doom and gloom—morning, noon, and night. Our mission is to drown out your values and keep you stuck. Our goal is to take over and control your life whenever we can. When you wake in the early hours, WANR will be there to make you aware of all the unpleasant aspects of your life, even before you get out of bed. We'll bring you all the things that you find most disturbing and distressing—anytime, anywhere. So don't forget that, and if you should try to forget us or tune us out, then we'll be sure to crank up the volume and broadcast even louder. So, please pay attention! And remember, Anxiety News Radio knows what's best for you—what you think and feel inside your skin can be really awful. So, just stay tuned and keep on listening. We know how to pull you out of your life in a flash and keep you stuck.

Just So Radio (WJSR)

Here's the message you could be tuning in to instead:

Wake Up! Anxiety News Radio is just a station—you can tune in or you can tune out! One thing is guaranteed though, whatever the time of day, you'll hear the same old stuff on WANR. If that's been really helpful to you, then go ahead, tune in and stay tuned. If not, then tune in more often to Just So Radio—WJSR. Here at WJSR, we bring you the news of actual experience, in the moment—all live, as it is, all the time. We won't bog you down with the negative spin that your mind creates, or leave you dwelling in the past or future that has yet to be. Living well right now is our business! So, at Just So Radio, we'll give it to you straight—color commentary about your experiences and your life just as they are. At WJSR, you won't find commercials trying to sell you the same old unhelpful thoughts that we know keep people stuck. Just So Radio brings you information about how things are, not how you fear they might be. At WJSR, we invite you, our listener, to step forward and touch the world, just as it is, and to touch your life, just as it is. Our business is to bring you into fuller contact with the world outside and inside your skin as we point you in directions that matter to you. And, we're entirely free! Our listeners tell us that tuning in to WJSR adds vitality to their lives and can even bring them joy. And, we get louder the more you listen to us. So stay tuned. Give us a fair trial and if you're not convinced by your own experience (please don't take our word for it), then WANR—Anxiety News Radio—is still there on the dial.

We suggest that you print the two parts of this metaphor on the front and back of a piece of paper and take it with you in your pocket, purse, or briefcase—whatever is most convenient. This way you have them handy when you're sick of WANR and are ready to tune in to WJSR. We also encourage you to listen to the messages of the two radio stations using the audio files available for download and notice the impact that each has on you.

Freeing Yourself from Your Mind Traps

Your mind and the simple language conventions you've learned over the years can play tricks on you that keep you stuck where you are. Recognizing them and making some simple and subtle changes in what you tell yourself can make a big difference in your life. Let's have a look at two insidious mind traps: yes-butting and buying in to your thoughts.

Getting off Your But(t)s

At some point you've probably said something like "I'd like to go out, BUT I'm afraid of having a panic attack." Snap—you just got caught in the "yes-but" trap.

Anytime you put "but" after the first part of a statement, you undo what you said; you negate the first part of the statement by denying it. This is the literal meaning of the word "but." "But" also sets up your WAFs as a barrier and problem you need to resolve before you take action. Let's see how this plays out with an example.

So when you say, "I'd like to go out, BUT I'm afraid of having a panic attack," you "undo" your interest in going out—and then you won't go out. You'll stay home because that "but" takes the "like to go out" away.

"But" also sets you up for struggle. Either the liking to go out has to go away or the fear of having a panic attack has to go away before you can go out. This is why when you use "buts" you often end up quite literally stuck on your butt. "But" makes going out or doing much of anything impossible. If you pay close attention, you may find that you use the word "but" many times every day as a reason for not acting on your values. This unnecessarily restricts your life, holds you back, and reduces your options.

Now imagine what would happen if you replaced the word "but" with "and." "I'd like to go out, AND I'm afraid of having a panic attack." This little change can have a dramatic impact on what might happen next. If you put it that way, you could actually go out *and* be anxious *and* be worried all at the same time. Most importantly, it would actually allow you to go out and do something vital even though you might feel anxious. It would also be a more correct and honest statement of what's going on for you in the moment.

Imagine how much more space you'd have in your life if, starting today, you were to say "and" instead of "but" every time a "but" is about to keep you stuck on your butt. How many more opportunities would you gain to do things? Getting off your but(t)s could be one of the most empowering things you've ever done.

Don't Buy In to Your Thoughts

You may have come across a saying that goes something like "Sticks and stones may break my bones, but words will never hurt me." But thoughts, evaluations, memories, and the like can hurt whenever you take them literally—when you treat them as if they were the same as sticks and stones in the real world. This is why it can be dangerous if you buy in to your thoughts.

You can learn to break this cycle. To do that, you'll need to recognize your thoughts and images for what they really are. For example, when you say, "I'll have a panic attack if I go out," you can think or say out loud, "I am having the thought that I'll have a panic attack if I go out." Or if you find yourself thinking, *If I don't learn to control my anxiety and worries, then things are going to go downhill for me*, you can say out loud, "My mind is feeding me the message that …"

You can apply the same strategy to scary images or feelings. With images you can say to yourself, *I'm having the image that I'm being attacked*. With feelings, you can say, *I'm having the feeling that I'm about to die* or *I'm having the feeling that* _____ [insert whatever you typically feel].

If you find this too cumbersome or difficult, there's an even simpler way of labeling. Whenever a thought comes up, whatever it may be, just label it *thinking* or *Oh, there's thinking*. Whenever an image comes up, just label it *picture* or *There's a picture*. And when sensations come up, just label them *sensations* or *There are sensations*.

Practice doing this deliberately and with any unhelpful thoughts your mind comes up with from time to time. This will give you space to see your thoughts for what they are—products of your mind that need not always be listened to, trusted, or believed.

Developing these new labeling and language habits is going to feel awkward at first. Just stay the course and keep practicing. These new skills will help you see thoughts as just thoughts, images as images, and feelings as feelings. This will give you the space you need to move forward when your WAFs show up. Even when the most scary and intense thoughts, images, or feelings are highly believable, they're still only thoughts, images, or feelings.

It takes a while before you develop these new habits. Every time you catch yourself yes-butting or buying in to thoughts, you can apply these techniques. And the more you do so, the more they'll help you create more space between you (the observer) and your mind, your experience, and your old history. It will help you become a more skillful and wise observer.

Riding Out Your Emotions

Imagine for a moment an ocean wave as it approaches the shore. It's steep and tall and hasn't yet crested into a breaker. Now imagine the wave nearing a group of gulls floating on the water. The birds don't fly away. They simply ride up the facing slope, round the top, and drift down the long back of the wave.

That's what you can learn to do with your WAFs too. All emotions are wavelike and time limited. They ebb and flow. Like waves, emotions build up, eventually reach a peak, and drift away. WAFs come and go in a similar way. They don't last forever, even if it feels as if they will.

We encourage you to ride the waves of your WAFs. You must initially face their steep leading edge. At this point, the waves are tall and scary. You may feel that they will go on forever and that they will overpower you, or that you may drown. Still, sooner or later the emotion reaches its peak, weakens, and starts to recede. You may feel yourself slipping down the back of the wave, the WAFs quieting.

That's how anxiety works if you don't try to control or block it, just allowing the waves to run their course. If you refuse to face and ride out a wave and instead try to fight it by swimming against it to get over it, it will throw you back and toss you around like a ping-pong ball. Then you're caught churning helplessly beneath the surface of the water, at the mercy of the full force of the crushing wave and undertow.

But if you swim or ride with the waves, or at least not against them, they will eventually carry you toward the safe shore. The same happens with your anxiety waves. Swimming against them and fighting them makes them bigger and seem more dangerous. Not fighting them and staying with them, or even just drifting along with them, takes much less effort in the moment. And, if you allow yourself a chance to experience that, then you'll learn that the anxiety waves will eventually crest and recede. That's how it works, even when you're faced with several waves coming and going, each lasting longer than you'd wish.

Listen to the audio of the following exercise with your eyes closed at http://www.newharbinger.com/33346 and try to imagine the entire scene at a beach.

EXERCISE: WAF SURFING

Right now you have a chance to learn to ride the wave of your worries, anxieties, and fears—your WAFs. If you're willing, then think of a recent situation where you felt afraid, panicky, nervous, worried, or upset. Visualize the scene and remember how you felt. Pause for a while before going on.

Notice the worrying and disconcerting thoughts. Perhaps you'll notice images of disaster too. Keep focusing on the upsetting scene as well as on the judgments you made about it and what was happening inside you. Let your anxiety rise till it's at least a 4 or 5 on a scale of 10.

Good—now go back to the white room like you did in chapter 5. Observe what your body might be doing. Notice the sensations and how your mind evaluates them. Simply label them all—*I am noticing* … Notice the sensations of warmth and of tightness. There's the thought that it's dangerous, that you're losing control. Just let your body and mind do its thing.

Do the same with worries, other thoughts, and images that show up—the old story line. None of them are right or wrong, true or false. Acknowledge their presence without trying to control or change them. Don't try to push them away. Simply label them and keep watching your mind and body.

In your mind, you can now ride the waves of your WAFs. You must initially face their steep leading edge. At this point, the waves are tall and scary. You may feel that they will go on forever and that they will over-power you, or that you may drown—and you keep on riding for a while. Be aware of the point where your WAF stops climbing. After a while you can feel it leveling off and starting to diminish. Experience the slow ride down the back of the wave. Accept wherever you are on the wave. Don't hasten to get past it. It moves at its own speed—all you can and need to do is let go and let it carry you.

You can watch your thoughts and bodily sensations entering and leaving the white room. And you can notice the progress of the wave. There's nothing more to do. Keep watching until the WAF has completely passed.

Using the Energy of Anxiety Wisely

Pema Chödrön (2001) describes an intriguing way you can use the energy of anxiety wisely. Emotions proliferate through our internal dialogue—what your mind is telling you about your anxiety. If you label those thoughts as "thinking" when you notice them and just observe what's going on, you may be able to sense the vital, pulsating energy beneath them. This energy underlies all of your emotional experience, and there's nothing wrong or harmful about it.

The challenge is to stay with this underlying energy: to experience it, leave it as it is, and, when possible, put it to good use. When anxiety arises uninvited, let go of your old story line about it and connect directly with the energy just below. What remains is a *felt* experience, not the story line your mind is feeding you about what's happening.

If you feel, and can stay with, the energy in your body—neither acting on it nor suppressing it—you can harness it in the service of actions that move you forward toward achieving your valued goals. The raw energy of anxiety is fuel. You get to choose to use that fuel for you or against you.

LEARNING TO ACCEPT YOUR ANXIETY

Mindfulness exercises are a way of learning that you cannot choose what comes into your mind and what you feel. You can only choose what you pay attention to, *how* you pay attention, and what you *do*. This is how you change your relationship with your mind, body, and world. The exercise below will help you do just that.

In this exercise, we're simply building on the skills you've been learning. What's new is the expanded focus of the practice. This time, you'll be actively and openly inviting into your awareness bodily sensations and unwanted thoughts, worries, and images so that you may learn to approach them in a more accepting and compassionate way. Just like the finger trap and tug-of-war exercises, this exercise encourages you to lean into anxiety rather than fight it or turn away from it. This will create space for you to feel your emotions and think your thoughts as they are, not as your mind tells you they are.

You'll practice opening up to uncomfortable feelings and thoughts rather than rushing to fix or change them. As you do that, you're dropping the rope and willingly making space for WAFs when they're present—because they're present anyway. And with that, you'll get more space to do the things with your life that you may have put on hold for a long time. Are you willing to do an exercise to help you do that?

If you are willing, we suggest you select a quiet place where you feel comfortable and distraction is limited. Let's call this your kind space, your peaceful place. Go through the exercise slowly and pause after each section. It will take about fifteen minutes.

The easiest way to do this exercise is by listening to the audio recording that is freely available online (see http://www.newharbinger.com/33346). After practicing with the audio for a week or two, you may prefer to practice at your own pace without the audio.

EXERCISE: ACCEPTANCE OF ANXIETY

Go ahead and get in a comfortable position in your chair. Sit upright with your feet flat on the floor, your arms and legs uncrossed, and your hands resting in your lap (palms up or down). Allow your eyes to close gently.

Take a few moments to get in touch with your breath and the gentle rising and falling of your breath in your chest and belly. There's no need to control your breathing in any way—simply let the breath breathe itself. As best you can, also bring an attitude of kind allowing and gentleness to the rest of your experience. There's nothing to be fixed. There's nothing else to do. Simply allow your experience to be your experience just as it is.

As you sink more deeply into this moment of just being where you are, see if you can be present with your values and commitments. Ask yourself, *Why am I here? Where do I want to go? What do I want to be about in my life?* Connect with the truth of it in your heart, and bring your awareness more fully to something you care about. Look to one of your values that has been difficult for you to act on because of the barriers. Rest in the truth of your experience with each natural breath, and become aware of what shows up that has been hard for you.

It could be a troubling thought, worry, image, or intense bodily sensation. Gently, directly, and firmly shift your attention on and into the discomfort, no matter how bad it seems. Notice any strong feelings that may arise in your body. Allow those feelings to be as they are and observe what your mind tells you about them. Simply hold your thoughts and feelings in awareness with a sense of curiosity and kindness. Stay with your discomfort, breathe with it, and see if you can gently open up to it and make space for it. With each new breath, imagine that you are creating more and more space for this barrier to simply be there. Simply allowing it to be as it is. Notice also who it is that is noticing all these thoughts and feelings … can you sense your silent observer?

If you ever notice yourself tensing up and resisting, pushing away from the experience, just acknowledge that and see if you can make some space for whatever you're experiencing with each new breath. Is this feeling or thought really your enemy? Or can you have it, notice it, own it, and let it be? Can you make room for the discomfort, for the tension, for the anxiety? What does it really feel like to allow it to be there, moment-to-moment? Is this something you *must* struggle with, or can you invite the discomfort in, saying to yourself, *I welcome you in because you are just a part of my experience right now?*

If the sensations or discomfort grow stronger, acknowledge that, stay with them, breathe with them, and allow them to just be. Is this discomfort something you *must not* have, you *cannot* have? Can you open up a space for the discomfort in your heart? Is there room inside you to feel that, with compassion and kindness toward yourself and your experience? Breathe and create more space in your heart center for you to hold all of you.

As you open up and embrace your experience, you may notice thoughts coming along with the physical sensations, and you may see thoughts about your thoughts. You may also notice your mind coming up with judgmental labels such as "dangerous" or "getting worse." When that happens, the practice is the same. Stay with them, breathe into them, creating more and more space within you to have what you are experiencing just as it is. Simply notice thoughts as thoughts, physical sensations as physical sensations, feelings as feelings— nothing more, nothing less.

Stay with your discomfort for as long as it pulls on your attention. If and when you sense that the anxiety and other discomfort are no longer pulling for your attention, let them go.

As this time for practice comes to a close, take a few rich inhales and slow cleansing exhales. Then, gradually widen your attention to take in the sounds around you. Take a moment to make the intention to bring this sense of gentle allowing and self-acceptance into the present moment and the rest of your day. Then, slowly open your eyes.

This exercise can be challenging—sometimes more so than at other times. This is the first time you're deliberately welcoming in your WAF experiences and practicing a new response to them. Don't let that challenge (a judgment) stand in the way of you doing the exercise again this week and in the weeks to come. It'll get easier over time.

Remember that mindful acceptance is a skill. Like a seedling, it needs to be watered to grow. The practice itself has many possible results, not just one. You may feel relaxed during or after the exercise, or you may not. You may feel tense and keyed up at some point, or you may not. You may experience sadness or regret, or you may not. These and other responses are just fine.

The best possible outcome of this exercise is when you find yourself better able to stay with your anxiety-related thoughts and feelings and ride them out rather than fight against them or push them away. So be kind with yourself as you do the practice. Remember, the ultimate purpose of being more accepting of your experience is that you can move forward with your life. Acceptance empowers you to do what you really want to do *and* experience whatever you may experience along the way.

It will be helpful to track your experiences with this exercise over the next several weeks, using the worksheet at the end of this chapter. This will give your practice some structure and give you a place to chart progress over time. We've included an example of how to complete the worksheet. You'll also find the worksheet on the book website at http://www.newharbinger.com/33346. Print out as many clean copies as you like.

LIFE ENHANCEMENT EXERCISES

Use this week to practice the exercises in this chapter, adding them to your self-care to-do list. Allow yourself opportunities to practice the Acceptance of Anxiety exercise (described above) at least one time each day. You can continue to do any of the exercises from earlier chapters. In fact, we'd encourage you to do them as often as you can. Play with them. Get good at using them. Look for opportunities to practice using them too. And above all, remember why you are doing this work. This is about what matters to you and living the kind of life you wish to lead. All of the skills are about helping you to create that kind of life, even if anxiety decides to come along for the ride now and then.

THE TAKE-HOME MESSAGE

Anxiety can be a monster crippling your life, or it can be a temporary experience that comes and goes pretty much all by itself. It's all a matter of how you respond to it. There's nothing in your head or heart that can keep you from doing what you want to do. You have choices. We hope that you're starting to experience that for yourself.

Everything in this chapter builds on skills you've been cultivating throughout the book so far. Every WAF moment can be an opportunity for you to learn a new way of responding. So continue to nurture your capacity to act with kindness, gentle observation, patience, and wholeness, and all with an eye on your values. You can't control the passengers that ride along with you on your Life Bus. What you can control is how you respond to them and whether you keep on moving north toward your values.

Facing My Anxiety, Getting On with My Life

Points to Ponder: Pain is part of life. When I shut down to WAF pain, I shut down to my life. Softening to my pain is the way to get my life back.

Questions to Consider: Am I willing to face, openly and honestly, my WAFs for what they are, and take them with me where I want to go? Am I ready to take a stand and accept WAF discomfort in order to get my life back?

ACCEPTANCE OF ANXIETY:
Life Enhancement Exercise Practice Worksheet

In the first column, record whether you have made a commitment to practice the Acceptance of Anxiety exercise that day and include the date. In the second column, mark whether you practiced, when you practiced, and how long you practiced. In the third column, note whether you used the audio file or not. In the fourth column, write down anything that came up during your practice.

Acceptance of Anxiety Life Enhancement Exercise Practice Form			
Commitment: yes/no Day: Date:	Practiced: yes/no When practiced? A.M./P.M. How long (minutes)?	Audio: yes/no	Comments
Commitment: (yes)/no Day: *Saturday* Date: *6/5/2014*	Practiced: (yes)/no Time: (A.M.)/P.M. Minutes: *15 minutes*	*yes*	*Was tough to be an observer, felt the pull of negative thoughts, physical tension; felt some scary sensations; had some space too. I'll work at being the board next time.*
Commitment: yes/no Day: Date:	Practiced: yes/no Time: A.M./P.M. Minutes:		
Commitment: yes/no Day: Date:	Practiced: yes/no Time: A.M./P.M. Minutes:		
Commitment: yes/no Day: Date:	Practiced: yes/no Time: A.M./P.M. Minutes:		
Commitment: yes/no Day: Date:	Practiced: yes/no Time: A.M./P.M. Minutes:		

CHAPTER 15

Bringing Compassion to Your Anxiety

Though we all have the seeds of fear within us, we must learn not to water those seeds and instead nourish our positive qualities—those of compassion, understanding, and loving-kindness.

—Thich Nhat Hanh

To open and awaken from the confines of anxiety and fear, you'll need to cultivate the conditions for your growth and freedom. No amount of willpower or brute strength will free you from your anxiety trap. As we learn from Thich Nhat Hanh, you need to nurture a new relationship with your mind and inner emotional life. This is the way to cultivate genuine happiness.

This new relationship is one where you decide to stop feeding the anxiety monsters and bullies on the bus. Instead, you greet them with compassion and loving-kindness. This simple idea is not fluff, for it now stands on a growing research base showing that learning to be kind to ourselves is one of, if not *the*, single most powerful antidote to suffering with anxiety, fear, and other forms of emotional pain. Period!

This work isn't easy and requires a conscious shift in perspective. You must decide to let go of the myth that your WAFs are your enemy—an enemy that must be defeated. You know by now that this fight has cost you dearly. You also know that you can't win it because you can never win a fight with yourself.

So here's an important question: Must anxiety really be your enemy? What if you were willing to approach anxiety with some compassion and kindness instead of with a declaration of war in your hand? If you did that, you'd find out—over time—that your worries, anxieties, and fears would become better travel companions. And you'd see that you can move *with* them, not *against* them.

Compassion and kindness can literally take the sting out of anxiety, panic, fear, and worry. This will transform your WAF roadblocks into something you can live with and move with on your way toward your value mountains. To develop compassion, you must cultivate your capacity for loving-kindness just like that of a mother toward her newborn child (Dalai Lama, 1999). Like a muscle, it is a skill that will grow with practice. The next exercise will help you do that.

EXERCISE: TRAVELING WITH MY ANXIETY CHILD

What if anxiety didn't look like the dark, menacing monster from the cartoon in the previous chapter? What if it looked more like the child in the cartoon below—like your child?

Perhaps you could treat this WAF child as you would your own child if he or she were acting out and being noisy. Think about how you might respond.

Some parents deal with the pulsating energy of their kids by lashing out, fighting, and screaming. The kids, in turn, bear the brunt of this unfettered negative energy as they take one punishment after the next. Many, in turn, will rebel and find ways to fight and resist right back.

Yet we know from countless research studies that these strategies are poor ways to encourage more appropriate behaviors. Parents end up feeling bad, tired, and frustrated, and the kids go on being kids, but now with frustrated, tired, and angry parents. Worse, the kids grow up learning to be harsh and very hard on themselves and others.

Other parents opt for a softer, yet firm, approach. They don't resort to fighting or punishing behavior simply because their child is behaving badly. They see through that first impulse (to react with negative energy), and instead, they redirect, refocus, and reconnect. They see their child as part of them. They wish for that child to know kindness and love, and so they respond in a way that shows that. They also act as a pack leader

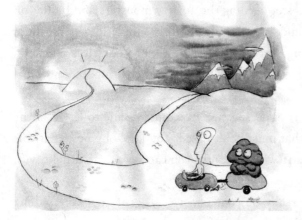

of sorts and take the child in directions the parent wants to go and in directions that are best for the child too. Research shows that this kinder way of relating is highly effective as a parenting strategy.

So what's your parenting strategy with your anxiety "children"? Do you yell, scream, and struggle? If you do that, has it worked? Or do you end up feeling worse—frustrated and tired out by the constant nagging? Do your anxiety children respond well to that, or do they continue to act up?

Perhaps it's time to refocus, reconnect, and redirect. After all, your WAF children are a part of you.

What would it be like for you to treat your WAF children with kindness and love? You'd still be firm. You wouldn't let them sidetrack you or get you tangled up in wild antics.

You'd also take those children with you. You'd do what you set out to do when you left home. Are you willing to do the same with your anxiety children, taking them with you as you drive into life?

PRACTICE ACTS OF KINDNESS AND TENDER LOVING CARE

We've found that people with anxiety disorders are very hard on themselves. They're often frustrated with how constricted their lives have become, so they get caught in the self-blame game. "Why can't I snap out of it? I'm so silly. I know it's all in my head. I'm angry at myself and I'm angry at the world. I hate my panic attacks—I just hate them."

Many people with PTSD, in particular, struggle with anger almost every day. They find themselves being hateful and angry at the perpetrator who abused them or the soldiers who committed war atrocities. They also blame themselves for not being able to "cope" better, or they wallow in shame, remorse, and regret for things they did or failed to do during the original traumatic event.

All this blaming and hating doesn't solve the problem. In fact, it creates the conditions for the problem to get worse. You probably know as much from your experience. What is needed here is for you to decide, perhaps for the first time, to change the way you relate with your mind, body, and experience. Instead of blaming and hating, you decide to take care of your own house—your mind, body, emotional life, and anything else that your old history throws at you.

There are only two ways to go here. You can create a house that is hostile and unkind or one that is full of kindness and compassion. But the most important part here is that it begins with you. You've got to learn to be kinder to yourself first and then to others if you want to stop being at war with your WAFs and your life. That's how it works.

Practicing acts of kindness toward yourself and others is a behavioral antidote to anxiety, anger, regret, shame, and depression. This practice will make it easier for you to stop fighting with your mind and body. It's a simple thing you can do to bring more peace and joy to your life.

How to Be Kind to Yourself

You'd like to be kinder to yourself, but maybe you don't know how to start. Here's something to do: make a commitment to practice at least one act of kindness toward yourself every day. Start each day with this commitment. Think about something you could do to be kind to yourself. These acts are particularly important when what we call *TLC problems* arise—when you feel tired/stressed, lonely, and are craving things like nurturing, praise, stimulation, food, or drugs. These TLC problems can be undercut if you remind yourself to meet them with compassion and kindness wrapped in tender loving care.

Compassion and kindness are not feelings. They're actions. Acting with compassion toward yourself and others means acting in a caring and loving way. You stop being a whipping post. If you're ready to make such a commitment, write it down on paper, or, better yet, share it with someone you care about.

You can attend to TLC problems by showing tender loving care toward yourself. This might involve taking time to practice meditation, reading a good book, going for a walk, listening to music, gardening, or preparing a good meal. You do this not because you deserve it. You do it "just because."

Valued living and being kind to yourself are related. Whenever you do something that moves you closer to one of your values, you're also being kind to yourself. Return to your Life Compass in chapter 13 and identify something you can do, however small, in the service of one of those values. Write it down in the space below. Then commit to doing it. Make giving yourself tender loving care every day a priority.

_____

_____

Make Your Mind and Body a Kind Space

Remember the chessboard and volleyball exercises we talked about in chapter 11. In those exercises you learned that you can be a player with a stake in each battle or you can be the board that provides a space for the game. In the next exercise, we'd like to help you practice making that space a kind space. You can listen along and download the audio version of the exercise at http://www.newharbinger .com/33346.

EXERCISE: LOVING-KINDNESS MEDITATION

Loving-kindness is soft and gentle. It is how you might handle a newborn child or the way you might touch and hold something fragile. In those moments, you open up and handle what you're given with the greatest care. You can do the same with anxious thoughts, worry, fears, and painful memories too. There is great strength and power in kindness.

Start by getting comfortable in your kind space. Sit upright, feet flat on the floor, arms and legs uncrossed, and palms, facing up or down, resting gently on your legs. Close your eyes and bring your attention to your breath as you've done with other exercises.

Continue to focus on each gentle inhale and exhale, simply noticing the rhythm of the rising and falling of your chest and belly. As you follow the soft flow of your breath, imagine a halo of kindness sweeping over you. It starts at your head and slowly moves, ebbing and flowing, past your face and then on to your chest and belly.

As it passes, feel the energy from the halo connecting with your heart. And, as it slowly passes down your head and trunk silently say to yourself on each inhale, *softening, opening, allowing, welcoming, kind, peaceful,* and *strong.* Continue as the halo gradually sweeps down past your hips, and with each rich inhale, silently say to yourself, *I am here now—awake, alert, spacious, and alive.* As the halo sweeps over your knees, repeat with each inhale: *softening, opening, allowing, welcoming, kind, peaceful,* and *strong.* When the halo reaches your toes, continue as you've done before but this time connect with the words *I am complete, I am whole, I am.* See if you can bring the intention of kind allowing to your experience as you imagine breathing in compassionate kindness.

As you do, bring to mind someone you know who is struggling and suffering. Perhaps it's a parent, a brother or sister, a friend, spouse, or coworker. It could be a child, an older person, or someone you've heard about in the news or on TV. See if you can imagine this person, present in the room with you now, suffering.

Now look into your heart and into your capacity for healing and kindness. Imagine that you could extend healing to the person you're thinking about; restore this person's mind, broken body, failings, hurts, struggles, and pain; and bring about wholeness. In your mind's eye and heart, see yourself reaching out to this person and offering kindness and healing. And then, extend your arms and offer that kindness and healing as you might a gift hidden in the cup of your hands.

In your mind's eye, see yourself wiping away this person's tears and extending love. Open your arms and wrap that person in your kind embrace—extend your heart. Allow yourself to connect your kindness with that person, who is no longer alone. You are not alone. You are united in your healing. By your generous act, you are sharing your capacity for kindness and healing. Stay with this person as long as you wish.

Continue to sit quietly with this moment in time. And when you are ready, gradually widen your attention to the sounds around you. Open your eyes with the intention to extend loving-kindness to yourself and others each moment of this day.

Kindness begets kindness. It's uplifting energy that will weaken the power of your judgmental WAF mind that's keeping you stuck. Kindness waters the seeds of compassion and acceptance in you. Many people find that their capacity for loving-kindness grows as they practice the loving-kindness meditation by bringing other people to mind—people they may respect or like, people they don't get along with particularly well, or people they don't know all that well. You can do the same as you develop this important skill.

Practice Kindness with Your Wounds

Being kind includes, foremost, practicing acceptance and compassion toward your own feelings, memories, and hurts. Many of us have old wounds from losses, unfair treatment by others, and sometimes even devastating abuse. When painful feelings, images, and memories come up, your first, instinctual response is to push them away. If you catch yourself doing that, please stop. This is a golden opportunity to embrace old hurts with compassion and acceptance.

Why should you do that? People who have been hurt continue to inflict pain on themselves and others because they haven't allowed their wounds to heal. If you don't take care of your wounds, you may pass them on to your children, spouse, friends, colleagues, and other people in your life. Hurt can be recycled many times.

For a moment, think about what you would do if something was physically wrong with you, like a bleeding knee or a problem with your stomach, your back, or your teeth. We suspect that you'd stop what you were doing and attend to your bleeding wound or sick organ. You'd never be rough with it, treat it harshly, or call it names. Instead, you'd take really good care of it. That makes sense. We suggest you do the same with your open WAF wounds—all those feelings of fear, panic, worry, and shame, along with all the anger and blaming you inflict on yourself and dole out to others.

To break the cycle of anxiety avoidance and life constriction, you have to start by taking better care of yourself. You do that by practicing being kind to yourself and by embracing anxiety with compassion. You do this by no longer buying in to all the thoughts your mind comes up with about you and your emotional pain—you stop being hard on yourself. Just as with your physical organs, your anxiety and emotional pain are parts of you. Even when you're in the throes of your WAFs, you can take good care of your anxiety. That's what embracing anxiety with compassion means.

You can take care of yourself, your anxieties, and your wounds by giving yourself loving-kindness. You don't need to rely on other people to do that for you. Thich Nhat Hanh (2001) developed a beautiful exercise to practice self-compassion. It is both powerful and simple. It shows you how you can take care of your WAFs as if they were your sick baby or child needing your love and attention.

EXERCISE: GIVING YOURSELF LOVING-KINDNESS

Remember when you were a little child and you had a fever? You felt bad. So a parent or caregiver came and gave you medicine. The medicine may have helped, but it was nothing like having your mom there. Remember that you didn't feel better until your mother (or other loving caregiver) came and put her hand on your burning forehead? That felt so good!

To you, her hand was like the hand of a goddess. When she touched you with her hand, freshness, love, and compassion penetrated into your body. The hand of your mother is alive in your own hand. Go ahead and touch your forehead with your hand and see that your mother's healing hand is still there. Allow the energy of your mother's loving and tender touch to radiate through your hand and into you. Bring that quality to your experience.

As with the finger-trap exercise, this is the time to take an unusual step and be open to what may happen. Here is what you can do: close your eyes, touch your forehead or your chest, and think of your mother's hand touching you when you were young and sick. You can also bring to mind anyone else who left you feeling good, loved, and cared for. The kindness of this caring person's hand is alive in yours. And you can give that kindness to yourself, right now and anytime, anywhere.

Practice Giving and Receiving Kindness

To build your kindness muscle, you need to practice. And what better time to do that than during your day when you find yourself walking. This next exercise builds on the mindful walking practice you did earlier, but with an important twist. We first learned about it from Sharon Salzberg, a well-known teacher in the art of cultivating compassion and kindness. This exercise is powerful when it is practiced regularly as part of your daily routine.

EXERCISE: EMBODY AND SHARE LOVING-KINDNESS WHILE WALKING

For this practice, all you need to do is walk at a normal pace, inside or outside. As you walk, you'll silently repeat a meaningful phrase—one that reflects a loving-kindness intention and wish for yourself. This personal kindness mantra ought to be simple and important to you. For instance, you may come up with a phrase such as *May I have peace*, *May I be kind*, *May I experience joy*, or *May I be free of suffering*.

Before moving on, come up with your own personal phrase:

May I _____.

As you walk and move about your day, silently repeat your personal loving-kindness phrase. And then, when you find your attention being pulled by something or someone outside of you, gently bring your aware-ness to whatever it was that caught your attention, and then silently extend your personal phrase to that object, person, or creature. For instance, if a tree caught your attention, you would then silently extend your phrase to that tree—*May this tree have peace*. If it's a stranger, do the same. If it's a memory, thought, or feeling, do the same. Even if it is an animal, car, or some other object, do the same. If this seems odd or strange, thank your mind for that thought and continue extending the phrase to anything that grabs your attention.

Then, after you silently extend your personal loving-kindness intention to whatever grabbed your atten-tion, bring your awareness back to yourself, and continue to walk as you repeat your personal kindness mantra silently to yourself (*May I ...*). Repeat this process of extending your phrase to yourself and then to anything that pulls your attention for as long as you wish.

This practice is a simple and powerful way to bring loving-kindness intentions into your daily life. It is best to do with an open mind because it can produce many possible results. The important thing is to practice without expecting any immediate outcome. Over time and with practice, loving-kindness will become more of a habit in your daily life.

So, are you willing to give this a shot? If so, then make an intention to practice this exercise as often as you can while you're walking during your day. Later, you can extend this exercise to times when you find yourself sitting or waiting in line.

Learning to Forgive Means Letting Go of Past Hurts

When people hear the word forgiveness, they often jump to conclusions. You may too. Your mind may tell you that forgiveness means condoning or forgetting past wrongs, or worse, ignoring the hurt and pain you may have suffered at the hands of someone else or even pain that was self-inflicted. You may see it as a sign of weakness or as something that you must feel inside before you take steps to forgive. None of these are true.

When the late Pope John Paul II met to forgive his would-be assassin, he wasn't condoning the wrong that was done. Instead, he was extending mercy and compassion. He was letting go of the burden he was carrying of being the target of a senseless act. The assassin still sat in prison for his crime. This is the essence of forgiveness—it's nothing more than letting go of a painful past so that *you* can heal and move on!

You and you alone can do this. And you do it for you because not doing it virtually guarantees that you will remain stuck, the victim, wanting and waiting for a resolution that may never come. If you look closely, you will notice that holding on to past hurts in the spirit of unforgiveness ultimately hurts you, you, you! It is a poison to your spirit and growth and does little for those who once wronged you. This is why it needs to stop.

Learning to forgive is the single most powerful way to soften the pull of your painful past. Studies report that the ability to forgive can be learned, and it improves health—physical, emotional, and spiritual. Those who learn this important skill report experiencing less hurt, stress, anger, depression, and illness; more energy, hope, optimism, compassion, and love; and a greater sense of well-being. These are the concrete benefits of forgiveness.

Beyond the benefits, letting go will give you the space to move forward with your life. No longer a prisoner of the injustices of your past, you can chart a new direction for yourself. From this point forward, you decide to let go of the old stories and attachments to the past and feelings of shame, anger, regret, and pain. You decide how you wish to move forward to create the life you want to have right now.

Below we describe a brief exercise that outlines four steps on the path to learning forgiveness as an act of letting go. You can listen to and download the audio version of the exercise at http://www .newharbinger.com/33346. The steps are as follows:

- **Step 1: Awareness**—waking up to hurt and pain as it is, without judgment or denial

- **Step 2: Separation**—softening using your observer self while inviting healing and change

- **Step 3: Compassionate witness**—extending compassion to your experience and others

- **Step 4: Letting go and moving on**—releasing grudges and resentment that fan the flames of your suffering, and then moving forward in your life in directions you want to go

EXERCISE: LEARNING TO LET GO OF GRUDGES

Take a moment to reflect on some past event that you continue to recycle over and over again in your mind. Look for a situation or event that leaves you feeling angry, hurt, resentful, bitter, and demanding justice. Get a piece of paper and jot down the details of the past transgression. Make it as detailed as possible.

When you're ready, close your eyes and bring the event to mind. Really get into it as best you can. What happened? Who did the wrong—you or someone else? How were you or others hurt? What didn't you get then that you are longing for now? Allow yourself several minutes to really open up to this experience.

Become aware of the pain that you experience about that past event. Allow yourself to experience the pain as it is. Where does it hurt now? See if you can face it squarely. What does it feel like? What does it look like?

Notice your mind linking your pain with judgment, blame, and negative evaluations. See if you can use your silent observer perspective to separate the judgment from the pain you are having now. Notice judgment as judgment, blame as blame, and bitterness as bitterness, without engagement. Simply watch and separate the pain itself and the suffering from the evaluations of the pain.

See if you can step back even further, as if you're watching this event play out on a giant movie screen. Imagine being in the audience, simply watching, as though you're someone seeing this drama unfold for the first time. See if you can open up your heart to be a compassionate witness to the actors in this scene. See who's doing the hurting. See who's receiving the hurt. See who's responsible for doing the hurting. See the person responsible for the felt pain, then and now.

Now kindly ask yourself this: Who's responsible for letting go now? Who has control over that happening or not happening? Who's in control over the resentment you feel now? Who is getting hurt, right now, by holding on to the memory of the past wrong? Who has the power to let go and move on?

The answer is *you*. You can let go of holding on to the wish and hope for a resolution. You can take the energy and effort focused on resolving, fighting back, or getting even and put it to more vital use. You can bring kindness to your experience by facing your pain squarely for what it is. Own it because it is yours, and then choose to let it go.

If you're willing to let the resentment and rage go, then do that. If you're having trouble doing that, then think about who's getting hurt by holding on—is it you or the person who once wronged you? Imagine what you'd do with your mental time and energy if you were no longer consumed by resentment and recycled rage. What would you think about instead? What would you feel? What would you do? Take time with this.

Put Kindness Toward Others into Action

In addition to being kind to yourself, be mindful of any chance you get throughout your day to act in a kind and compassionate way toward others. These acts of kindness could take many forms. You might practice saying "Please," "Thank you," and "You're welcome," more often. You might open a door for someone, offer a helping hand, extend a smile to a stranger, or let a driver merge into traffic. Give a hug or a kiss to a loved one. Show understanding, compassion, and forgiveness when you feel hurt and the urge to strike back.

The point of these activities and other acts of kindness is that you're doing something loving and personally uplifting for the sake of doing so—"just because." You're expressing the value of kindness and compassion. Doing so may feel contrived at first, but don't let this feeling get in the way of your commitment to act kindly. You don't need to wait to feel peaceful and loving before you decide to act in a kind and loving way. You can just do it regardless of what you feel.

Look for moments when you can share. Watch for times when you can show care and moments when you can offer gratitude or extend warmth. Look for times when you can offer hope, love, or a helping hand. Do this when you'd rather shut down, tune out, or explode. These are the moments when the benefits of practicing tender loving care with your hands, feet, and mouth are needed most and when they will benefit you and others most.

With practice, acts of kindness will become automatic and bring with them an increased sense of peace, love, and trust. You'll find that people will be more likely to gravitate in your direction when you practice acts of kindness. This outcome can only enrich your relationships. In fact, several studies show that practicing acts of kindness will benefit you by increasing your overall sense of happiness! Be mindful, however, that you may not always get kindness in return. The point is that *you* are taking charge by being kind and loving. This is something *you* can do.

Regardless of the target or the outcome, kindness and love are fundamentally about you! Nurture them. Develop them. Make them the core of your being and how you choose to live.

LIFE ENHANCEMENT EXERCISES

Focus on nurturing a new relationship with your anxious mind and body. Make an intention to be patient and kind with yourself and practice acts of kindness for yourself daily, including time for the important work you are doing with this workbook. Look for ways to uphold your values as an act of kindness toward yourself and your life. Remember that you control your Life Bus!

For this week, expand your self-care to-do list with a deeper focus on practicing exercises that nurture tender loving care toward yourself and your WAFs:

- Starting today, do something kind for yourself every day—however small that something may be.

- Be kind to your WAFs by practicing acceptance and compassion toward your feelings, thoughts, memories, and hurts. You can do this by practicing the Acceptance of Anxiety exercise (from chapter 14) and at least one of the loving-kindness exercises (from this and earlier chapters) at least once each day.

- Nurture your capacity for forgiveness—*let go* of the resentment and regret associated with past wrongs committed by you or others. Drop the rope!

- Integrate acceptance in your daily life by continuing to practice labeling of thoughts and feelings without getting tangled up in them. Whenever uncomfortable thoughts and feelings show up, notice them, label them, let them be, and move on with whatever you were doing. If the emotions are intense, take a moment to practice WAF surfing (described in chapter 14). Then move on.

THE TAKE-HOME MESSAGE

Although WAFs feel like monsters, they're more like kids. Like most kids, they respond better to tender loving care than to reprimands, rebukes, or harsh punishment. You can learn to bring more compassion to your worries, anxieties, and fears by practicing acceptance of your thoughts and feelings instead of trying to get rid of them. And you can practice kindness to yourself and others. Do this every day. Even small acts of kindness matter. Over time and with regular practice, compassion and kindness will become a habit. And they'll take the sting out of anxiety, panic, fear, and worry. This will make it easier for you to stay on the road to your value mountain without being steered off course.

Learning to Bring Compassion to My Anxiety

Points to Ponder: Anxiety is not really my enemy. I can learn to bring more compassion and kindness to myself and my experience. Kindness and compassion are shown by my actions—how I relate with my mind and body and my life. They will help me heal and move with my anxiety instead of remaining stuck, struggling with them.

Questions to Consider: Am I willing to meet my WAF children with friendliness and compassion? Am I willing to give kindness and forgiveness to myself and others so that I can move on and reclaim my life?

CHAPTER 16

Developing Comfort in Your Own Skin

When we come to that compassionate awareness that is not afraid of the fear, that can embrace the fear, we are able to heal the wounds of the child and the adult and begin to live the lives we've always wanted to live.

—Cheri Huber

Everything you've been learning in this book up until now has prepared you for this moment: to embrace, perhaps for the first time, the fears and anxieties that have kept you stuck for so long.

You might be thinking, *Oh, here it comes—they're going to ask me to face my fears*. In a way, this is true, but this isn't about white knuckling your way into and through your discomfort for its own sake, or about proving something to yourself. This chapter is bigger than that. It's about facing your life— what you care about—while staying with your discomfort and bringing compassion to that experience. This is probably the kindest thing you can do for yourself.

And you won't be doing this naked, without any tools. Those tools are the skills you've already been practicing to help you to make a choice to be kinder, more compassionate and mindful, and less prone to get caught up in struggle with your bodily discomfort.

The exercises in this chapter are simply additional opportunities to practice flexibility and softness with unpleasant bodily sensations that have tended to keep you stuck. You can think of it as learning to stretch like athletes, who need to do this regularly to maintain flexibility and lessen the chance of injury. Life also calls each of us to be flexible. When you tighten around your pain, you risk injury to the most precious commodity of all—your life.

GETTING WITH YOUR PAIN, LIVING YOUR LIFE

Pain is part of living well. When you shut down to pain, you shut down to life. When you open up to life, you must open up to pain in all its forms. This is how it works. To have it all, you must be willing to have it all—the good, unpleasant, and sometimes ugly.

We're pretty certain that your WAF bodily discomfort is linked with doing what you care about—living out your values. In fact, if you look closely, you'll see that as you take a step in a direction you want to go, you'll probably get something that you don't want to have—unpleasant bodily sensations. These sensations are the barriers we talked about in chapters 13 and 14.

The solution is simple—to move into your life, you need to let go of the urge to act on your WAF discomfort while moving into and with your feelings and bodily sensations, just as they are. This can be difficult to do, just like many other things in life that are potentially good for you. Think about that for a moment.

Recall some vital and important things that you do now and that were once difficult to do. Think simple and expand out. What was it like when you first learned how to eat with a fork and knife, or to use a toilet? How about when you first started learning your ABCs, writing letters of the alphabet and eventually your name? How about learning how to read or use money? Go further.

Consider the steps involved in first starting an exercise routine, playing an instrument, riding a bike, hitting a baseball, starting a career, driving a car, all the way up to navigating your daily routine and your varied roles as friend, teacher, partner, spouse, or parent, and more—learning to love, share, care, give, and forgive.

You should see that your life up until now has been a journey of small moments. The things that you do and want out of life often start out seeming difficult or impossible. And to do the things you want to do calls on you to move with and through difficult moments, often many times. Had you not done that, you might still be wearing a diaper, be illiterate, or need to be spoon fed by someone else. To get the life you want, you must open up to difficulty now and then.

A powerful way to learn to open up to difficulty is to stop avoiding pain and chasing pleasure. This rat race is the root of much unhappiness. The path out of it is doing the opposite. You invite in the discomfort you are feeling anyway and give away what's good and joyful. You breathe in the discomfort and receive it and breathe out and away what you so desperately want and think will bring relief. You're doing this for every person out there, and in so doing, you're doing it for you.

If you let the words go—drop the story line—and just feel the discomfort and sit with it without getting tangled up with it, you share what we all share. That's what compassion really means. Experiencing this sense of shared humanity has tremendous healing power—as Pema Chödrön (2001) tells us, it's the path out of misery and into vitality.

Breathing in pain and breathing out relief is the basis of an ancient form of meditation known as *Tonglen* (meaning "giving and receiving"). Welcoming your pain and giving away good may strike you as odd. It goes against the grain. This is precisely why it can be so powerful. When you embrace what you don't like, you transform it. That transformation will release you from attachment to pleasure seeking, fear, and self-absorption, and it will nurture your capacity for love and compassion. The next exercise will help you develop this important skill.

EXERCISE: EMBRACING THE "BAD," GIVING AWAY THE "GOOD"

Start by getting yourself comfortable in a place where you'll be undisturbed for five to ten minutes. You may sit on the floor or in a chair. Sit upright with your palms up or down on your lap.

Now, close your eyes and gently guide your attention to the natural rhythm of your breath in your chest and belly. After a few moments, bring to mind something painful or hurtful, perhaps a recent event or a time in which you felt very anxious. Then, with your next inhale, visualize taking in that negativity and painful upset. Breathe in the discomfort with the thought in your mind that what you're feeling in this very moment is being felt by millions of people all over this world. You're not alone with this. This anxiety has been felt by countless numbers of people from the beginning of time.

Your intention here, for yourself and others, is for you and them to be free of the suffering, the struggle, blame, and shame that can happen with the pain that you and they experience. With that intention in mind, on each exhale, breathe out relief, joyfulness, and goodwill. Do it slowly with the natural rhythm of your breathing. Continue to connect with your pain as you breathe in, and with each out-breath, expend goodwill and a wish that others may find relief from the suffering they get caught in when they experience hurt and discomfort.

If you find breathing in anxiety gets too heavy or tight, you can imagine breathing into a vast space, or that your heart is an infinite space. Imagine breathing into your heart, making it bigger and bigger with every out-breath until there's enough space for all the worries, anxieties, and concerns. With each out-breath, you're opening up your whole being so you no longer have to push the worries, anxieties, and fears away—you're opening your heart to whatever arises.

If you find your mind wandering or you feel distracted, just kindly notice that and return your attention to the intention of welcoming in your pain and hurts, and releasing goodwill and kindness. Continue this practice of giving and receiving for as long as you wish.

Then, when you're ready, gradually widen your attention and gently open your eyes with the intention of bringing this skill of kind observing to your experiences throughout the day.

You can also practice Tonglen in everyday life. Whenever anxiety shows up, you can remind yourself, *Other people feel this too. I'm not alone with this.* It will help ease the sense of isolation and burden of feeling that you're alone with your WAFs.

When you notice yourself getting anxious and not wanting to be, you can practice on-the-spot Tonglen for all the people out there who, just like you, get caught in the struggle by pushing their discomfort away when they notice it. Right then, wherever you are, you can start breathing in—acknowledging the discomfort—and breathing out and giving away a sense of peace and calm. With every moment you're willing to stay with uncomfortable anxiety, you learn more and more not to fear it.

As you witness and accept your WAF discomfort and hurt, you'll be moving with and through what may seem difficult. As you do that, you'll be making room for compassion, kindness, and forgiveness. In the process, you'll continue to soften and learn several new things:

- You'll develop greater honesty about your experience. You'll learn to acknowledge bodily discomfort and other unpleasant sensations, without engagement, as you feel them.

- You'll nurture the courage to do nothing, to just sit with your WAF discomfort. This part is critical. You'll learn to stop running from yourself, and you'll develop comfort in your own skin.

- You'll continue to develop your capacity to observe your experience just as it is (the observer perspective). Watching without judgment and engagement will allow you to disentangle yourself from what your mind and body are doing. This will give you space to act in ways that matter to you rather than reacting. This stance will free you to let go and move forward in your life.

So when your mind gives you *This is difficult* or *This is too much,* kindly recognize those thoughts as a signal that you are on the path of something new and potentially vital. To help you along, we'll give you lots of opportunities for practice in this chapter and the next using FEEL—Feeling Experiences Enriches Living.

FEEL EXERCISES

FEEL exercises have one purpose only—to help you engage your life to the fullest. They're a natural extension of the exercises you've been doing up to this point.

Here, you'll get a chance to practice being an observer of your WAF bodily sensations, just noticing and experiencing them as they are while meeting them with a quality of kindness and compassion. When you do that, you'll be defusing the urge to avoid, run, or fix what your body is doing. Instead, you'll have the room to focus on what you want to do, what you want to be about, and where you want to go. As you get better at feeling, your life will grow.

FEEL Steps, in a Nutshell

The steps are straightforward. The first step to any of the exercises is to flip your willingness switch to on—fully. Remember, you can control this switch. And unless you choose to turn it on, you'll continue to get what you've always got.

The second step is to think about what you care deeply about—your values. Having your sights on your values—what you want to do and where you want to go—will allow you to practice a new response to the bodily discomfort that has stood between you and your life for so long. You'll want to have your Valued Directions Worksheet and Life Compass handy and look for places where bodily discomfort has stood between you and your valued intentions.

The third step involves gently bringing on bodily sensations that normally send you into a tailspin and keep you stuck. As you practice just noticing the bodily discomfort without acting on it, and bring to the experience a sense of kind allowing, you'll be letting yourself off the hook. This part calls on your observer self and mindful acceptance skills.

To sum up, FEEL exercises involve you making a choice for willingness, experiencing your bodily discomfort with gentle kindness and allowing—always with an eye on the things you care about and want to do. You'll have opportunities to create and watch bodily discomfort show up and then to practice letting that discomfort be as it is. As you do that, you'll be learning new skills that will transform discomfort *difficulty* into discomfort *vitality*.

Importance of Practice and Pacing

All of the exercises require practice, practice, practice. You'll be walking into familiar territory—you know the discomfort. You know what's there. What's new is this: approaching your dark discomfort with the bright light of a kinder and more compassionate response. This more skillful way of relating needs to be nurtured—and it can happen over time.

Take it slow. Don't rush through the exercises. It's best to repeat them several times in one sitting and then again over several days. Practice at home first. Find a place in your home to do the practice and make it your kind space. As you develop the skills, you can put that practice into action in your daily life. Let willingness and compassion be your guide.

It's okay if your willingness switch seems to toggle on and off during the exercises, at least early on. The important thing is that you recognize that and are willing to keep going the next time. When you are able to keep your willingness switch in the on position with minimal or no disruption, then you're ready to move on to another exercise.

A Word of Caution

We're pretty certain that you'll experience some discomfort as you do the exercises. And we're pretty certain that your old history will be right in your face—urging you, begging you, to stop, pull out, or run. The results of many research studies show that if you stick with the exercises in this program and allow your old history to do its thing without doing what it says you should do, then you'll get some relief.

That relief may take several forms. Some people experience it as peace. Others report feeling less anxious or fearful. Many more feel like a burden has been lifted. They tell us the discomfort is still there once in a while. And sometimes that discomfort is very intense. But underneath all of that, they notice a profound shift in the experience of WAF discomfort. They are no longer fighting with it and, without the fight, the WAF loses its edge. And they notice that letting go of the struggle with their bodily discomfort has given them relief in the form of newfound freedom.

Don't do the FEEL exercises for the purpose of chasing emotional goals—like feeling less anxious, keeping panic at bay, or stopping your mind from doing its thing. We talked about these familiar dead-end goals early on. They are more of the same stuff that hasn't worked. The quality of your anxiety will likely change, but paradoxically this is most likely to happen when you least chase it.

The goal of FEEL exercises is to help you develop comfort and kindness in your own skin—to take the stance of being the chessboard or volleyball court and not of being one of the struggling teams. This shift in perspective will free you up to live better with whatever your body and mind may be doing.

Anxiety will take a backseat because you'll be spending less time with your WAF discomfort *and* more time focused on and engaging your life *with* your discomfort. That's how it works. That's how you get your life back. And that's the path to thinking and feeling better too. You can't experience peace so long as you remain in a fight with your mind and body.

FEEL EXERCISES FOR YOUR BODILY DISCOMFORT

The exercises below will help you practice being with and moving with the barriers you listed on your Valued Directions Worksheet and the Life Compass in real-life situations. Before going on, take a moment to review these worksheets and look for places where avoidance or struggle with your bodily discomfort has stood between you and what you wanted to do—your values.

We've found that people benefit most when they do all of the exercises. The reason is that each exercise provides you with skills to undo potential barriers. And doing all of them gives you a chance to practice developing flexibility with different forms of bodily discomfort. Again, you're learning to stretch.

The worksheet below is to help you track your progress with the exercises. You'll find a copy of the worksheet online at http://www.newharbinger.com/33346. You'll want to print several copies and have them handy for your practice.

FEEL* BODILY DISCOMFORT WORKSHEET

Date: _____ Time: _____ a.m./p.m.

0	1	2	3	4	5	6	7	8	9	10
Low					Moderate					Extreme

Exercise	Sensation Intensity (0–10)	Anxiety Level (0–10)	Willingness to Experience (0–10)	Struggle with Experience (0–10)	Avoidance of Experience (0–10)
Staring at a Spot	_____	_____	_____	_____	_____
Spinning	_____	_____	_____	_____	_____
Head Between Legs	_____	_____	_____	_____	_____
Shaking Head	_____	_____	_____	_____	_____
Breath Holding	_____	_____	_____	_____	_____
Breathing Through Straw	_____	_____	_____	_____	_____
Fast Breathing	_____	_____	_____	_____	_____
Fast Walking	_____	_____	_____	_____	_____
Jogging in Place	_____	_____	_____	_____	_____
Climbing Steps	_____	_____	_____	_____	_____
Other Aerobic Exercise	_____	_____	_____	_____	_____
Staring at Self in Mirror	_____	_____	_____	_____	_____

* Feeling Experience Enriches Living

How to Do the FEEL Exercises in Seven Simple Steps

All of the FEEL exercises follow the format below. You'll want to have a watch or clock close by as you do them. Remember to apply all of the skills you have been learning up to this point as you do each exercise. Here are the steps:

1. **Identify a valued domain.** Get an index card or small piece of paper and write down one of your important values. Before each practice, take a moment to connect with that value and keep it in your mind as you do the exercises. Think of the things you want to do in one important valued area. Later, you can switch to another valued domain and repeat each FEEL exercise with your intentions in mind for that area.

2. **Practice a FEEL exercise.** Start the exercise and continue it for thirty to sixty seconds beyond the point at which you first notice sensations of discomfort, or five minutes beyond the point at which you might experience disturbing thoughts or images.

3. **Apply your mindful acceptance skills.** Continue to simply observe, with kindness and gentleness, for one to two minutes after you stop each exercise. Simply observe each sensation, one at a time, and make space for what you're experiencing.

4. **Chart your progress.** Complete the FEEL Bodily Discomfort Worksheet to record your reactions and progress right after you do each exercise.

5. **Reflect on your practice.** Gently reflect on the exercise you just did. Look at your ratings. Did you experience unwillingness or high levels of struggle, or avoidance? If so, try repeating the exercise more slowly. As you do, watch for sticky judgmental thoughts such as *This isn't working* or *I can't stand this anxiety anymore.* See if you can simply notice these thoughts from your observer self perspective. The next time you do the exercise, approach it from an observer perspective, and when sticky thoughts show up, notice them, and gently say to yourself, *I am having the thought that this isn't working* or *My mind is feeding me the thought that I can't stand this anxiety anymore,* or *I am having the thought that this is too much.* Or simply label them all as "thinking."

6. **Repeat FEEL exercises.** Practice is critical for skill development. So repeat the exercises during your home practice sessions. Shoot for at least two to three repetitions of an exercise per practice session when you start out. Allow yourself a mindful rest period between exercises where you can sit comfortably and just notice your thoughts and sensations as they are.

7. **Review your ratings on your FEEL Bodily Discomfort Worksheet.** You'll be ready to move on to a new exercise when you notice that your willingness rating is *yes* and your struggle and avoidance levels are at 3 or lower. These ratings are your benchmark for progress. This is why recording your reactions is so important.

Keep the seven FEEL steps handy as you first do the exercises. Commit them to memory.

Physical Health Check

If you haven't done so already, do check in with your doctor to see that you are physically able to do the exercises. Most involve mild-to-moderate physical activity. If you suffer from any of the following health conditions, we strongly suggest that you *not* do the FEEL exercises until you've talked with your doctor.

- Asthma or lung problems

- Epilepsy

- A heart condition

- Physical injuries (neck, joint, back)

- Pregnancy

- History of fainting/low blood pressure

Should your doctor recommend against you doing one or more of these exercises, you can still practice the ones that have been approved for you. If your doctor recommends against all of these exercises, you can still practice applying your mindfulness skills and taking the observer perspective when you experience intense physical sensations as part of your regular daily activities. Remember that the goal is to practice staying with discomfort in all its forms without getting tangled up in it, whenever and in whatever form the discomfort may take.

EXERCISES: BEING WILLINGLY DIZZY

This set of exercises will help you practice mindful acceptance with sensations of dizziness, unsteadiness, or vertigo. The experience of dizziness will be different for everyone. It's an experience that occurs when you move your head and body through space at a rate too fast for your brain's balance system to keep up with.

Some people experience lightheadedness, a sense of imbalance or floating, and nausea. These are all expected reactions. And there are several ways that you can create them yourself:

- **Staring at a Spot.** Position yourself about one to two feet from a nearby wall. Find a small spot on the wall and stare at it for about two minutes. Try to resist blinking as much as you can. Then, turn away quickly and focus on something else in the distance.

- **Spinning.** Using a swivel chair, spin yourself round and round as quickly as you can by pushing off of the floor as often as needed. Do this with your eyes open. You can then vary this by spinning while standing up with arms outstretched.

- **Head Between Legs.** Get in a sitting position. Place your head between your legs (at the knees) and hold that position for about thirty seconds. Then sit upright quickly. Do this gently if you have a history of back problems. You can play with this exercise by repeating it from a standing position.

- **Shaking Head.** From a standing position, move your head back and forth and from side to side, slowly, with your eyes open. Do that for at least thirty seconds or until the sensations of dizziness are first noticed. Again, do this in a way that is steady and not too vigorous. Then stop and focus straight ahead.

To start, get set up in your kind space where you won't be disturbed and have a clock or watch nearby. Be sure to position yourself in a spot where you won't fall or hurt yourself during the practice. Select the first dizziness activity and then follow FEEL steps 1 to 7 as you practice. Stay with and repeat that exercise until you notice that you are able to be with any discomfort without needing to stop or resolve it (willingness rating yes, and struggle and avoidance levels at 3 or lower). Then, move on to the next dizziness exercise and so on.

It is best to keep your eyes open as you do the exercises. It's fine if you need to sit down between practice sessions. Just watch that you don't immediately go to sitting or lying flat on the floor as a default coping strategy. If you can remain in a standing or sitting position while dizzy, you'll notice that the sensations will pass without you having to do anything about them.

Being willingly dizzy may have been hard for you. The experience can readily make anyone feel like they are losing touch with reality. The experience is not harmful to you, and the discomfort does pass. Congratulate yourself for practicing a new response to it.

EXERCISES: BEING WILLINGLY OUT OF BREATH

The exercises in this section allow you to practice making room for discomfort with the experience of feeling out of breath, short of breath, or with sensations coming from your heart and chest, such as heart flutters and chest tightness. Along with those sensations, some people experience lightheadedness, dizziness, a sense of detachment from themselves, blurred vision, tingling, or numbness in areas of the body.

These experiences are normal. They happen as a consequence of what we do—many activities have the potential to bring them on. They are a natural byproduct of our normal blood-gas balance getting out of sync, specifically the balance of oxygen and carbon dioxide. Your body is set up to restore this blood-gas balance without effort on your part.

You can willingly bring on these sensations with any of the FEEL exercises below:

- **Breath Holding.** For this exercise, simply take a deep breath and hold it for as long as you can. Start by doing the exercise while sitting down with your eyes open. You can then vary it by doing it longer the next time, while sitting, and then standing with eyes open or closed. Play with it. Be willingly creative with your discomfort.

- **Breathing Through a Straw.** For this FEEL exercise, you'll need to get a hold of some inexpensive straws. During the practice, breathe through the straw while you pinch your nostrils closed with your free hand. See if you can do it for at least thirty seconds the first time, and work up from there. You can vary this exercise, as you may have done with breath holding, by doing it with eyes closed or open, while standing or sitting, or even while walking up and down stairs. The important thing is to take it slow. When you can be with the discomfort without pulling out from it, you are ready to gently up the ante in terms of length or new variations.

- **Fast Breathing.** Just about everyone has had the experience of being out of breath. When you breathe too quickly or too deeply, you take in too much oxygen relative to the carbon dioxide in your body. The technical label for this is *hyperventilation*. Though you may typically experience this response as beyond your control, you can bring it on by taking rapid inhales and exhales at a pace of about one breath every two seconds. When you first do this exercise, start in a sitting position. Take in a deep breath and then exhale fully, and repeat. Use a watch with a second hand and see if you can do it for at least sixty seconds at first and then work your way up to two or three minutes. This exercise is a powerful way to create a host of uncomfortable sensations that can keep you stuck and off track. And it is a great way to practice a new, more mindful response to them.

Before moving on, take a moment to review your practice and your progress on the FEEL Bodily Discomfort worksheets. Are you making a conscious choice to turn on your willingness switch and leave it in the on position? Are you meeting the discomfort that you are producing with a new, less engaged, and softer response? As you did the exercises, were you keeping your values in focus? Take stock. It's okay if this doesn't come easily. And there's no need to rush. Be kind and patient with yourself. These small moments will add up to something new in your life.

EXERCISES: BEING WILLINGLY AEROBIC

Engaging your life requires action in the form of aerobic activity. If you've avoided activities, including exercise, because of the potential for WAF discomfort, then it's time to practice willingness by deliberately feeling the physical arousal that must happen within your body as you get moving. You'll see that there are many ways you can do that, and most have the added benefit of being good for your health. Here are a few:

- **Fast Walking.** Walking engages your entire body. You can do this exercise indoors or outside. Start slow and work up to a fast and comfortable pace. As we describe in FEEL steps 1 to 7, allow enough walking time so that you're able to notice and experience bodily WAF discomfort. It's best to do this exercise without other distractions (such as listening to music). When you can willingly be with your body while walking, you can then add the headphones.

- **Jogging in Place.** This will give your heart rate and respiratory system a boost. And it can be practiced in your kind space at home. Let FEEL steps 1 to 7 be your guide.

- **Climbing Steps.** Simply go up and down a few steps, over and over again, until you begin to notice bodily discomfort. You can then increase the number of steps and duration of practice (such as two steps, five steps, ten steps, a flight or several flights of stairs).

- **Other Aerobic Exercises.** The list of possible aerobic FEEL exercises is only limited by your imagination, and includes anything that gets your body going. You could apply them while doing household chores such as vacuuming, cleaning, mowing the lawn, or raking the yard, or in the context of swimming, going for a hike, shopping, running errands, sexual activity, or taking a bike ride. Just follow FEEL steps 1 to 7 as you play with the possibilities.

All of the aerobic FEEL exercises get you up and moving. And all are good for you in more than one way. They'll buy you a renewed sense of freedom and increase your vitality, range of options, and more. Remember to keep your values in view as you move into your discomfort—your values and life are the whole point of why you're doing these exercises in the first place.

EXERCISE: STARING AT SELF IN MIRROR

This exercise is about learning to be willingly present with yourself. Most of us don't like what we see when we look at ourselves in the mirror. There's always something about our bodies that could be different or better. The same is true of our sense of who we are—the part of us that is more than our hands, eyes, breasts, hips, or feet. It can be uncomfortable to see yourself exposed. Learning to be with yourself, just as you are, involves embracing your vulnerabilities and imperfections. This skill is particularly important in your interactions with other people.

This exercise involves looking at yourself in front of a full-length mirror for two to five minutes. The exercise is more powerful if you can do it undressed and fully exposed. Just like the earlier exercises, it will probably bring up some things for you that are uncomfortable.

Start by standing fully naked in front of a mirror so that you can see your entire body. Take a moment to look at yourself, really look. What do you see? What's it like to stand with yourself, unmasked, just as you are? Just notice any sensations coming from your body. See yourself from a kind perspective—there's nothing to be fixed, no need to hide anything. You are you.

Then shift your attention to your head and face. Notice the top of your head—your hair and skin. What does it really look like? Study it, noticing the textures, shape, and colors. Then gradually move to your face—eyes, nose, mouth, and cheeks. See if you can look closely into the perfection of your eyes—the colors, depth, and textures. Are those eyes something to be disliked or hated? What do you want to do with your seeing eyes, hearing ears, or your lips and mouth? See if you can allow yourself to be with your experience and let your mind do its own thing.

Then gradually move your attention to the area just below your chin. Slowly scan the midsection of your body—inside and out. What do you see as you gently focus on your shoulders, chest, belly, and each arm and hand? What do these parts of your body look like? Notice colors, textures, shapes, contours, and sensations from this region of your body.

Each is a part of you. Each has its own story to tell. What is your mind telling you about them now? Perhaps there is regret, shame, embarrassment, humiliation, or thoughts such as "too big," "too small," "ugly," "beautiful," "wrinkled," "smooth," "attractive," or "unattractive." What are you experiencing on the inside? Can you be with your body and mind just as they are—just as you are? Must you hide from yourself? Allow yourself time to just notice the labels your mind may be giving you and then see if you can focus back on the raw, unedited experience of you.

Continue your body scan slowly as you move your attention down to your feet and toes. Notice any inner discomfort that may show up. See if you can be with your discomfort as you spend this time with you. Is there anything about you that must be fixed?

Allow yourself to be with you just as you are—whole … complete … unique … perfectly imperfect … and vulnerable … like everyone else.

WHEN FEELING BODILY DISCOMFORT GETS TOUGH

This section is for times when you find yourself experiencing high levels of unwillingness, struggle, or the urge to avoid or stop your practice. This isn't a time to cave in to what your mind might be feeding you. What you need to do here is to take your practice more slowly and with greater simplicity of focus. So instead of being with the entire experience, bring your kind attention to two or three bodily sensations, one at a time.

EXERCISE: STAYING WITH INTENSE BODILY DISCOMFORT

Start with one bodily sensation that is particularly difficult for you. As you bring your attention to this sensation, simply acknowledge it: *There is tension*, *There is fast breathing*, *There is my heart beating*, or *There is dizziness, lightheadedness,* or *There is the sensation of heat or cold*.

Acknowledge the presence of the discomfort, open up to it, stay with it, breathe with it, and bring kindness to it. As in the Chinese Finger Trap and Acceptance of Anxiety exercises, this is the perfect time to lean into the discomfort and invite it in rather than struggle with or move away from it.

If you need to, you can slow the process down even more. To do that, close your eyes for a moment, allowing _____ [insert the uncomfortable sensation] to be what it is, a feeling in your body, nothing more and nothing less. Ask yourself a few key questions:

- Where else have I experienced this one sensation? Maybe it was when you were mowing the lawn, or outside on a hot day. Maybe it happened during a pleasant surprise, or in the course of otherwise mundane life activities. Notice here that you've had this sensation before and then move on to the other questions.

- Is this something I need to push away from, or can I acknowledge its presence and make room for it? Can I make space for it?

- What does this sensation *really* feel like? Where does it start and where does it end?

- Must this particular feeling be my enemy, or can I just have it as a feeling, a sensation?

- Is this sensation something I must not or cannot have? Even if my mind tells me that I can't have it, am I willing to open up a space for it in my heart?

- Is this something I absolutely must struggle with, or is there room inside me to feel all that and stay with it? Can I make my inside space a kind space?

As you make space for each sensation, one by one, you may notice that your mind is feeding you all sorts of labels—old F-E-A-R (False Evidence Appearing Real) labels—like "dangerous," "getting worse," or "out of control." When that happens, simply thank your mind for such labels and then gently shift your attention back to watching and noticing with gentle curiosity, openness, and compassion.

This exercise is a good reminder that you can control where you put your attention and you can choose to meet your discomfort with a quality of softness instead of hardness. You don't need to like what you are feeling in order to be willing to have it.

You may also reframe your "Don't do it" mind by using some of the mindfulness strategies, metaphors, and exercises that you learned in the previous chapters to help you move with barriers. For instance, this is the time to practice getting off your but(t) by transforming "I want to get better BUT … this is too hard … too much … too difficult" into a more honest and correct statement, like "I want to get better AND I'm thinking this is too hard." Remember that you drive your Life Bus and can control your relationship with sensations that your body dishes out from time to time!

LIFE ENHANCEMENT EXERCISES

For the next two weeks, commit to making the following activities a priority on your to-do list:

- Practice Tonglen and the FEEL exercises in this chapter for your bodily discomfort. If possible, do some every day. Make sure you record your commitment and progress with them.

- Practice the Acceptance of Anxiety exercise (introduced in chapter 14) once a day, with or without the audio.

- Practice mindfulness skills and taking an observer perspective when anxiety shows up during daily life activities, and don't leave out your practice of loving-kindness and acts of tender loving care.

THE TAKE-HOME MESSAGE

Facing your discomfort with a kind willingness is the first necessary step out of anxiety and into a more vital life. Developing comfort in your own skin is something you can choose to do—anytime, anywhere. You need to practice this important skill—it needs to be nurtured. When you choose to be with your WAF discomfort, just as it is, you are letting yourself off the hook. Situations or triggers that evoke discomfort—many of them associated with what you care about in life—will be less likely to get you sidetracked from what you want to do and where you want to go. This discomfort vitality is how you'll get your life back. Look for it instead of waiting for it to look for you. Practice and play with the exercises.

Facing My WAF Discomfort Is Vital and Liberating

Points to Ponder: It's easy to duck, run, and hide from bodily discomfort. The harder and more vital path is to face my discomfort openly and honestly for what it is—plain old physical, mental, and emotional pain. Approaching my discomfort with kindness and compassion will result in discomfort vitality and freedom from fear.

Questions to Consider: Am I willing to experience unpleasant bodily sensations and not let them stand between me and what I want to do? Am I willing to face my discomfort as it is, accepting myself with all my flaws, weaknesses, and vulnerabilities? Are these sensations really my enemy?

CHAPTER 17

Developing Comfort with Your Judgmental Mind

There are only two ways to handle tense situations: you can change them, or you can change the way you look at them. There is enlightenment to be had in changing the way you look at things.

—Paul Wilson

Your mind can be your greatest friend and your worst enemy. It all depends on what you do with it. There's nothing packed between your ears that can do you harm. Thoughts are just thoughts, ethereal, without form or substance. Things that you might imagine or visualize in your mind are like that too. They can seem quite real, but when you look at them, you'll find that there really isn't much to them at all.

This chapter is an opportunity for more growth and change, a chance to expand your practice by stepping back and watching your critical mind for what it is—a machine whose job it is to produce thoughts, images, memories, judgments, and evaluations (more thoughts), and to connect them with you, your body, your experiences, and your actions. Often these body-action-mind (BAM) connections can serve you well: they help you do what you care about doing. But at other times, they can really keep you stuck—BAM!—not doing what you care about.

Using the perspective of your observer self will help you see that these barriers to your life need not be barriers at all. You have a choice to do something else when your mind baits you with fuel for your suffering. Practicing compassion with your catastrophic mind is a powerful way to defuse all this activity and give you clarity and freedom to make more vital choices and take more vital actions.

YOUR MIND MACHINE

Your mind is constantly at work, producing a never-ending stream of thoughts. It creates. It evaluates. It solves problems. It helps you make sense of your experience. And it can create futures that haven't happened or pull you into a past that once was. It is the instrument of love and kindness and the fuel for anxiety, hatred, blame, and self-loathing. This is what a mind does. It's remarkable, really.

Your mind machine will always be doing its thing as long as you are alive. Yet you have choices in how you respond to it. You don't have to buy in to everything that your mind does. You can step back and watch. You don't have to take the bait.

The exercise below, shared with us by ACT colleague Richard Whitney, will give you a better sense of what we mean.

EXERCISE: UNHOOKING YOUR JUDGMENTAL MIND

Our minds work like a good fly fisher whose job it is to catch weary trout by managing to trick them into taking the bait. Good fly fishers take time to match their artificial flies to the insects that trout are feeding on. And they carefully present those flies with each cast. When they get it right, the trout can't tell the difference between a real insect and the fake fly. The trout sees it floating by, buys that the fly is real, bites, and gets hooked. The trout then finds itself in a fight for its life.

Here, let's just imagine that one of those trout is you. Just like a skilled fly fisher, your mind creates thoughts, worries, and images that look like carefully crafted flies—just the ones you will bite on. Your mind casts them out onto the stream of life, again and again, here, there, and just about anywhere. They seem so real to you that you "buy" them.

So you bite and get hooked. Perhaps it's on the "Wingless Nutcase" or the "Blue-Winged Panicker" or the "Soft-Hackled Worrier." You may even get snared by the "Hopeless Dun," the "Out-of-Control Dragonfly," or the "Mad-and-Angry Streamer." Once you're hooked, there's nothing left to do but struggle. The struggle sets the hook deep. You're now in a fight for your life, being pulled in directions you don't want to go.

There's one important difference between a fly fisher and your mind: your mind can only tie flies on barbless hooks. Your mind will tell you there is a barb on the hook and that you can't get off, and it also feels like you can't get off. But if you pause from the struggle and observe the hook more closely, you can see that the hook really has no barbs. You can let go of the hook.

As you swim in the stream of life, flies are floating by on the surface all the time. As you get better at recognizing them as barbless hooks—*Oh, that's just another WAF fly floating by; I don't have to bite*—you'll get hooked less often. At other times, your mind will trick you again, and you'll bite. Getting hooked once in a while is part of being human. The skill is in noticing that you've been hooked. Once you do that, you can then make a choice to let go and move on.

Thoughts Are Just Words Too

Our minds tend to take words literally, and before we know it, the thought has become the "real thing" in our mind—no longer just a thought or words. If we can step back a little and begin to notice the thought as just a bunch of words, we can open our minds to more than the automatic conclusion we draw from those words.

This next exercise, inspired by an activity developed by our colleagues Matthew McKay and Catherine Sutker (2007), will help you see for yourself that thoughts are just words.

EXERCISE: DEMOTING YOUR WAF MIND PLAYFULLY

Let's start with the word "spider." When you think "spider," what does it look like in your mind? Can you see it crawling? You may even feel a little anxious or disgusted if spiders scare you in real life. Now sit somewhere near a clock. Say that word "spider" out loud, over and over, as fast as you can: "Spider, spider, spider …" Do it for exactly forty seconds.

When you're done, reflect on what happened to the meaning of the word after forty seconds. Did it still make you feel creepy (if you did feel creepy) and did it continue to summon the image of the spider? Did the words start running together? For many people, the word just starts to sound like an odd sound—"ider, ider, ider …"—and the meaning dissolves during those forty seconds.

This is a useful exercise for helping you see that the products of your judgmental mind can create an illusion of WAF monsters that are really not monsters at all. The monsters are words, linked with images and sounds, and with meanings that we assign to them. When you understand that about language, you can alter your relationship with your unpleasant thoughts, feelings, and images.

Right now, go back to your Valued Directions Worksheet and Life Compass from chapter 13. Look at one of your important values and the WAF barriers that seem to stand in the way. Select one barrier and give it a one-word name, like "worry," "panic," "anxiousness," "aloneness," "space," "airplane," "sadness," "death," "dirtiness," "sickness," "heights," "crashes," or "crowdedness." You may also bring to mind a negative word that you think about yourself, like "unattractive," "stupid," "worthless," or "boring." It might even hurt or make you mad to think this word.

Now say that word out loud as fast as you can for about forty seconds. Does it still sound as believable? Can you see how it's also just a word, a sound with no meaning or truth?

You can create even more space by doing the following: Say the thought out loud and *slowly*, like "wooooooorrrrrryyyy," "stuuuuupid," or "unreeeeeal." Say it in another voice—as a child or an old person, as Minnie Mouse or Donald Duck, as someone intoxicated, or as a grumpy person. Notice what happens as you add a playful quality to the thoughts.

To add another layer of play, you can put your thought to music. Take the thought and sing it to yourself. Put it to the melody of a favorite holiday tune, children's song, or whatever song you'd like. Start with something simple like "Jingle Bells" or "Row, Row, Row Your Boat." See what happens to the thought as you put it to music.

This is a powerful exercise. You can do it anytime or anywhere. As you practice it, you will develop your capacity to get unhooked and to see thoughts, evaluations, and the stories you may tell yourself as just mere thoughts. Some of it might even make you laugh.

Your Mind as a Person

We've all met some people we didn't like very much. You have too. They may annoy you. They may even scare you, revealing your deepest fears and vulnerabilities. Their words and actions are unwelcome, perhaps hurtful, and yet they prod you in ways that hurt. And you end up feeling bad.

Your mind can be like one of these people—bullying you and taunting you. It shows up uninvited and its labeling is unwelcome. Here, you can benefit from getting some perspective. Simply asking yourself, *Who's telling me that right now?* can be a useful start. But it can also be helpful to make this more concrete. The next exercise will help you do just that.

The exercise was created by John's wife, Jamie, and emerged naturally during her therapeutic work with people struggling with significant anxiety and depression. We share it with you now because it can be a useful way to create space between you and what your mind feeds you.

EXERCISE: WHAT KIND OF PERSON IS MY MIND?

Begin by getting in touch with your WAF mind. Focus on the key unsettling messages your mind feeds you about you and your life before, during, or after you're anxious or afraid. Now get out a sheet of paper and let's see what this mind of yours would be like if it were a person you just met. Go ahead and imagine this for a moment.

On the piece of paper, describe what this person is like. What kind of personality does your WAF mind have? What kind of person are you dealing with here? Is this a caring, loving person? Is this someone you'd like to spend time with? Would you want to be friends or have this person over for dinner?

Once you have the personality of your WAF mind down, go ahead and fill in some details. Is this person male or female? How old is he or she? What is this person's appearance (face, body, clothing)? How does this person carry him- or herself?

Now go further. How does this person sound? Loud? Opinionated? Boastful? Negative? Nagging? Does the person speak with an accent?

Get it all down in a paragraph or two. And once you have it, stop. Step back and read what you wrote down. Who is this person? Give the person a name. Take time to reflect.

If your WAF mind were the character you just created, would you really want to spend so much time with, listen to, and defer to this person? When Lisa, a bank teller, did this exercise, she identified a number of WAF thoughts that her mind tormented her with—"worthless," "wrong," "broken," "unlovable," and "scared." She then created a character who represented her WAF mind.

Her character was a short, frail, seventy-eight-year-old woman from Brooklyn, New York. She carried several bags and was dressed right out of the 1930s. She wore a loose-fitting green and purple dress, a thick fur coat all year long, heavy green eye shadow, and lots of rouge on her cheeks. This character spoke with a sharp Brooklyn accent and wore a set of false teeth. She was crotchety, loud, and always seemed to be complaining. Lisa gave her the name "Crabby Abby."

When Lisa created this image, she actually began to smile. Every time Crabby Abby opened her mouth to go off on one of her rants, her false teeth would fly out and land on the ground. The image of Crabby Abby's false teeth popping out every time she opened her big mouth made Lisa chuckle. Beyond that, Lisa began to see her thoughts in a new way.

She asked herself if she really wanted to spend lots of time listening to Crabby Abby. Her answer was clear. No! In fact, Lisa actually felt bad for Crabby Abby, who was no fun to be around. She seemed so sad, bitter, and miserable. From this point on, when Lisa noticed her mind feeding her unhelpful thoughts, the image that came to mind was Crabby Abby with her teeth popping out of her mouth every time she tried to say something to bring Lisa down.

Lisa experienced a profound shift of perspective. She saw her mind as a person she did not have to spend time with or listen to. It even made her laugh. And, she also began to feel compassion for Crabby Abby when she showed up. This exercise gave Lisa a renewed sense of freedom.

Your Mind Machine and Your Values

We said that your mind can be your worst enemy and your greatest friend. The way to tell the difference is by first noticing what your mind

You can choose to stay hooked or let go.

is telling you and then asking yourself this: *If I listen and do what my inner voice tells me right now, will I do more or less with my life in this moment? Will it bring me closer to or further away from my values? What does my past experience tell me?* If the answer is *less* and *further away* and you do what your mind says, then you won't move forward. You'll remain hooked, struggling, and stuck.

So what are you to do? The answer is to do something radically different from what you have done before. This means watching, with mindful compassion, your mind's hooks and choosing to let them be just thoughts, brief moments in time, not nets that keep you trapped. The exercises below will help you do more of that.

FEEL EXERCISES TO UNHOOK YOUR JUDGMENTAL MIND

The FEEL exercises below build on what you practiced in chapter 16. If you need to, go back and review the basic FEEL steps and guidelines. The only difference here is that you'll be practicing being with your judgmental mind—your WAF thoughts, images, memories.

You'll want to be mindful of the thoughts, images, or memories that you listed as barriers to your values. So take a moment to review your Valued Directions Worksheet and the Life Compass. Look for places where avoidance or struggle with your mind has stood between you and what you wanted to do—your values.

As you did in chapter 16, begin each FEEL practice by bringing an important life area to mind. Write that area of your life on an index card and list some of your values and intentions—the things that matter to you and what you want to be about in that area. Connect with what the card says and keep it close by as a reminder of why you're doing the exercises. Let your willingness switch be your guide!

The exercises in this section are meant to help you get back behind the wheel, driving your Life Bus in directions you want to go. These exercises build on everything you've been learning up to this point in the book. They provide you with opportunities to stay with your judgmental mind and do something kinder with it.

We encourage you to work with all the exercises to expand your skill base the most. It's fine if just a few exercises seem to resonate with you. To get to that point though, you'll need to allow yourself time with each of them.

You can use the worksheet below to chart your progress with the FEEL Thought and Imagery exercises. You'll see that it's similar to the FEEL Bodily Discomfort Worksheet you used in chapter 16. You can also download the worksheet from our book website (http://www.newharbinger.com/33346). Print several copies and have them handy.

FEEL* THOUGHT AND IMAGERY WORKSHEET

Date: _____   Time: _____ a.m./p.m.

0	1	2	3	4	5	6	7	8	9	10
Low					Moderate					Extreme

Exercise	Sensation Intensity (0–10)	Anxiety Level (0–10)	Willingness to Experience (0–10)	Struggle with Experience (0–10)	Avoidance of Experience (0–10)
Bubble Wand	_____	_____	_____	_____	_____
Kind Allowing with Disturbing Images	_____	_____	_____	_____	_____
Difficult Thoughts and Urges Cards	_____	_____	_____	_____	_____
Stand Silently with Urges	_____	_____	_____	_____	_____
Leaves on a Stream	_____	_____	_____	_____	_____
Other _____	_____	_____	_____	_____	_____
Other _____	_____	_____	_____	_____	_____

* Feeling Experience Enriches Living

FEEL Exercise for Nagging Worries and Doubts

This exercise is quite long, and it's one of the most important ones in this book. Set aside ten to fifteen minutes for it. We recommend that you start by listening to the audio recording of the exercise on our book website (http://www.newharbinger.com/33346). You can follow along, or you can read through the script a few times first and then close your eyes and do the exercise.

EXERCISE: BUBBLE WAND

Go ahead and get in a comfortable position in your chair. Sit upright with your feet flat on the floor, your arms and legs uncrossed, and your hands resting in your lap (palms up or down, whichever is more comfortable). Close your eyes and take a few deep breaths. Allow your body to rest without drifting off to sleep. Bring an intention of kindness to this practice.

Now bring into your awareness a recent situation where you found yourself in a bout of endless worry. Perhaps it's a situation you know all too well or one you wrote down on your LIFE worksheets over the past weeks.

Really work to bring this experience into your full awareness and right into the room with you. Make it as real as possible. Continue to visualize the situation until you can notice a wave of unpleasant changes sweeping over your body and mind. Allow yourself to connect with the experience. Relive every bit of it as best as you can. Keep doing so until you're at a point where you feel taken over by anxiety and tension and a strong desire to do something about it.

Now, we want you to go more deeply into this experience. Imagine that you have a large bubble wand like the kind that kids sometimes play with at the beach or in the park. Go ahead and fill the wand with bubble soap. Then look within you and notice all the elements of the unsettling experience. Start by locating one of the most obvious judgments or worrisome thoughts.

For each one, take your bubble wand and sweep it through each worry thought. Trap each thought in a giant bubble. Then, one by one, notice each thought in its bubble and label it as you watch each drift upward in the gentle breeze—*There goes worrying … what if-ing … second guessing … judging … blaming … shaming … criticizing.* Keep watching the bubbles go higher and higher until they're out of sight. Then take a few slow, deep breaths.

Allow yourself to go more deeply into this experience. See if you can find the next thought underneath the first worry. For example, if you worry about not having enough money to make ends meet, then you might gently ask, *And if that were true, then what?* Watch what your mind comes up with. Perhaps it's the thought *I won't be able to pay my bills.* Notice that thought and place it in a giant bubble and watch it float upward. Follow this with *And then what?* Keep going with an attitude of gentle curiosity and kind allowing.

As you go more deeply into your worry, you'll likely notice more physical sensations in your body: heart pounding in the chest, feeling shaky, trembling hands, shortness of breath, feeling hot, or the sensation of an upset stomach. There's tension everywhere. You may feel like you're about to pop. As that unfolds, notice your impulses to respond and label these sensations one at a time: *There is my impulse to shout … run away … shut down … struggle … make a fist … lash out … point my finger … or stop this exercise.*

Your task now is both simple and difficult: Do nothing! Sit with these thoughts, sensations, and impulses. Feel the restless energy in this situation. Sitting still and doing nothing is the last thing you want to do, and it's the wisest thing you can do: Say nothing. Do nothing. You want resolution now, and there isn't any.

The energy of anxiety and worry works like a big ocean wave—just allow yourself to ride with it as each wave comes and goes into and out from your awareness. Watch as the wave rises until it reaches its peak, staying strong and powerful for a while, and then eventually settling back down and drifting away. Continue to sit still with the energy in this situation and let the worry wave run its course.

Then gently return to the worry situation and take a final inventory. What are you left with here? What do you see? If you look closely, you'll see two things: the pain and hurt that fueled your worry to begin with and your values.

See if you can turn your attention to the pain and hurt underneath the worry. Give that pain and hurt a label. If you have a hard time identifying the hurt, ask yourself, *What would I have left to feel if I didn't get caught up in worry in this situation?* Take a moment to really take stock.

Perhaps you see hurt, fear, abandonment, loneliness, inadequacy, loss, guilt, vulnerability, or shame. There is no need to trap these feelings or cover them. They're part of you and belong to you without being you or defining who you are. Just allow them to be. Make space for them.

As if they were open wounds, take care of them by bringing kindness, care, and compassion to your experience and to this moment. Forgive yourself for burying and rejecting your pain for so long, for acting in ways to push it from view.

If at any time you feel like stopping and stepping back inside your worry armor, thank your mind for that option and simply return to your experience. If you notice judgment or resentment popping up again, place these thoughts into their own bubbles and let them go, floating upward.

Next, gently turn your attention to your values lying close by. Which ones do you see? Pick one or two that are important to you. Now ask yourself this question: *If worry and doubt are between me and moving in the direction of those values, am I willing to have them and still do what matters to me?* If you're willing, worry is no longer a barrier. It's just a thought.

Now think of a situation where worry had gotten in the way of you acting in accord with your values. Then go ahead and imagine yourself doing what you value and bringing your hurt and pain with you.

That probably feels strange and it also feels vital because you're moving toward what you care about in life. Here, you're exerting control where you truly have it. Take time to really connect with this. This is what it's all about!

Then, when you're ready, gradually widen your attention to take in the sounds around you in the room you're in. Take a moment to make the intention to bring this sense of compassion and forgiveness into the present moment and to the rest of your experience on this day.

Doing this exercise isn't easy. At first, you may have trouble taking an observer's perspective. Don't beat yourself up over this or other "failures" or difficulties. Being compassionate isn't about perfection. Continue to do the work, be patient, and relax with yourself. Commit to doing the exercise again tomorrow and again the next day. Do the best you can.

Repeat the same worry episode once a day until you can more readily adopt your Silent Observer Self perspective as you stay with the negative energy and hurt that shows up for that episode. Then move on to different worry episodes and cycle through the same process as before.

Continue practicing this exercise with worry episodes until you can stay with the bodily discomfort and hurt (using compassion and forgiveness), with minimal entanglement in judgment. This may take several days or even weeks. The key is this: stay on the path!

FEEL Exercise for Disturbing Images

Being able to imagine—to visualize—is a great gift. We can paint in our mind's eye portraits of experiences that once were or that may be, and we can do this anytime and anywhere. We can also create "realities" that aren't real and treat them as if they were.

Our minds can turn any word into an image, and we can also put most images into words. Think the word "sunset" and you may find yourself being able to see one in your mind. Read the word "jerk" and you may be able to visualize a person who treated you or others poorly.

You have these capacities and need them. These same processes are at work when you experience joyful and serene images and thoughts and when you experience disturbing or fearful thoughts. Here's a powerful way to learn to hold your WAF images more lightly.

EXERCISE: KIND ALLOWING WITH DISTURBING IMAGES

Start by generating a few sentences describing troublesome or disturbing WAF images. Here are a few examples:

My children drowned in the bathtub, and it was my fault.

I feel sick to my stomach, and my heart is pounding.

I'm living on the streets because I'm incompetent, weak, and unable to think.

I'm in a psychiatric ward because I'm crazy.

My hands are shaking, I'm disoriented, and nobody understands me.

I'm being attacked and I'm frozen in fear.

If my husband's health gets worse, we might lose our home or he might die.

You may be having difficulty coming up with images. If you've suffered a past trauma, the images you may have are hard to open up to. Or if you're on constant worry autopilot, you may find it difficult to imagine anything because you're so caught up in a stream of worrisome thoughts. And if you've struggled with disturbing obsessions, you may find your images particularly nasty and unacceptable. You may even believe that thinking a thought or image may make it come true.

These are normal reactions for many people. In each instance, though, you'll need to ask yourself whether the reaction is serving you well or not. So if you've tended to blot out or shut down to thinking about upsetting images, you may ask yourself if "not thinking" is working for you.

What does your experience tell you? Will more of the same—shutting down, closing up—get in the way of your effort to change in more vital ways? Can you flip your willingness switch on? We know you can. You simply need to decide to do it and see how it goes over time. Are you willing to create that list now? If so, continue.

Once you have your list, go over it with both eyes fixed on willingness. For each image, ask whether you are 100 percent willing to have the WAF image just as it is. Remember, it's okay if you don't like it or if the image makes you uncomfortable. The willingness question is not about liking it. The question is, are you open to having that image and the discomfort that goes along with it, without doing anything about it?

Next, get settled in a quiet space, your kind practice space. Close your eyes and become centered on the breath. Then, when you're ready, select an image that you're 100 percent willing to have, and hold that image gently in your awareness.

Recognize the image as an image and label it as such: *I am having the image of* … Bring kindness and compassion to the image as if you were holding something that you care about deeply. As you do, notice that these passengers on your Life Bus are just thoughts and images. You, not they, control the gas pedal, brake, and steering wheel. You, not they, control what you do.

Allow yourself to bring an attitude of kind allowing to the image for at least five minutes beyond the point at which the image is vivid. Then you may move on to the next image or plan that for your next practice. It's best to stay with one image until you can do it with your willingness switch in the on position most of the time. Then you're ready to move on to a different image.

Go through all the images you rated as ones you'd be willing to have, and then practice with the ones that you were unwilling to have. Be patient and take your time. Follow FEEL steps 1 through 7 from chapter 16. Track your progress with the FEEL Thought and Imagery Worksheet.

If you continue to have difficulty bringing kindness to your unpleasant thoughts and images, you may use prompts from newspaper stories or look to photographs or movies to help you practice simply being with unpleasant imagery without trying to resolve it in any way.

FEEL EXERCISES TO DEAL WITH CUT-AND-RUN URGES

We know how difficult it can be to face your discomfort squarely. You've had lots of experience doing just the opposite—pulling out, pushing away, or tuning out. The urge to act is powerful. It's a well-practiced habit for you. And it's natural that old cut-and-run urges show up as you consciously choose to move into your discomfort with an eye on doing what you want to do in your life. Anxiety News Radio wants you to tune in 24/7.

What you need to do is be patient and kind with yourself. Old habits may die hard, but they'll die much harder if you continue to rehearse them again and again. Remember that when you step in the direction of something you want, you'll gain vitality in your life but risk discomfort. Along with that discomfort will be the old urges that have kept you stuck.

Up to this point in this book, you've learned skills to go against the old urges. Instead of pulling out of your discomfort, you're moving into it. Instead of hardening to your discomfort, you're softening to it. Instead of seeing the world through the blinders of your critical, judgmental mind, you're learning to see your mind for what it is.

The next exercise (Hayes, et al., 2012) can be enormously helpful during those times when you find yourself trying to resist urges and other unwanted WAF thoughts.

EXERCISE: PUTTING DIFFICULT THOUGHTS AND URGES ON CARDS

This exercise can be done anytime and anywhere WAF thoughts and urges show up. All you need are some small pieces of paper or index cards. When the WAFs show up, simply label them, placing each thought, worry, sensation, urge, or image on its own card.

Next, look at what you put down on the card. If we asked you to describe what you see, what would you tell us? You're first reaction is probably to say, "I see the words …" Or, maybe you see an emotion. But here, we want you to get more granular. What do you actually see on the card? Just focus on what is there and not what your mind tells you is there.

If you take a moment and just focus on what your eyes see, you will eventually notice that you see words, letters, and ink. That's it. If you write down "I am incompetent" and look, you will see words, letters, and ink. If what you wrote was "I am a banana" you will see the same thing—words, letters, and ink. All thoughts are made up of the same stuff.

A moment ago the thoughts and urges were inside your head. They probably seemed really hard and heavy in there. Now they're out, exposed, and you can look at them. Now see them for what they are. What happens when you turn your life over to the words, letters, and ink on the card? Notice that you have a choice to do what the card says and struggle, or you can allow what you wrote to be just as it is … a thought … a sensation … an image … an urge to act. Just words, letters, and ink.

To get a sense of the struggle, place the card with the thought or urge on it between your hands and push your hands together really hard. Do this for at least thirty seconds and then stop. Gently place the card on your lap. Notice the difference in effort between pushing against the thought or urge compared to the experience of the card gently resting on your lap.

You can practice holding your thoughts and urges by carrying them with you. To do that, place the cards in your pocket, purse, or briefcase as you go about your daily activities. Notice that you can move with them. Once in a while you can take them out and look at them, but make sure you don't get hooked by what they say—just look and observe. Remind yourself what you are really looking at on the card—words, letters, and ink. Notice that you have a choice here: you can either choose to engage them or engage something else in your life. If you look to your experience for advice, you will know what to do. It's time to trust your experience, not your mind hooks.

We suggest putting your thoughts and urges on cards and taking them with you wherever you go every day for as long as you wish. If you like, you can change the cards from time to time. Some people we've worked with tell us that they prepare a stack of index cards. Then, every morning, they shuffle them and pick four or five different cards and take them along for the day.

Remember, every time you happen to touch or read a card during the day without getting tangled up in what it says, or doing as it says, you're honing this important skill. The cards will be there anytime you wish to attend to them, just as your old history is always with you.

The next exercise will give you more practice being with your WAF urges and not doing what they compel you to do. This exercise can be helpful during your FEEL practice and anytime that the urge to cut and run shows up.

EXERCISE: STAND SILENTLY WITH URGES

Old urges to act will show up in a flash, and it can be difficult to remember that you have other options. So let's keep it simple: *in the heat of the moment, do nothing and practice patience*. Just be still with what you experience in that moment. Here's what you can do specifically.

Say and Do Nothing

You do have a choice here: You can do what your mind and body compel you to do. Or you can make a choice that seems ridiculous and as unnatural as pushing into the finger traps—you can choose to act with patience. You can stop, be still, and wait until the hardness of the stirring, raucous, and searing energy gradually softens and drifts away.

You aren't suppressing here. You're just being honest with the fact that you're uncomfortable or hurt or sad or lonely or fearful or whatever you're experiencing at the moment. And you stay with it, without feeding it or reacting to it. This will give you time to think about what you really want to be about in that moment and what you want to do moving forward.

Watch Your Mind Machine as an Observer

We guarantee that the mind machine will be in overdrive doing its old thing. Don't get tangled up in what it's doing or respond to it. Just watch what it's doing from the compassionate observer perspective and meet that stirring energy with gentle acceptance. You don't need to get hooked. This will give you space to consider other, more vital options.

Ride the WAF Tiger

This is really tough. Sitting with the discomfort and doing nothing while you feel like exploding or running is like riding a wild horse or a tiger, and it's very frightening. In that moment, bring attention to the physical experience of anxiety. Is there pressure? Is there tightness or contraction? Where, specifically, do you feel it? Does it have a shape?

Here, perhaps for the first time, you can make a choice to sit and stay with the raucous energy and not do what you've always done. And you can do so in your daily life. Once you are still, you can bring compassion and curiosity to the energy and pain.

Look deeply into your experience without attempting to resolve it, fight it, or suppress it, and without acting on it. As you look, see if you can find the pain. Once you locate the pain, as in the previous exercises, look more deeply into it. And then let it be.

Approach this act of patience with softness and curiosity. You do have a choice to hold on here or to let go. This quality of patience is very much like the practice of extending forgiveness.

We mentioned resolution and relief earlier. Doing what your WAF urges compel you to do will bring no lasting relief. Doing something new by doing nothing at all can bring a sense of enormous relief, relaxation, and connection with the softness and tenderness of your heart.

The next exercise is another opportunity to develop space between your judgmental mind and your experience. Again, the easiest way to practice is to download the audio version from the book website (http://www.newharbinger.com/33346).

EXERCISE: LEAVES ON A STREAM

Start by getting centered and focus on the breath as you've done before. Just notice the gentle rising and falling of your breath in your chest and belly. There's no need to control your breathing in any way—simply let the breath breathe itself. Allow your eyes to close gently.

Then, after a few moments, imagine that you're sitting next to a small stream on a warm autumn day. As you gaze at the stream, you notice a number of large leaves of all colors, shapes, and sizes drifting along, each at its own pace, one by one, in the slowly moving current. Allow yourself to simply be there for a moment, watching.

When you're ready, gradually bring your awareness to what's going on inside you. As you do, gently notice and label each experience that shows up—thoughts, feelings, sensations, desires, and impulses. Pay attention to what's happening in your mind and body and then label what's going on. Perhaps one of those thoughts is "I don't have time for this."

As the thoughts, feelings, sensations, desires, or impulses come along into your mind, notice them and gently place them one by one on each large leaf passing by. Observe as each leaf comes closer to you. Then watch as it slowly moves away, drifting along as it carries the contents of your mind and body out of sight downstream. Return to gazing at the stream, waiting for the next leaf to float by. Continue placing each thought, feeling, memory, or impulse on its own large leaf. Watch each one as you let them just float away downstream.

When you're ready, widen your attention to take in the sounds around you. Open your eyes and make the intention to bring gentle allowing and self-acceptance into the rest of your day.

Do the Leaves on a Stream exercise every other day for a couple of weeks. As you get better at it, you can start practicing it during real-life experiences with your eyes open. You can also allow yourself to take the perspective of the stream, just as you did in the chessboard exercise. Being the stream, you hold each of the leaves and notice the thought, feeling, sensation, desire, or impulse that each leaf carries as it sails by. You need not interfere with them—just let them float by and do what they do until they are eventually carried out of sight. And notice how you're learning to be an observer.

LIFE ENHANCEMENT EXERCISES

For the next two weeks, make the following activities a priority on your self-care to-do list. And do them with your values and your life in mind:

- Practice the Acceptance of Anxiety exercise (from chapter 14) once a day, with or without the audio.

- Practice the exercises in the "FEEL Exercises to Unhook Your Judgmental Mind" section; record your commitment and progress with them using the FEEL Thought and Imagery Worksheet.

- Practice the exercises in the "FEEL Exercises to Deal with Cut-and-Run Urges" section; record your commitment and progress with them using the FEEL Thought and Imagery Worksheet.

- Practice mindfulness and observer skills and also kindness when anxiety shows up. Remember: do the best that you can.

THE TAKE-HOME MESSAGE

Developing comfort with your judgmental mind is one of the most powerful ways to end your WAF suffering. The acceptance exercises in this chapter and the entire book let you experience that your WAF flies are always on barbless hooks. You and you alone can choose to let go, even after you've been tricked into biting. The take-home message here is that if you stop struggling, you can get off the hook. This will give you freedom to swim in the direction of your values.

My Mind Is Not My Enemy

Points to Ponder: My mind is not my enemy. It is what I do with it and because of it that can hurt me.

Questions to Consider: Am I willing to face my painful thoughts, memories, judgments, and urges as they are? Can I take the bold step to let go and bring compassion, kindness, and forgiveness to my hurt and pain? Am I willing to make room for something new?

CHAPTER 18

Making Peace with a Difficult Past

Even though you may want to move forward in your life, you may have one foot on the brakes. In order to be free, we must learn how to let go. Release the hurt. Release the fear. Refuse to entertain your old pain. The energy it takes to hang onto the past is holding you back from a new life. What is it you would let go of today?

—Mary Manin Morrissey

You have a past. Everyone does. It is full of moments—dark, bright, and neutral. And, most of us remember very little of it. Still, you know there's much more to your past than that small bit you can remember. Some of it is sweet, and other parts are bitter, even extremely so. What you remember can leave you feeling more alive, or torn apart and wounded. And, your memories and their impact on your life right now depend quite a bit on how you respond to them—friend or enemy—in every crucial moment of your life.

In chapter 11, you learned that all moments of your past are parts of the vessel that we call you. But you are not the history you've had. You are not the experiences that ended up in your vessel. This distinction is important to understand. You were there before the sweet and dark moments you lived through. You were there before the hurt you endured, the trauma you suffered, or even the mundane moments you've lived through. And you are here right now with a life of possibility ahead of you.

Sometimes we get wisdom from remembering past trials and traumas we have endured, and we leverage that to live more wisely and fully now. You may discover an inner strength, a renewed appreciation for life, and an inner resolve not to repeat the hardships you endured. Often though, painful memories have the opposite effect. They keep us stuck in the past, reliving old wounds that do not serve us well from this point forward in our lives.

There are many ways to get stuck in the past. Maybe you've been trying to figure it out, make sense of it, or understand. Or, maybe you relive traumas you endured during combat, or at the hands of someone else—a parent, a stranger, or a once-trusted friend or partner. You may remember and be overwhelmed by guilt and shame. Or, you may be attached to the good moments, the way things once were, wishing that they would return again as they were. In these moments, we forget the simple truth that life is about change, time is always moving forward, and nothing remains the same.

It's very hard to go forward in life when you're always looking back. Imagine you're in your car headed somewhere—maybe to the store, work, or a friend's house. You can look forward through the windshield and backward through the rearview mirror. Now imagine trying to go where you'd like to go with your eyes fixed on the rearview mirror, focused on what's behind you! What do you suppose would happen? You'll eventually crash and end up hurting yourself and even other people. It's the same deal with life. When you spend lots of time living in the past, you'll end up crashing again and again.

All this doesn't mean that you forget your past. You don't ignore the rearview mirror driving your car. It simply means that you learn to acknowledge your past as the past, noticing what it may teach you, and then use that as you move forward. The key is to keep your eyes and heart looking forward from right where you are, in the present. This is the only way to get where you want to go in life.

The past cannot be changed. The future has yet to be. All we really have is the present. And it turns out that learning to be present is a powerful way to break free from the hooks and snares of your past. In fact, the present is the only place where you can ACT to change your life. You've got to be in the driver's seat, right now, to guide your Life Bus in the right direction.

We're going to help you learn to do this in a way that honors your past, however painful. In fact, the larger message of this chapter is about finding a way to make peace with your past—to simply allow it to be as it was, and not get drawn into the drama over and over again and pulled out of the present.

The first exercise in this chapter will help you ground yourself in the present, right where you are. We'll then move on to an exercise that will help you learn to observe and carry your history forward without getting tangled up in it. After that, we'll walk a bit more deeply into the stories that your mind has created about you, and the trials, traumas, and difficulties you've lived through. And, you'll practice being less attached to the story line. We'll close with an exercise that will help you bring kindness and gentleness to your old wounds.

Before going forward with the next section, we'd like you to pause and center yourself as you've done so many times before. Remind yourself of why you are here and the important work you're doing to reclaim your life.

EXERCISE: YOUR PAST AND YOU

Let's start off with a simple exercise that will teach you something about how the mind works with memory. We're going to share two numbers. Ready? 4—3. Now don't write them down. Just respond to the next questions silently to yourself. What were the numbers? Suppose we were to ask you ten minutes from now, do you think you could tell us what the numbers were? What about if we asked you at the end of this chapter? Suppose we made it worthwhile to you, like, say you'd get a million dollars if you can tell us the numbers ten years from now. Do you think you could do it? We bet you could. What were the numbers again?

Let's step back and look at this. How many seconds did it take us to give you that history that became a memory? Maybe ten seconds? And now you have two numbers, with no real significance, swirling around in your head. And, notice that you didn't choose to have those numbers in your head. We gave that history to you. And now, they're in there and can be remembered by you.

What Is a Memory Anyway?

Painful memories are reminders of what once was. That's it. They have no real substance. They can be linked to all sorts of things going on inside you and can be triggered by situations happening in the world around you. Yet the memory is just that—a collection of images, thoughts, physical sensations, and emotions. These can show up in an instant. The hurt you reexperience is real, but the source of that hurt is now only your mind doing its thing. A painful memory is not the same as the hurtful or life-threatening event you once endured. This can be hard to grasp.

If you step back, you'll see that the memory hurts and seems real, but there's nothing you can do now to undo it, change the outcome, or bring about any resolution. And there's nothing you need to do either. The event is in your past. You are in the present. This is what we mean when we say, "Painful memories are not the event." The only thing repeating now are thoughts and the emotional pain. What is not repeating is the actual event, although your mind works hard like an experienced Hollywood film director to make it as real as possible.

What Goes In, Stays In

Your painful past may show up over and over again. That's because we are all historical creatures—we all come into the world like an empty bucket. Over time, your life bucket collects many different kinds of experiences—some you choose, and others just happen. And, you'll continue to collect experiences for as long you're alive. Nothing is subtracted or deleted. What goes in, stays in. Some of it you'll remember easily; other experiences not so much. But it's all in there.

You've seen that your mind and body are always producing thoughts and sensations that you have little control over. Memories are like that too—they can pop into your awareness without much effort. Just like "Little Miss Muffet sat on a _____." You probably don't use the word "tuffet" on a daily basis, yet we're pretty sure the word "tuffet" popped into your mind. We can't even remember when we first learned that. Still, it's part of our history.

And, memories often include images—things you can see as if you're watching a movie. These images are often smeared with the mind's endless judgments, accompanied by strong bodily sensations and emotions, some pleasant and others heavy and dark.

And you know what? Being able to remember can be a wonderful gift too. Even painful or traumatic experiences can be used wisely to help you move forward and avoid past mistakes. Or, maybe your past can be used to appreciate what you have and to maximize the time you've been given. But that's not easy to do.

Getting Hooked on Your Past

It's far easier to get hooked on the past—painful moments in your life bucket that you'd rather dump out, or pleasant moments that you cling to and want to keep around. Maybe it's combat, or an accident, a rape, loss, abuse, regrets, missed opportunities, or choices that you wish you could undo. It may be a difficult childhood, or anger and resentment at how your parents and friends treated you. Recalling some of these experiences leaves you with an overwhelming sense of guilt or shame. You may also linger with wonderful past experiences and feel loss and sadness that they're missing from your life now. It's all in the mix. And, there's absolutely nothing wrong with being able to remember the good, bad, and ugly moments you've lived through. Without that ability, you wouldn't learn and grow.

It's okay that you don't like remembering some of your past. Everyone has things they would rather forget. Some have worse things than others do—but everyone has something. But getting hooked on the past and dwelling there is a trap. The next exercise will show you why.

EXERCISE: STUCK STIRRING A BUCKET OF SHIT

Imagine that you're sitting next to a large bucket with a heavy wooden ladle. This bucket is your past. You try to resist opening the lid, but for whatever reason, the lid pops off. Now, you find yourself staring down into the bucket, only to find that it's full of shit and it really smells awful. So you start stirring, hoping that this might somehow lessen the smell.

In a way, getting hooked on the past is like getting caught stirring a bucket of shit, around and around, with your mind telling you, *You can't go forward because of the pain you lived through.* Or, *You don't deserve to go forward.* Or, *You're just damaged goods, so why bother?* You may even think, *Maybe if I stir long enough I will figure this out and make it go away.* And still, you sit and stir the pot, going back, reopening old wounds, regrets, painful experiences. Maybe you think that if you stir the shit long enough, something will change. But truthfully, no amount of stirring is going to turn shit into sweet ice cream. If anything, it's just going to stink all the more and make a mess. And, you end up exhausted from all that stirring too.

Here's something else to notice—all of this remembering, reliving, and stirring is happening right now, in the present. This is important to notice. There is no time machine to go back. Time only goes forward, and you have to go forward too.

What's needed here is for you to acknowledge the past as the past, drop all the unhelpful stories about you and your past that your mind baits you with. Then, you'll be able to focus on where you are, right NOW, what you want to do, right NOW, and how you can move toward what matters, right NOW.

And, from the present, you can learn to notice remembering for what it is—your mind thinking—and then meet that experience with gentle curiosity and kindness. That's how to free yourself from your mind's attachments to the past, and all of its traps and snares. And, you do that without forgetting or condoning the wrongs or challenges you endured. Instead, you decide to learn from it, open up to it, honor it, and carry it forward in ways that dignify your life as it is now. So, if you're willing, let's get started.

DEFUSING FROM A DIFFICULT PAST

When a painful or traumatic memory pops into your awareness, it's easy to get pulled out of the present in a flash. When this happens, the first thing you need to do is pause, take a few slow deep breaths, and notice what's happening. You're remembering, which is just another form of thinking. And notice that you're doing it NOW, from the safe refuge of the present.

We know that this can seem hard at first. If you tend to get lost in a whirlwind of thoughts about your past, or find that the traumas you've endured seem to pull you out of the present or even right out of your body—like you're in another place—then you know what losing your sense of grounding feels like. It's like having the rug pulled out from under you. That can be scary and make it hard to do what matters in the present moment.

So, if you're willing, let's do an exercise that will help you ground yourself wherever you are and regain your ground when you've been snared by thoughts from your past. All you need for this exercise is about five minutes. Download the audio file from the book companion website at http://www.newharbinger.com/33346 and follow along. With practice, you'll be able to ground yourself without the audio.

EXERCISE: GROUNDING IN THE NOW

Start by removing your shoes if you can, and get in a comfortable position, sitting upright and breathing naturally. Or, if you prefer, you can do this exercise standing, with knees slightly bent.

Once you're ready, close your eyes and bring your attention to your breath. Notice where you feel your breath most strongly. Perhaps it's in your chest, abdomen, or nostrils.

Now bring your attention to your feet. Feel them contacting the floor and ground beneath you. Notice the sense of pressure of your body against the earth below.

Go ahead and wiggle your toes for a moment, and then scrunch your feet into balls by curling your toes downward toward the ground. Notice the movement of the small bones of your feet, and the soft tissue between the bones. Allow yourself to bring all of your attention to these movements. And notice that you can notice them.

Next, bring your awareness to how your feet feel, and notice any sensations there, like tension, relaxation, pain, pressure, warmth or coolness, or even no sensation. Again, noticing that you can notice them.

Go ahead and gently press your feet into the ground beneath you. Become aware of feeling a strong contact with the ground. Then ease up, allowing your feet to contact the floor naturally.

Now, imagine that your breath is passing in and out through your feet as you take a deep, rich inhale … and then a slow exhale. On the next in-breath visualize the pores of the soles of your feet breathing in and filling your body with the solid foundational energy of the earth beneath you. On your out-breath, feel your feet discharging this energy back into the earth, creating strong roots.

Continue on like this—grounding to the earth and where you are now. Notice the dynamic connection between you and the earth and your surroundings. And, if you find your attention wandering, bring it back to your feet, deeply breathing in and out through them and feeling the grounding earth connection …

As this time for practice comes to a close, direct your attention back to the room. Notice the sounds in the room, the feeling of your body as you sit or stand, the temperature of the air, the position of your body, the smells in the room, the feeling of the air on your skin.

And notice that you're here in the now—present, alert, and alive. When you're ready, gently open your eyes and carry this grounding presence with you into the present moment and the rest of your day.

Practice this exercise as often as you can, wherever you are. If you have an injury, then modify the practice by focusing on a part of your body that you can breathe through as you contact the chair, bed, or floor below you. Use the audio to guide your practice until you can remember it, and then do it on your own. It will help you stay present and give you skills to regain your ground when you find yourself being pulled into your past by a difficult memory. Grounding is also a useful way to show up to your life and values right where you are.

You can also ground yourself by engaging your five senses intensely—you can taste something that's strong like a lemon or black coffee; smell something that is pungent like cologne, perfume, soap, or your pet's fur; touch objects that have unique textures, shapes, or weight; or look at something bright, stark, or unusual—a picture or something in your environment. You can listen too—focusing on sounds that stand out in your environment.

Engaging your senses this way will also bring you back to the present. Just be mindful about why you're doing this. It's easy to use your senses as a clever way to turn away from painful memories, but that just puts your memories in charge of your Life Bus and gives them more power to steer your life off track. Instead, engage your senses with your life in mind—as a way to come back to the NOW so that you can act on your life and values now. Just practice these grounding strategies and see what works best for you.

THE MANY STORIES OF YOU

We talked earlier about the metaphor of the chessboard. You are the board upon which the pieces of your past and present experience come and go. Each game has its own character and strategy, but the board never changes. One board might host a thousand struggles; one board might hold the moving pieces (thoughts and feelings) of a lifetime's challenges. Still, the board is not the game. You are not your memories. You are much bigger than your past.

Your mind will pull you to get tangled up in the pieces of your past, and will build a story about your past and you, much like a director works with the scenes when putting together a movie. Your mind, like the director, is selective and tells one kind of story, even if there are many possible stories in there.

To see how this plays out, suppose you wanted to make a film about the wonders of Africa. So, you set out with your film crew and shoot lots of footage. You capture shots of landscapes, wild animals, colorful plants, interesting foods. You capture the scenery and vistas, colorful dress, and tribal celebrations.

But that's not all. You also shoot footage of animal carcasses, poachers, warring tribal factions, men and young boys carrying assault rifles, babies and young children starving and thirsty, illness and disease, famine, starvation, and extreme poverty. Your crew records stories of abuse, rape, drought, hardship, and natural disasters. But remember, you're making a film about the wonders of Africa. So, back in the studio, you review the footage, cut out all the nasty images, and leave them on the cutting room floor.

Your mind does the same with your past too, except that it tends to keep all the nasty stuff and cut out the rest. So, if you've lived through trauma, hardships, and pain, your mind will focus on those in creating your life movie, and leave the rest, even years' worth of wondrous footage, on the cutting room floor.

In a way, your mind is trying to protect you—if you've lived through traumatic and painful experiences, your mind's most important task is to help you avoid that happening again. But the mind doesn't know how to do that in a balanced and life-affirming way. And, the one-sided "darker" story it's feeding you may be severely limiting your life now and for years to come.

But you have a role here in crafting your life movie and in how much to buy in to what your mind tells you. The dark story of you, the one that you may relive and be haunted by now, is one story that could be told. And, if you look, other stories could be told too—moments of sweetness and beauty, joys and triumphs, some parts neutral and other parts uplifting and special.

To craft your whole story, you have to be willing to look back and see what's being left out, and that means looking at moments of both darkness and light. And, you have to be willing to let go of the current story and allow yourself to get curious about other stories that could be told, using all of your experiences up until now.

The next writing exercise will help you do that. All you need is willingness, some curiosity, a bit of lightness, some paper, and something to write with. Don't forget why you're doing this either. This is about breaking free from the shackles of your past, honoring your history, and moving forward in ways that are in alignment with your values. You'll need about fifteen minutes, but you can go longer if you like.

EXERCISE: THE DOCUMENTARY OF YOU

Let's start by writing about the life movie that your mind feeds you most often. Imagine that you're watching your past on a big movie screen. What experiences and events make up your story? What events or experiences does your mind gravitate toward and use to tell the story of you?

Your Life Movie—Take 1

Go ahead and write one paragraph describing what your mind naturally comes up with. It's okay if the things you come up with include mostly dark moments from your past. It's okay if that's not the case. Just write it all down as if no one will know. Let it pour out. No editing. When you're ready, continue reading.

Now pause and take a few slow breaths, and then read, slowly and out loud, what you wrote down. As you do, be mindful that you can observe the script, just like the chessboard observes the game. Notice the words, letters, and ink describing your past and you. What kind of story is being told? How old is it? And, how does it grab and hook you? Is there anything in there that you absolutely cannot think about NOW? Is there anything you're experiencing now that's really your enemy? Just notice, and see if you can open up and be a kind and impartial observer. Don't rush this. And, when you're ready, continue reading.

Your Life Movie—Take 2

Now, we'd like you to write another script. Keep the facts in there from Take 1—the experiences that actually happened or you lived through. But this time, we want you to add to the story. What experiences are missing? What else could be added? Think of experiences that your mind is leaving out, small moments even, or experiences you may remember with a bit of effort. Neutral, sweet, or dark, it doesn't matter. And, it doesn't matter whether they fit with the original story line. In fact, look to experiences that might seem trivial or out of place, like eating a hamburger, taking a hot shower, or watching a movie. Just look to add to the script with experiences that are part of your history, however small. Give yourself at least five minutes to write and rewrite. This story should be longer than the first. Once you have it down on paper, move on and continue reading.

Again, pause, take a few slow grounding breaths, and then read aloud what you wrote down. Notice the words, letters, and ink on the page … just observing what's there with a sense of kindness, curiosity, and gentleness. What kind of story do you have? Is it old? Does this more complete story grab and hook you in the same way as the first? Is there anything about the script that you cannot have or experience NOW? Take a few moments reflecting, and then when you're ready, continue reading.

Your Life Movie—Take 3

Now, if you're willing, we'd like to invite you to go ahead and repeat this exercise at least one more time. Again, keep what you have in Take 2, and add to that with experiences you've had. Think as small or as large as you wish. And, allow yourself to add in experiences that may be far removed in time—distant past or more recent experiences. Then, rewrite the script by adding to it—don't take anything away. This story should be longer than Take 2. Give yourself about five minutes to write, and then when you're done, continue reading.

Again, give yourself a few moments to pause, breathe, and then read aloud (not silently) what you wrote down as an observer. Notice the words, letters, and ink on the page—again, observing what's there with a sense of kindness, curiosity, and gentleness. What kind of story do you have now? Is it old? Does this more complete script grab and hook you in the same way as the first or second one? Is there anything about the story that you cannot have or experience NOW? Take a few moments reflecting, and then when you're ready, move on and continue reading.

This exercise can be challenging at first, and that's okay. Your mind seems to prefer to keep it simple and nasty. It won't like it when you make your life story fuller, richer, and truer to all that you've witnessed and experienced.

Go as far with this exercise as you're willing to go. Each time you rewrite and add to the documentary of you, you'll notice that there's more to you than the one-sided "dark" story your mind gives you. The story of you will continue to be written for as long as you're alive. The trick is to observe your experiences, looking for bits that your mind leaves out or ignores. Look to see what's useful from your past in guiding your life from this point onward.

MAKING PEACE WITH YOUR PAST

We'd like to end this chapter with two exercises that will help you change your relationship with your past—moving from one that is adversarial to one that is kind, gentle, and peaceful. Both are available for download from the book companion site at http://www.newharbinger.com/33346. We suggest that you follow along with the audio first, and later you may do the exercises on your own.

The first exercise will take you back in time to a younger you—a you who was there before the trauma or painful memories you may be struggling with now. The second one will help you practice the skill of letting go and healing old wounds from your past.

Both exercises will teach you how to be kind to yourself and your old wounds. We're not going to say that this will be easy to do at first. But if you stick with it and practice a few times over this week, you may notice that your past loses some of its power to steer your Life Bus off track. You can heal yourself. You'll need about ten minutes for each exercise.

EXERCISE: BEING KIND WITH YOUR OLD WOUNDS

Begin by getting yourself in a comfortable position. Sit upright and allow yourself to get grounded with a few slow breaths in … and out, from the earth below you, up your torso, and then back out through the soles of your feet, rooting strongly in the earth below.

Now bring to mind a memory that you've been struggling with for a very long time. See if you can put yourself in that situation. Where were you? What happened? What were you doing? What were others saying or doing? Watch it as if it was unfolding on a giant movie screen. See if you can give yourself permission to be present with this experience as fully as you can. Notice how you reacted then. And, notice how you may be reacting to the memory now.

Slow things down as best you can … and notice the thoughts as thoughts, images as images, physical sensations as sensations, emotions as emotions … just as they are. Watch and gently observe parts of your experience as they come and go, as you take the perspective of the chessboard. There's nothing to do but notice. You don't have to take sides … just stay with this experience as best you can and breathe.

When you're ready, release that difficult image with a large grounding breath in and out through your feet, and then imagine an earlier time in your life—one long before the difficult memory. Go back as far as you can remember … to a time in your childhood when you remember feeling good. See if you can visualize that younger you—notice your face and eyes as a child, your hair, what you were wearing, and how small you were. And, notice where you were, what you were doing, what you were experiencing that left you feeling whole and complete, even if that sense of feeling good was short-lived.

Now, imagine that younger you is standing in front of you now, and comes over to sit on your lap. That younger you has no idea what the future holds. Only you know. And, you know what that child will eventually experience in life because you've lived through it.

As you hold that younger you on your lap, you pause and notice each of you looking into the other's eyes and heart. As you look, what advice would you share with him or her, knowing all that you know about what this younger you will face in the future? How would you respond to that younger you? What does that little child need from you? What does he or she need to hear from you? Take a moment to hear your words as you look into the eyes of the younger you from very long ago. And notice that you were there then, and that you are here now too.

Linger with this experience for a few moments. When you're ready, allow yourself to slowly come back to an awareness of sitting where you are right now … see if you can bring a sense of kindness to your experience now and to any old wounds that you remember. As you do, hear the words that you shared with the smaller you and extend them to your experience now. Sense any gentleness and compassion you may have felt with the younger you and bring that to yourself and your experience now. What do you need to give yourself right now?

As this exercise comes to a close, make one last gesture of kindness with both hands. Place one hand on your chest and the other on your belly. Let them gently rest there as you hold yourself kindly. Sit this way as long as you wish—just caring for yourself, being with yourself, giving yourself comfort, rest, and support. Gently remind yourself that you're more than what you lived through, however difficult or painful it may be to remember. Stay in this moment as long as you wish.

Then, when you're ready, take a final grounding breath or two and gently open your eyes, with or without tears, it does not matter. Simply allow yourself to come back to the present, with the intention to bring kindness to yourself, your history and old wounds, and your life.

This exercise can be quite powerful. You may have felt strongly while doing it. You may notice that you were moved to tears. You may also notice a sense of numbing out or hardening, finding it difficult to extend kindness to yourself as you would to a younger you. You may have also noticed a sense of peace, as if a weight was lifted off your shoulders. You may have had a different experience too and that's okay.

But the key insight to connect with here is the fact that you were there before the dark history you lived through, and that you have the power to change your relationship with your past. You can choose to open up to your old memories in a kinder, peaceful, and more loving way. In fact, you have an abundant capacity to do just that. Nothing from your past can rob you of that, unless you allow that to happen.

This is the time to take control over the life you wish to create from this moment forward. The past is behind you. It isn't helpful to continue stirring the pot, reopening old wounds. Listen to the words you shared with your younger you. There is wisdom in those words. There in those words, you will find your heart. You can extend them to yourself right now and for each moment to come.

This is a critical moment. Your brain and nervous system have no delete button. This means that normally what goes into the mix, stays in the mix. What you can do now is change the mix by adding something new to it. You do that by doing something new with your painful memories when they show up. That something is compassion and forgiveness.

Before beginning the next exercise, we'd like you to find a candle, and a quiet, comfortable place where you can set it up. Light the candle as a symbol of your commitment to let go and forgive. This candle represents someone or an event that caused you pain or hurt. You will be focusing on the flame as you go through each step.

This exercise is likely to be difficult for you at first. Steps 3 and 4—bringing compassion and letting go as you extend forgiveness to the source of hurt or pain—are particularly tough. Be gentle with yourself if it feels like it's too much or too difficult. Your mind will give you all sorts of reasons why you shouldn't do it. Acknowledge these doubts and apprehensions about extending forgiveness and see whether you can be willing to have them for the sake of living the life you want.

It takes practice to cultivate forgiveness. Give yourself time. If you've suffered trauma and you experience a lot of painful memories and images, we suggest you do this exercise every other day for several weeks. You can either listen and follow the instructions using the audio at the book companion website (http://www.newharbinger.com/33346), or record the text below in your own voice at a slow pace and then listen to it. You could also try both options and see which works better for you.

There's one final thing to keep in mind before you start. Forgiveness doesn't mean condoning what happened to you. You may ask, "Why should I forgive those who harmed me?" or "How can I forgive myself when what I did was clearly wrong?" The answer is simple and practical: forgiving yourself and others is the only path to healing.

> *Forgiving yourself and others is the only path to healing.*

If you don't let go and forgive others for the harm they did, they and their deeds will continue to haunt you, harm you, and have a hold on you. Every moment you hang on to your resentment, you hurt yourself one more time. So by not forgiving, you hurt yourself. Remember, this practice is for you, not for people or circumstances that once hurt you!

EXERCISE: THE CANDLE OF FORGIVENESS

Go ahead and light the candle and then get in a comfortable position in your chair. Sit upright with your hands resting in your lap. Your legs can either be uncrossed or crossed, whatever is more comfortable. Allow your eyes to focus on the candle flame and simply watch it.

As you watch the flicker of the candle flame, bring your attention to the gentle rising and falling of your breath in your chest and belly. Like ocean waves coming in and going out, your breath is always there. Notice the rhythm of the breath in your body with each passing inhale … and exhale. Notice the changing patterns of sensations in your belly as you breathe in and as you breathe out. Take a few minutes to center yourself as you breathe in and out.

Step 1: Become Aware of the Wrong and Hurt Beneath the Painful Memory

Now allow your awareness to shift to a painful memory or traumatic event. See if you can allow yourself to visualize the scene fully as if you were watching a movie in slow motion. What happened? Who else was there? Watch the flame as you acknowledge the painful situation unfolding in your mind's eye. Focus on your breathing as you watch the situation unfold. See if you can slow the painful situation down, slower and slower with each passing breath.

As you do, bring your attention to any sensations of discomfort that show up. As best you can, bring an attitude of generous allowing and gentle acceptance to your experience right now. See if you can make room for the pain and hurt you had then and that you may be reliving now. Soften to it … as you breathe in … and out … in … and out.

As best as you can, open up to all of it: the hurt, pain, sadness, regret, loss, and resentment. Allow yourself to become aware of your hurt and painful emotions, and simply acknowledge the hurt you experienced and the hurt you may have caused. There's no need to resist or fight or blame. Simply acknowledge and become aware of your experience.

Step 2: Separate Hurtful Actions from Your Hurt and Its Source

Visualize the person or event that inflicted the hurt. As you begin to do so, allow the person or event to drift over and become the candle. If it was you, then see yourself as the candle. Focus on the candle and continue to visualize the person or situation that hurt you or caused the hurt. Now remember and visualize what happened. As you focus on the candle, notice what your mind machine is doing with the images and sensations that show up.

You might see your mind making a judgment ... blaming ... having feelings of sadness ... bitterness ... resentment. As these and other thoughts and sensations come into your awareness, simply label them as you did in previous exercises—*There is judgment ... blame ... tension ... resentment*—and allow them to be. Bring a gentle and kind awareness to your pain and hurt as you breathe in ... and out ... in ... and out ... slowly and deeply.

Next, create some space between the actions that made you feel hurt and angry and the person or situation that created them. If it helps, you can visualize the action that hurt you as the flame, and the person or situation who committed the hurt as the candle. If you were the source of hurt, then let your actions become the flame and you the candle.

Notice that the flame is not the candle. The actions of the person who hurt you are not the same as the person who committed them. As you breathe in and out, give yourself time to connect with this difference. Then, bring each hurtful action into the flame one by one and notice it, label it, and then see the difference between the hurtful action and the person. Visualize what was done, not who did it.

After you spend some time noticing each action, allow it to disappear up into the smoke, leaving the candle flame. Keep watching any tension, discomfort, anger, hurt, or whatever else your body may be doing. Make room for what you experience as you return your attention to your body and your breathing. Don't change or "fix" anything.

Step 3: Bring Compassionate Witness to Your Hurt

Next, bring your attention back to the human being in the candle—the perpetrator of wrongs against you, or those you may have committed yourself. Notice how he or she is also a human being and vulnerable to harm just like you are. At a basic human level, the two of you are not that different.

See if you can allow yourself to take that person's perspective as a compassionate witness and see what life might be like through his or her eyes. Connect with that person's hardships, losses, missed opportunities, poor choices, faults and failings, hurts and sadness, and hopes and dreams.

Without condoning his or her actions, see if you can connect with that person's humanity and imperfections as you connect with your own humanity and imperfections, hardships, loss, pain, and suffering.

As a compassionate witness to this other human being, see if you can connect more deeply with that person, even if that person is you, as another human being. Notice the offender's thoughts and feelings, knowing that you've also experienced similar types of thoughts and feelings. What might it be like to have lived the life of the person who offended you? As best you can, bring an attitude of generous allowing and gentle acceptance to what you experience now.

Step 4: Extend Forgiveness, Let Go, and Move On

Now see if you can bring into awareness what your life would be like if you let go of all the negative energy you are holding on to—your grievances, grudges, bitterness, and anger. What would it be like to let go of the effort needed to shut out this painful experience from your past? Connect with the reasons behind why you want to be free from the painful memory, the anger, or the desire for revenge.

Allow yourself to visualize a new future, full of the things you've missed out or given up on by resisting the memory or holding on to your unwillingness to forgive. See if you can connect with your future without forgetting what happened in the past, and without carrying the weight of bitterness, anger, and resentment toward the person or event that hurt you.

Allow yourself to take the courageous step forward in your life by letting go of the memory, your pain, your anger, and your resentment. Take time to really connect with this relief as you imagine separating from the resentment and bitterness you have carried for so long. Allow all of it to drift away with each out-breath, and with each in-breath, welcome in peace and forgiveness as you continue to breathe in … and out, slowly and deeply.

When you're ready, bring into your awareness how you have needed other people's forgiveness in the past. Imagine extending that forgiveness to the person who hurt or offended you. What could you say to that person? As you think about this, notice any discomfort showing up and what your mind is doing here.

If the thought *The person doesn't deserve that* or *I don't deserve that* shows up, just notice that thought and gently let it go. Return your focus to your breathing as you remind yourself that kind and gentle acts of forgiveness are for you, not for others.

Imagine the burden being lifted from you as you choose to extend forgiveness. Allow yourself to connect with the sense of healing and control that comes along with this. As you give the powerful gift of forgiveness, notice some budding feelings of softness where before there was only hardness, hurt, and pain.

Embrace this moment of peace as you return to the image of the person who offended you, even if that person is you. Gently extend your hands as you say, "In forgiving you, I forgive myself. In letting go of my pain and anger toward you, I bring peace and freedom to myself. I invite peace and compassion into my life and into my hurt and pain. I choose to let go of this burden that I have been carrying for so long." Repeat these phrases slowly as you extend forgiveness.

Stay with and simply observe and label whatever thoughts and feelings come up as you offer this act of forgiveness. Sense the emotional relief that comes when the burden of a grudge is melting away. See if you can notice the peace and feeling of inner strength that comes about as you extend compassion and forgiveness in this moment.

Then, when you're ready, bring your awareness back into the room, to your body, and to the flicker of the candle flame. Finish this exercise by blowing out the candle as a symbolic gesture of your commitment to forgive and let go and of your readiness to move on with your life.

LIFE ENHANCEMENT EXERCISES

We all have something in our past that can haunt us and keep us stuck. So, as you work with the exercises in this chapter, be mindful that you're learning new skills that will help you break free from the bondage of your past so that you can create a new future. This week, we suggest that you spend time with the exercises in this chapter. Do them at your own pace. They need not be done all at once. And be mindful that you are doing this work in the service of living the kind of life you wish you have from this point forward. Remember that the pages of your Life Book from here on out have yet to be written. They can be a repeat of the past, or something truly new. You get to decide what goes in there.

THE TAKE-HOME MESSAGE

Your mind is set up to recall events over and over, particularly the nasty ones. That's what modern psychology teaches us. But keeping your eyes fixed on the past is no way to live. You don't need to live your life as a victim of your past either—as living proof of all the terrible wrongs that were committed against you. This just hurts you again and again.

All memories you experience are about a past that once was; they show up right where you are, often without much effort on your part. The important lesson and skill is to learn that you are not your experiences. You are more than your past. You also have control over how you carry all those memories forward from this point onward. There is no going back to undo, get rid of, or replace what came before. All you can do is learn to let go and learn from what you've lived through. Making peace with your painful past is how you'll gain the freedom now to keep yourself moving forward toward the life you really want for yourself.

Making Peace with My Past So I Can Move On

Points to Ponder: My past is my past, and over much of it I had very little control. *I* was there before the trauma and dark moments and I am here now—I am. I cannot change what happened, but I can learn from it, make peace with it, and decide to move forward and become the person I wish to be.

Questions to Consider: Am I willing to make peace with my past? If not, then what is getting in my way? Am I living my life as a victim—as living proof of past wrongs? Is this serving me well? Am I willing to look forward and carry all that I have lived through into the new life I wish to create? Can I take the bold step to let go and bring compassion, kindness, and forgiveness to my hurt and pain? Am I willing to make room for something new?

CHAPTER 19

Moving Toward a Valued Life

The journey of a thousand miles must begin with a single step.

—Chinese proverb

The journey of your life is made up of the steps you take—what you do. Each and every step will move you either toward or away from what matters to you. The key is to step and step wisely, for in these steps you will create the conditions for genuine happiness.

Wise steps are those that are guided by your values—that shining light in the sea of life that we talked about in chapter 13. Values, as you learned, act like a beacon. They point you in a direction toward what's important. This is crucial when you feel pulled and pushed around in a sea of worry, anxiety, panic, and doom and gloom. The next step is to take control of your actions and start moving in vital directions by focusing on specific goals. Goals are like destinations that you'll visit along the journey toward living out your values.

The wonderful thing about values is that they can give a very personal meaning to your life. The key to living out your values is to break them down into incremental steps. Living a rich life is all about taking steps, however small or large, each and every day, toward achieving your goals and living your values. You must commit to taking those steps. You do that by setting goals and following through with action.

By taking charge of your behavior, you take charge of your life. Are you ready and willing to take these steps?

SETTING AND ACHIEVING GOALS

Go back to the Life Compass you completed in chapter 13. Now is the time to decide which of these value areas and intentions you want to have more of in your life right now. Choose a value that has been difficult for you to act on. Perhaps you put this aspect of your life on hold because of anxiety-related barriers. This would be a good place to start. If you sense that you're not yet ready to confront barriers in this important life area, then choose a different area and make that your ready-and-willing starting point.

For now, we'd like to walk you through one area to give you an idea of how the process works. Later you can go through the same steps for the other value domains on your Life Compass. Once you've chosen a value, write it down on the top line of the Value and Goals Worksheet that appears at the end of this chapter and on the book companion website (http://www.newharbinger.com/33346).

Be SMART with Your Goals

George Doran (1981) developed a very effective five-step behavioral program to help people achieve goals. He called them SMART goals. Though Doran developed the program for people in business, it has been used widely and successfully in ACT (Harris, 2008) to help people, just like you, do more of what matters to them. For purposes of this workbook, we've tailored SMART goals just a bit. Let's go over these steps one by one:

1. **S**pecific—Identify concrete goals on your path.

2. **M**eaningful—Set goals that matter to you and reflect your values.

3. **A**ctive—Select goals that you are able to accomplish yourself and that add to your life satisfaction and vitality in some way.

4. **R**ealistic—Set goals that are reasonable given your life circumstances.

5. **T**ime-framed—Be able to make a commitment to the day, time, and setting where you plan to take the step (and don't forget to pat yourself on the back after you complete a step!).

The last important piece here involves practice. Once you set a SMART goal, practice taking the steps to live out your values in situations that have been difficult for you. Below, we'll walk you through how to do just that.

Identify Concrete and Achievable Goals

As you start thinking about goals, you'll find that some are short-term goals you can attain in the near future. Others are long-term goals you'll only be able to attain further down the road. Both types of goals are important, and achieving one may lead you to the next.

For instance, suppose you value your health and one of your valued intentions is to increase your fitness level. So you commit to walking each day. Your long-term goal might be to walk to a telephone pole one mile from where you live. Between your house and that pole are a number of other poles, all spaced about the same distance apart. A short-term goal here might be getting to the first pole. The next day you commit to getting to both the first and the second pole, and so on. If you keep at it, you'll eventually reach the pole at your one-mile marker—your long-term goal. This is how short- and long-term goals work—they get you moving on a valued path.

To get and stay moving, it's important that you avoid ending up on a dead-end street. Setting goals is all about workability (Hayes & Smith, 2005). If you don't make your goals workable in the context of your life, it's unlikely you're going to get very far down the path of your values. Choose achievable, obtainable actions that can realistically fit with your life. Doing this makes it much more likely you'll actually be able to live your values every day.

In the space below (or on a separate sheet of paper), write down some goals related to the first valued intention you chose to work on from your Life Compass. Be sure they are concrete and specific.

To help you get concrete, ask yourself this: *What would other people see me doing? How would they know I have done something new?* Focus on what you can do with your mouth, hands, and feet. And, be sure it's something you could then tick off your to-do list:

_____   _____

_____   _____

_____   _____

We suggest that you start with one or two goals. One should be a short-term SMART goal—something you can start working on this week. Then ask the following questions for each goal to make sure it's achievable:

- Is the goal **specific** (concrete, practical)?

- Is it **meaningful** (reflects what truly matters to me)?

- Is it **active** (something I can do and have control over)?

- Is it **realistic** (does it work with my current life situation)?

- Is it **time-framed** (can I put in on my calendar and do it)?

And, above all, does this goal lead you in the direction of your valued intention? Does it express what matters to you, what you want to be about and become? If you can answer "yes!" to these questions, then you've set a good SMART goal. If you said no, then go back and rework your SMART goal—think small. What tiny step could you take that would express your values and move you into the life you wish to lead?

Once you have your SMART goal down, write it in the left column of the Value and Goals Worksheet at the end of this chapter. You'll also find a copy of the worksheet on the book companion website at http://www.newharbinger.com/33346. If necessary, revise and clarify the goal until you get a "yes" answer to each SMART goal question. You'll want to have several blank copies of this worksheet handy for other valued intentions that you'll want to work on later.

Identify Steps and Arrange Them in Logical Order

Having settled on goals, you've put the first guideposts on your road map. Now focus on the incremental steps you need to take to get there. Start with the short-term goal and break it down into smaller intermediate steps. Think of each step you need to take to attain your goal. Then write those steps down in the space below (or on a separate piece of paper):

_____   _____

_____   _____

_____   _____

Now think about a logical order for the steps. What needs to happen first before the other steps can follow? If no particular order is necessary, then start with the easiest step. Copy the steps into the Value and Goals Worksheet in the order in which they need to be completed. You can go through the same procedure for other goals you've identified.

Let's look at two examples. Suppose your goal is to change jobs and eventually become a manager with a large corporation rather than the small outfit you're currently working for. This goal, in turn, includes smaller specific actions, such as brainstorming ideas, checking relevant newspapers and Internet sites for postings of managerial jobs, networking, updating your resume, setting up an informational interview at a company that interests you, and submitting a job application to a potential new employer. Notice that the interview depends on the other steps happening first, including plain old brainstorming ideas.

Here's another one. Let's say you want to work on spending more quality time with your spouse or partner. This goal may be approached via several steps, such as doing something once a week with your partner that you both enjoy, perhaps going to a movie or a show, dining out, going away for the weekend, taking a bike ride together, or spending quiet time at home talking. Notice that there's no logical order to the steps in this example. What's important is that you do these things regardless of how you feel at the moment.

Make a Commitment and Take the Step

Now it's time to make a commitment. Are you willing to commit to the values explored in chapter 13 and to the behavioral and life changes they imply? If so, commit to a day and time to begin step 1 on your Value and Goals Worksheet. Tell someone else that you've done so. Then, no matter how you feel at that time, do it. This is all about action and doing something different with your life. Unless you take action, nothing will change. You'll continue to get what you've always got.

Write in the date when you achieved each step. Put a gold star on the chart if you want to. Make sure to congratulate yourself: give yourself credit for what you've accomplished, no matter how small the step was. Review your Value and Goals Worksheet frequently. It'll give you valuable feedback on how you're progressing and will encourage you once you start ticking off your goals.

To give you some ideas about how to break down a goal into intermediate steps, take a look at the two examples below. They both refer to the same value—parenting. However, due to the nature of each individual's anxiety problem, the barriers and strategies are somewhat different.

■ Jill's Valued Goals

Jill, a thirty-seven-year-old mother of two daughters, has suffered from panic disorder and agoraphobia for over fifteen years. She's missed every school concert and special occasion that involved being in a crowded school auditorium or gym. Here's how she completed a section of her Value and Goals Worksheet. Note how some steps can and should be repeated to provide more opportunities for practice.

VALUE AND GOALS WORKSHEET

My value: _Being a good and supportive mom with my kids_

Goal I want to achieve: _Attending my daughter Mary's school concerts_

Steps toward achieving my SMART goal	Barriers	Strategies	Date(s) completed
1. Go to quiet place every other day and imagine myself being at next school concert.	Stress of knowing that eventually I'll have to attend the concert	Practice FEEL exercise & Silent Observer Self skills. Make a list why attending concert is important for living out my values.	9/15 9/17 9/19
2. Attend an outdoor concert with family.	Fear of everyone around me knowing that I'm nervous and may have a panic attack at any moment	Practice watching my mind as an observer. Practice WAF surfing if panic arises.	10/15
3. Sit twice in empty auditorium to become familiar with the surroundings two weeks before concert.	Fear (thought) that I'll feel so anxious that I won't be able to make it through the concert when people are around	Practice watching thoughts and feelings as an observer—from acceptance exercises. Keep eyes on value of being a good mom and supporting my kids.	11/1 11/14
4. Go to two rehearsals when few people are around.	Fear of not being able to escape without interrupting the rehearsal	Practice FEEL exercise & Silent Observer Self skills. Watch thoughts, feelings, and images. Remind myself of value.	11/20 11/28
5. Attend daughter's school concert.	Fear (thought) of embarrassing Mary if I have a panic attack during the concert	Let thoughts be, and focus on Mary's performance and the value of being a supportive mom. Practice WAF surfing if I feel panic.	12/10

It took Jill almost three months from taking the first step to completing the last one. This is fine. Some people move faster, and other people need more time. It really doesn't matter how long reaching any of your goals takes you. The only thing that matters is that you stay on course and move in the direction you want to move in—at your own pace and with both patience and persistence.

■ Eric's Valued Goals

Below is the example of Eric, a forty-two-year-old father of a son and a daughter. Eric was diagnosed with obsessive-compulsive disorder at the age of nineteen. Here's how he completed a section of his Value and Goals Worksheet. Again, note how Eric was doing just fine at his own pace, and that he repeated some steps to provide more opportunities for practice.

VALUE AND GOALS WORKSHEET

My value: _Being an active and engaged dad (and good role model) with my kids_

Goal I want to achieve: _Doing at least one outside activity per week that kids and I like_

Steps toward achieving my goal	Barriers	Strategies	Date(s) achieved
1. Make a list with my kids of activities we'd like to do together.	Stress of leaving the house and going outside my comfort zone	Drop the rope. Make a list of all the reasons why it'll be good for me and my children to do more outdoor activities.	6/1 6/5
2. Practice sitting outside in the grass three times and just noticing the urge to wash my hands and clothing without giving in to the urge.	Anxiety of having germs all over my body and not being able to wash myself	Put disturbing thoughts and urges on cards. Imagine intrusive thoughts and worries as leaves floating down a river. Be kind to myself and remind myself that I can live out my values and be anxious at the same time. I can be willing.	6/15 6/18 6/21 6/25
3. Do two low-anxiety-provoking activities or outings (different one each week).	Worries about children not having a good time because of my anxiety	Look at worries as thoughts; use bubble wand—just WANR again. Remind myself of how activities help me live the life I want for me and my kids.	7/2 7/14
4. Do two activities or outings that kids like. May bring on medium anxiety (different one each week).	Fear of not being able to reduce my distress if there are no sinks nearby	Drop the rope in tug-of-war with urge to wash, continue to do what I'm doing, and take the urge with me. Sit with it and do nothing—ride the wave.	7/21 8/5
5. Do two activities or outings that kids like and may provoke considerable anxiety (different one each week).	Fear of getting sick from all the germs at public places	Use an observer perspective when it feels like anxiety is going to overwhelm me, and practice urge and anxiety surfing when it gets strong. Focus on the moment and the value in the action.	8/15 8/20

Practice Living Your Values in Difficult Situations

The two sample worksheets also give you a good idea of how to practice living your values in difficult situations. It's quite likely that the old WAFs are going to show up as you embark on your road to valued living. The FEEL exercises in the previous two chapters were meant to prepare you for how to move with barriers in difficult situations. In fact, all of the exercises in this book are in place to help you gain the freedom to live your life. Now it's time to apply all the skills you've been learning.

KNOWING YOUR BARRIERS

All along you've been working to get clear about barriers that get in the way of living your life. Most of the barriers we've covered arise from within you. But there's another set of obstacles that can trip you up. We call them external barriers, like lack of money, time, skills, or necessary information to do what matters. Others may involve conflicts between your goals and what other people want, need, or expect.

The good news is that it doesn't really matter if the barriers are inside or outside of you. What's most important is that you develop a plan, as Jill and Eric did, for how you'll approach and move with them. The next exercise will help you to anticipate barriers and challenges that might get in the way of you acting on your value-guided SMART goals. That way you can come up with a plan, using all the skills you've been practicing so far, to approach them so that you keep yourself moving in ways that matter.

So, let's take a moment to settle and get clear about the barriers you might face as you act on your value-guided goal. Listen to the audio from the book companion site at http://www.newharbinger .com/33346 as you do the next exercise.

EXERCISE: ANTICIPATING BARRIERS

Just take a moment to close your eyes and bring to mind one of your valued intentions—the things you care about in your heart and want to be about. Sink into the sweetness of that—the sense of lining up with your core. If that's hard to do, imagine for a moment that nothing gets in your way and that you're free to do what you really, truly care about. See yourself being about something that matters in your heart.

Now, see yourself living out those intentions as if watching yourself on a giant movie screen. Focus on the very first step or two just as you decide to act. Notice where you are. Notice what you're saying. Notice what you're doing with your hands and feet. And, if other people are involved, watch how they might be responding to you. And now, take an inventory of what's showing up inside of you.

Observe what your mind is telling you. Is there judgment of you, or the situation, or other people? Do you notice blocking thoughts, like *I can't do this … it's too much*? Or, discouraging thoughts, like *nothing matters*

… so don't bother. Or, maybe your mind is conjuring up images of catastrophe, old wounds, doom and gloom, or maybe it's telling you something else like *I don't have enough time.* Just notice what's there and take stock.

Now move on to what's going on in your body. What are you feeling? And, if that's still difficult for you, see if you can notice any sense of hardening, closing down, or pulling back. As you observe, notice what's showing up just as it is, like *I'm noticing hardening, tensing,* or *shutting down.*

And, see if you can detect any physical sensations in your body such as tension, energy, your heart pounding, or maybe holding your breath or breathing really fast. Just take stock of that too and observe it as the chessboard would.

Now look and see if your mind is commanding you to do something. Is it telling you to cut and run, turn away, lash out, or give up? Just notice these urges and impulses and ride the wave.

And, if we've left anything out, just notice what that may be in your experience. It could be thoughts, emotions, sensations, or urges to act or react. Look to the barriers you've been working on to guide you here. Some may arise within you, others may be external to you.

And now, let's come back to where you are right now, and allow yourself one or two deep breaths in and out. And then, slowly open your eyes.

Use what you learned from the imagery exercise we just did, or look to your past experiences, to get clear about the barriers that may show up as you step in directions that matter. As part of this, lay out the barriers you might face as you complete the Value and Goals Worksheet. Then look to the skills from this book that you've found helpful. And, as Jill and Eric did, write down the skills you plan to use to keep yourself moving forward if and when your barriers show up.

Maybe it's dropping the rope, mindfulness, grounding, taking the observer perspective, writing thoughts on cards, saying to yourself *I'm having the thought that …,* or any of the other skills. Remember, look to the exercises, metaphors, and images that you've found helpful so far.

We encourage you to take your time with this part. It's really important that you have a plan to approach your internal barriers in a new way. If you don't, you're putting yourself at risk of falling back into old patterns that didn't work before, and that probably won't work in the future. As we've talked about in previous chapters, if you do what you've always done, chances are you'll get what you've always got.

THE REWARDS AND CHALLENGES OF LIVING YOUR VALUES

The next two exercises will help you get in touch with the immediate challenges and rewards that living your values can offer you. As you follow along with the audio from the book companion website (http://www.newharbinger.com/33346), focus on the immediate positive impact of acting on your goal and appreciate that it may be both hard to do *and* rewarding at the same time.

EXERCISE: GETTING IN TOUCH WITH THE REWARDS OF LIVING MY VALUES

Go ahead and close your eyes and take a few slow breaths as you center yourself. Now bring to mind the valued intention you've been working with in the previous exercise. Once you have that value in mind, see yourself acting on that value just as you wish *and* with nothing standing in your way. You're free of barriers and successful in doing what you set out to do.

Notice what you're doing and sink into the sweetness of this moment, this experience, just as you might linger with a beautiful sunset. What does success feel like on the inside? Notice any thoughts, emotions, and physical sensations. See if you can touch a sense of satisfaction, a sense that you're doing something good for yourself and your life too.

Stay with this image, and when you're ready, shift your attention to the world around you—the people, the events, and the environment that surround you in this scenario. What's different? Become aware of how people in the situation are reacting to you and to what you've accomplished. How does it feel to be freed up from an old barrier? How does it feel to freely do something you've been afraid to do? Notice how the situation changes for the better because of what you did in the service of your values.

Stay with this exercise, this experience, for as long as you wish. And, when you're ready to wrap up, open your eyes, and then grab a piece of paper and jot down all of the positive outcomes you discovered during this exercise. Let them serve as a reminder to you of what is possible as you embark on your journey with the Value and Goals Worksheet.

In the next exercise, we'll ask you to shift your awareness to what's possible as you act on your values in situations where one of your WAF barriers shows up. This exercise will help you see how you can uphold your values even when it is difficult to do so.

EXERCISE: CREATING A SUCCESS STORY

Get comfortable and take a few slow, deep breaths. Allow your eyes to close gently. And, when you're ready, bring to mind one of your values that's been difficult for you to act on because of your anxiety barriers—you can use the same value as before or a different one. When you have it in mind, imagine that you're taking just one step to act on that value. See the very first thing you'd say or do as if you're watching yourself on a movie screen. See your actions and hear your words.

As you do, see and hear how others respond to you as you watch the scene unfold. What are they saying? What are they doing?

And then kindly observe any barriers that show up inside you. See if you can notice emotions that seem to block you from taking another step to support your values. Notice any thoughts that are trying to thwart your path. Do the same with any physical sensations in your body. Continue to watch and observe your thoughts, feelings, and physical sensations without resistance. Open up to them, allow them to be, however scary or unpleasant they might seem. Notice the wave of emotion and remind yourself that sooner or later it'll crest and then recede. So stay and ride it out. As you do, be kind with your mind and body and experience. Soften to the barriers with each breath, creating more space for you to be right where you are.

Now, come back to the scene and see yourself completing what you set out to do. Sink into the satisfaction of doing what you care about, and every good thing that happens for you, for others, and for your world. Notice any sense of sweetness in that. Acknowledge that you did something good for yourself and your life by having a clear intention to act and following through, even as you had to face emotional pain and other barriers along the way.

Both of these exercises are ways to help you turn your attention to what you can do, and what's possible in your life. Every barrier has the same message: you can't have this, or don't do that. But there's no way to do what matters when you listen and buy in to your mind telling you *You can't do it!* We saw this play out with one of our sons, Aidan, during Little League.

At the time, Aidan was in a real batting slump. He was really hard on himself about that too. When he'd take batting practice, he'd quickly get frustrated and say, "I can't hit this stupid ball." This got to the point where he stopped swinging at pitches during games, and it became a chore to drag him to the field for batting practice.

In a way, Aidan was in an impossible situation. He was trying to get up to the plate and hit a ball while listening to his mind tell him how much he "can't hit." How's he going to hit the ball when he's focused on not hitting?

So, after explaining the situation to Aidan's coach, we came up with a solution: Aidan was asked to imagine himself getting up there and hitting, what it might be like seeing himself making contact with the ball, and the joy and satisfaction that may follow from that. This is what brought him out of his batting slump! You can do that too. But you need to have a clear image of what it is you want to do, where you want to go, and the possible rewards of acting in ways that matter to you. That's why SMART goals are so important. They are the steps along the path into the life you wish to create. Just be sure you give yourself time to practice as much as you need.

LIFE ENHANCEMENT EXERCISES

Practice valued living by following the steps outlined in this chapter. Use the Value and Goals Worksheet to plan activities and to prepare for the difficulties and barriers that may come up along the way. Start with one value and a set of related goals. Later, you can work on other values and goals in a similar fashion. Practice the exercises that will help you visualize and make contact with the rewards of living out your values, even when WAF barriers show up. Also continue to practice any of the earlier mindful acceptance and observer skills exercises as often as possible, including kindness toward yourself, when anxiety shows up during the day. Every exercise in this book will help you move in directions that matter to you.

THE TAKE-HOME MESSAGE

To change your life, you'll need to commit to changing what you do, pure and simple. You can get back on the road to a valued life by focusing on your values, setting goals, and then taking action no matter how you feel. Acceptance, compassion, and kindness will be your friends when you deal with barriers that will undoubtedly come up.

Putting My Values into Action

Points to Ponder: I can live my values by setting concrete and achievable goals one day at a time. Making commitments and practicing living my values—even in difficult situations—is what life is all about.

Questions to Consider: How can I put my values into action every day? How can I break up my goals into small steps so I can keep on moving?

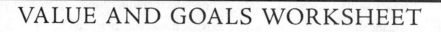

VALUE AND GOALS WORKSHEET

My Value: _____

Goal I want to achieve: _____

Steps toward achieving my goal	Barriers	Strategies	Date(s) achieved
1.			
2.			
3.			
4.			
5.			

CHAPTER 20

Staying the Course and Living Your Values

Where you end up isn't the most important thing. It's the road you take to get there. The road you take is what you'll look back on and call your life.

—Tim Wiley

As we learn from Tim Wiley, life is not a destination. It's a journey—and that journey is what you will look back on someday and call your life. This way of looking at things demands a shift in focus.

When you started this book, you may have been looking to tackle your anxieties and fears first, so that you could then be happy and thrive once you started feeling better. We hope that you've learned by now that this is not the path to genuine happiness. In fact, it is a recipe for more suffering.

This is why we've encouraged you to put your attention on learning the skills for changing your relationship with your mind and body first, with the purpose of making the most out of the life you have and in ways that you care about. This shift in focus is exactly how you create genuine happiness. And yes, you deserve to be genuinely happy. You cultivate genuine happiness by practicing being gentle, kind, mindful, and defused, and by being more willing, open, and allowing with your mind, body, and everything your history throws at you. These are the skills that will create genuine happiness and peace. We hope that by now you are starting to connect with this basic truth—a truth that is now supported by quite a bit of research as we discussed in the prologue.

So here, we'd like to congratulate you for all the work you've done and will continue to do. You've come a long way! But there is still more to do—fortunately, your journey isn't over yet. And we truly want you to keep yourself moving forward in ways that matter to you, long after you put down this book.

To do that, you need to be ready for the old WAF barriers to show up, because they will. They'll try to stop you from getting where you want to go and doing what you want to do. The risk of getting sidetracked by these barriers is great. So, as we bring this book to a close, we'll review some of the key strategies to keep on moving with the barriers that will spring up along the way and to approach setbacks and slipups gently, with kindness and compassion.

HOW TO KEEP ON MOVING

As you embark on your journey of putting your values into action, there will be new obstacles, doubts, and setbacks. The old WAF obstacles and barriers will show up too. At times, you won't put your commitments into actions. Sometimes you'll slip into old WAF habits. Once in a while you may take longer to reach a goal than you had hoped. All of this and more is just fine. We all move at our own pace.

The most important thing is that you keep yourself moving forward in vital ways. You can draw upon the strategies and skills you've learned in previous chapters when discomfort *difficulty* threatens to get in the way of discomfort *vitality*.

Practice Your Skills

The first and most important recommendation we can give you is to keep on practicing the skills you learned in this program. You've had to practice to develop them. And, like all skills, you have to use them to keep them. One of the main reasons people fall back into old, familiar, and unhelpful habits is that they stop using the skills and exercises in programs like this one.

So, make a commitment to practice an exercise or two daily in a quiet place, and use your skills in your daily life. Download the audio exercises from this program and make them part of your daily routine. The practice doesn't have to be long or drawn out—even five to twenty minutes a day can be helpful. The key is to keep the skills alive by using them. The more you use them, the more they'll become a habit that will make it easier to keep yourself moving forward and living the life you want to live.

Recommit to Action After Breaking a Commitment

There will be times when you make a commitment to take some action in support of your values, and then for whatever reason you fail to follow through. Many times, if you look, a lack of follow through will come back to old and new barriers showing up. We're pretty sure that the passengers on your Life Bus will be shouting things like "You'll never make it!" "You'll just make a fool of yourself!" "You're going to get hurt!"

Following through with a commitment is difficult when WAFs are right in your face. But here, it's crucial to remember that you can always recommit to taking actions that support your values and your life. Expect that you'll experience barriers, uncertainty, and doubt, and that your mind won't always offer helpful advice. In fact, your mind will likely offer up all of your fears and doubts, trying to keep you from taking action. During these times, come back to this key question: *Am I willing to commit to this chosen activity 100 percent in the service of my values?*

This is a choice only you can make, and we hope you will, again and again. Knowing that you're bound to experience discomfort and doubt, are you still willing to commit to this or that activity 100 percent and go through with it? Remember, commitment isn't something you can merely try or do halfway. You either make the commitment or you don't.

We're not asking you to commit to success or any other particular outcome like "being in a steady relationship by July 1st" or "feeling better and less anxious." Many outcomes are beyond your control. They lie somewhere in the future and can only be known *after* you've put your new skills to use. We're only asking whether you're willing to commit to doing something that will work for you *and* taking all those passengers with you on your Life Bus. Will you do that and mean it?

The commitment means that you choose to do something, and then follow through right where you are, in the present moment. It doesn't mean that you'll never fall short, because we all do from time to time. And when that happens, learn from it, pick yourself up, and then recommit to some action, and mean it.

GETTING BACK ON TRACK IS WHAT COUNTS!

Remember, a valued life is built on SMART goals, one step at a time, one moment after the next. Each day offers another opportunity to take action on your SMART goals. Your commitment is that if and when you do break a commitment, you'll recommit and mean it once again, and that you'll do what you can to stay on the path of your values.

Your choices and actions ultimately determine what happens with barriers and setbacks on your road to valued living. At times, all of us will fail to live consistently with our values. What happens then is critical. You make a choice. Learn from the experience. Pick yourself up. Let go of buying in to the "failure" judgment and being strangled by it—just put it on a card and take it along. And then make a renewed commitment to take actions that move you in life directions you care about.

When you let a WAF barrier stop you from time to time, don't slide into thinking that this means that WAFs will take over your life again. That won't happen unless *you* allow it to happen. It's your choice to either give up or recommit to small actions that make your life meaningful—and then put those actions into practice. So long as you do that and keep moving, you'll be truly living a life that expresses your values.

This entire book has been about helping you make choices—every day and every moment of your life—that will keep you moving in the direction of those values. If you've worked the exercises so far, then you're not the same person you were when you first cracked open this book.

Move with Barriers and Setbacks

Remember that you don't need to overcome WAF barriers before moving forward on the road to living your values. You don't need to get rid of them. And, you don't have to change them either.

The key is to acknowledge the barriers and move *with* them—take them with you for the ride. Let your values show you the way. Make room for all the unwanted stuff. Don't let it stop you from doing

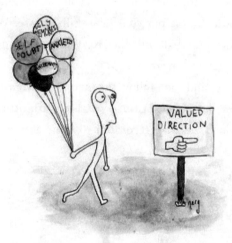

what's best for you. Keep on nurturing your willingness to have what you have, and stop running from yourself.

Focus on changing your relationship with your mind, body, spirit, and life right now, in this moment and then the next. You and you alone are the driver of your Life Bus. To have the life you want, you need to keep yourself in the driver's seat and carry all the passengers with you, pleasant and unpleasant. Unpleasant passengers will be the most challenging, but there are other passengers too—ones who need your attention, because they'll remind you of what you care about and want in your life.

When in doubt, do the opposite of what WAFs seem to be telling you. Don't listen to Anxiety News Radio; tune in to Just So Radio by watching what's going on from your kind and gentle observer perspective. Cherish the moment as it is! It too will pass.

And don't miss watching what's going on inside you with some kindness and compassion. Nurturing friendliness and willingness will make it easier to move with your WAFs. They are not your enemy but more like a wounded child who needs some loving-kindness. Take care of that child. Embrace it. Take it with you on your journey.

Don't Let the Mind Machine Trap You

The mind machine won't stop its chatter just because you've made a commitment to act and to take your WAFs with you when they show up. Sometimes you'll fall short of being accepting and following through with your commitments. Your judgmental mind may scorn you: *Stop all this acceptance and commitment BS. You just can't do it. The only thing you should accept is that you're a failure at acceptance and commitment!*

When your mind is throwing this and other old, sticky stuff at you, it's important not to get tangled up in all that chatter. This is just another example of your mind doing what minds do all the time: creating thoughts and evaluating. It's just more "blah, blah, blah."

Ask yourself if the "blah, blah, blah" is really helpful to you. Do you need to listen to and trust all the thoughts your mind feeds you? Must you argue with "blah, blah, blah"? Or can you make room for whatever your mind comes up with and let it be? This will free you up to move on with your life, no matter how strong or powerful the feelings are, no matter how loud the thoughts get. These are the times when you need to watch and expose your mind machine in action, as you've learned to do in the earlier exercises.

Here, the practice is always the same: willingly acknowledge and observe your mind doing its thing, without struggling with it or buying in to everything it comes up with. This is how you can gradually learn to drop all the old story lines your mind loves to feed you. This will position you to use your mind wisely when it serves you well.

Over time, you'll get better at noticing when you're hooked, coming back to right where you are, and asking if your mind is being helpful or not. This important skill will help you move forward with your life, no matter how loud the thoughts get.

Watch for Idleness and Fill It with Active Vitality

When you just sit on your hands and don't do anything that's in line with what you truly care about, you create a big void in your mind. And your mind will do what it can to fill this empty space, often with judgments, criticisms, and old barriers. You've probably noticed this yourself. These times can be high-risk situations for getting hooked. Idleness is a great setup for WANR.

You have two ways to go here. One path is to get mired in whatever shows up and do nothing. The other is to welcome what shows up and get moving. We think the latter option is better for you. Doing something vital will clear out the old junk and make room for something new.

So when you're stuck with nothing to do except swim around in a sea of thoughts, emotions, and physical sensations, pause, and ask yourself this: *What do I want to be about right now?* Think action! Then, go and do something, anything, that's in line with what you care about. That's how to make your life grow.

Practice Flexibility

Every time you do something new, different, or out of your comfort zone, you're practicing flexibility in your life. You expand and grow—you become less narrow, less rigid, more open, and more adaptable. And you set yourself up to get the most out of your life. You learn new things.

There are several ways to practice flexibility. Here are a few suggestions:

■ **Freshen up your mindfulness and meditation practice.** You can do this by switching between the different types of exercises in this book and on the book's companion site (http://www.newharbinger.com/33346). You can also practice the exercises in places other than your usual, special kind space in your home. In addition, you can find new exercises in many books, online, and on CDs. Or you can create new exercises yourself.

■ **When you're stuck in a rut, step out of that rut and do something new.** One of our clients noticed he'd been stuck in such a rut. Every time he'd go out to dinner, he'd order the same thing—steak. It didn't matter where he went. He finally decided to consider the whole menu of options and choose something different. He now enjoys crab. Life is like a menu too. It gives you many offerings. Look for them, step out of your ruts, and follow your bliss.

■ **Continue reading and learning.** Check out the list of further readings and helpful internet resources provided on the book website (http://www.newharbinger.com/33346) to expand your knowledge about mindfulness, meditation, and the ACT approach to anxiety and other related concerns.

■ **Feed your mind and life with uplifting news and experiences.** If you're the type of person who's glued to the news, the Internet, social media, or other sources of stimulation, it might be a good idea to cut loose. Give yourself a break—quiet time away from the negative noise of the world around you. Turn off the TV, the cell phone, and the radio, and do something you value. Stillness creates opportunities for peace and gives you space to think and move. You can fill that stillness with something other than negative news coming from your old history or the media. Fill it with valued action, uplifting information, beautiful nature, music, or art. The most effective way to dispel darkness is to bring light into the room rather than try to chase darkness out of the room.

■ **Nurture a spirit of playfulness with your mind, body, and life.** Kids are masters at the art of play, and we seem to lose that as we grow up. But study after study shows that adults who practice being more playful with themselves and others, and make time for fun and play, are generally happier and healthier, and live longer too. Perhaps you've left play on the back burner for a very long time. That's fine. There are lots of ways you can practice bringing it to the front. Think about the things you like to do that are playful and fun, and see if you can build a spirit of play into your life. You can also bring the spirit of playfulness to your mind and emotional life. You may be pleasantly surprised at what it offers you.

Build Your Willingness Muscle

Life is asking you whether you're *willing* to open up to the difficulties you face inside, and in the world around you, in the service of living a life that matters and is important to you. You already have a sense of what willingness is like. It's not the absence of fear, but the decision that something else is more important than the fear. So willingness takes courage. You decide to step, and step with your arms wide open. You'll never be certain about what you may find, but you can rest in the sweetness of knowing that you stepped in ways that uphold what matters to you.

You now have a new perspective and a set of powerful skills that will allow you to carry and move with your barriers in the service of living a valued life. You don't have to be someone other than who you are, or have a history other than the one you've had, to create the life you wish to lead.

You control your willingness switch, and you can choose to flip it on, and then make that choice again and again. When old WAFS try to take over your Life Bus, ask yourself, *Am I willing to engage in my life now, whatever that might bring, in the service of doing what matters to me?*

Are You Moving Forward or Backward in Your Life?

Whenever you encounter barriers and you're unsure whether your planned action is good for you, ask yourself one simple question: *Is my response to this event, thought, feeling, worry, or bodily sensation moving me closer to or further away from where I want to go with my life?* Below are some variations of this crucial question:

- If that thought (emotion, bodily state, memory) could give advice, would the advice point me forward in my life or keep me stuck?

- What advice would my value _____ [bring to mind a core value of yours] give me right now?

- What would I advise my child or someone else to do in this situation?

- If others could see what I am doing now, would they see me doing things that I value?

- In what valued direction have my feet taken me when I listened to this advice?

- What does my experience tell me about this solution? And what do I trust more—my mind and feelings, or my experience?

Asking questions like these when faced with adversity and doubt is far more helpful than listening to what your unwise WAF mind comes up with or what the surging impulses seem to be telling you. The answers will remind you that past solutions have not worked: you now have the opportunity to choose to do something different.

EMOTIONAL DISCOMFORT IS YOUR TEACHER

WAFs, along with other emotional pain and hurt, are not your enemies. They are your teachers. Think about that for a moment. Without experiencing disappointment, you'd never learn to hold your expectations about the future more lightly. Without the hurt and frustration you receive from others, you'd never learn kindness and compassion. Without exposure to new information, you'd never learn anything new. Without fear, you'd never learn courage and how to be kind to yourself. Even getting sick once in a while has important purposes—it strengthens your immune system and helps you to appreciate good health.

Moments of adversity and pain provide you with opportunities for growth and change. They teach you important skills. They give you perspective on life. You need them. They offer you great opportunities to expand your response-ability when faced with pain, hurt, or feelings of inadequacy, loneliness, or sadness.

When these feelings show up, they'll pull your eyes off of what you can control and make you focus on what you cannot control. Start by looking at what you're doing, and then be response-able. Focus on what you can control to have your needs met and to keep you moving forward in directions that you care about. This is something you can do. Be specific here and write down a plan that keeps you moving forward even in the face of adversity.

We suggest you apply your compassionate observer skills to each of your painful experiences when you have them. You can choose to open up to and embrace them when they show up and bring compassion and forgiveness to them. The payoff is this: your emotional pain will no longer be fertile soil for your WAFs and won't sidetrack you from moving in directions you care about. You will also create the conditions for genuine happiness to grow within you!

A MEANINGFUL LIFE IS BUILT ONE STEP AT A TIME

Sitting still with your WAFs and not getting all tangled up with them is one of the toughest parts of practicing courage on a day-to-day basis, and so is letting go of the internal dialogue and struggle. Over time, you'll get more skilled—so long as you keep practicing loving-kindness toward your own slipups, limitations, and all-too-human inability to be perfect.

Begin each day with this commitment: *today, to the best of my ability, I'm going to act with kindness and courage.* Then follow that with an intention to make your day a value-rich day. In the evening, go back and examine your day with loving-kindness. Don't beat yourself up if your day ends up being filled with some of the same old things you've always done. Look for the new and vital things you did do that day.

Compassion, softness, flexibility, and courage are skills and powerful antidotes to suffering. Recognize that you're only human and that you're going to make mistakes and experience setbacks. You're never going to be able to be courageous and accepting all the time; and still, you keep moving in directions you care about, one day at a time.

What matters is that you are taking steps to bring acceptance and compassion to yourself and your worries, anxieties, and fears. The small steps eventually add up. Sooner or later you'll find that loving-kindness and patience will become habits in your life. Give yourself time. Working through this book in the span of several weeks is not the end of something. It is the beginning of a new chapter in your life. It takes months to become really familiar with the exercises so that you can readily move and keep on moving in valued directions. And the work is not over with this book. Your life journey takes a lifetime.

The important thing is to keep practicing the skills you've learned in this book. By now you will have found out which exercises and metaphors have been particularly helpful in getting you unstuck and moving forward. Revisit them and focus on them.

You could also start doing one or two exercises that you haven't tried yet and see what happens if you practice them for a while. It may also be helpful to keep reflecting on your remaining WAF sticky spots—thoughts, images, memories, bodily sensations, urges, and situations that tend to get you stuck—and then focus your mindful acceptance and observer self practice on them. If you ever feel discouraged, we suggest you revisit your epitaphs and particularly focus on your Valued Life Epitaph—you could even rework or expand it.

It's risky to make changes. Things sometimes do go wrong or don't turn out as intended. Yet the biggest risk in life is taking no risk at all. There are few things in life that are certain. The future is, by definition, not knowable. Most choices involve risk for this very reason. Choosing to play it super safe is a surefire way to guarantee that nothing will change. You can count on that. And if nothing changes, you'll end up going where you've always headed before—a place where you're stuck, suffering, and waiting for your life to begin. Risking living your life, while you can, is risky business, but the payoff is huge—you'll get more of what you want. You'll risk living out your dreams.

THE LIFE QUESTION

We'd like to end with what we call the "life question." It's by far the single most important question life is asking you when you're faced with barriers, problems, and pain.

At those times, STOP, take a deep breath or two, and ask yourself this simple life question: *Am I willing to take all that life offers and still do what matters to me?*

We all need to face this question squarely and be willing to answer it, one moment after the next, for as long as we're alive.

And, it turns out that "yes" is the only answer that will help you create a life in line with your values. "No" means only one thing: you're choosing NOT to live the life you want. Whenever you find yourself answering "no" to the life you want, remember, you can always choose to change your answer, to take a bold step on a new path, and to risk doing something new to get a different outcome in your life.

THE CHOICE IS YOURS

When you first opened this book, you were probably looking for a new gold shovel that would finally dig you out of your anxiety hole so that you could get on with your life. We've done our best to show you that this isn't necessary. By now, we hope that you're experiencing this for yourself and doing what the image to the right shows. Remember that image from chapter 1? If you need to, go back and review that cartoon series and reflect on just how far you've come.

The most rewarding thing you can do to create a life that matters is to put each moment of every day to good use. How you decide to use your precious time and energy from this day forward is up to you. You don't have to conquer anxiety when it shows up or endure it with brute force of will. Instead,

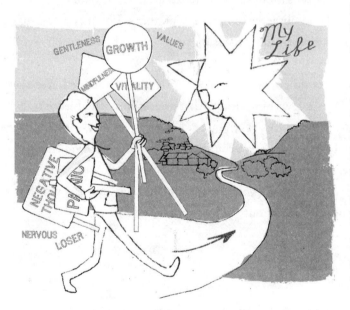

you can apply the skills of acceptance, compassion, and observing to whatever is going on. These skills are your friends to help you stay on track.

It's your choice. Use your time wisely. There's no going back, no way to carry over until tomorrow the lost moments of today. In the end, it all adds up to what you'll call your life. Make the most of it. Make it about something bigger than your anxiety. We know you can do it. You have the skills. Continue to nurture them. Allow them to grow. Make your values a reality. This is what matters and what, in the end, leads people to say, "Now there was a life lived well."

Staying the Course for the Long Haul

Points to Ponder: I can live my values *and* take my WAFs along for the ride. My greatest barriers are those that my mind creates. I need not let them stand in the way of where I wish to go with my life.

Questions to Consider: How can I best keep on moving with my barriers toward a valued life? Is what I am doing now moving me forward or backward in my life? Is what I am doing now what I want to be about?

Further Readings and Internet Resources

Here we list suggestions for further reading if you'd like to learn more about the ACT approach to anxiety and other related concerns. We particularly recommend the book by Steven Hayes and Spencer Smith for more examples and suggestions about how to use ACT in your life. There are several other good ACT books on the subjects of anxiety, worry, trauma, and depression, many of which are published by New Harbinger Publications.

We also recommend that you check out books, such as the one listed below, by Pema Chödrön—a great source of strength, courage, and practical advice on how to approach emotional pain with its most powerful antidotes: compassion and patience. Books by Thich Nhat Hanh, Tara Brach, and Jeffrey Brantley contain practical advice on achieving self-transformation using mindfulness and on nourishing the positive seeds in you and in others, while starving the negative ones. Books by Deepak Chopra (such as the one listed below) will help you connect with your true self and the I Am presence in you. Deepak offers easily accessible advice on mantra meditation and spiritual practices to help you gain more peace; see also Norman Rosenthal's book on transcendental meditation.

Lastly, the Internet is a hub for resources on mindfulness and exercises that will help you cultivate peace of mind and kindness of heart. We've listed a few sites that provide text and audio exercises. Use them to enrich your skills and expand your practice.

FURTHER READINGS

Brach, T. (2004). *Radical acceptance: Embracing your life with the heart of a Buddha.* New York, NY: Bantam Books.

Brantley, J. (2003). *Calming your anxious mind: How mindfulness and compassion can free you from anxiety, fear, and panic.* Oakland, CA: New Harbinger Publications.

Chopra, D., & Simon, D. (2004). *The seven spiritual laws of yoga: A practical guide to healing body, mind, and spirit.* New York, NY: Wiley.

Chödrön, P. (2001). *The places that scare you: A guide to fearlessness in difficult times.* Boston, MA: Shambhala Publications.

Dyer, W. (2012). *Wishes fulfilled: Mastering the art of manifesting.* New York, NY: Hay House.

Eifert, G. H., & Forsyth, J. P. (2005). *Acceptance and commitment therapy for anxiety disorders: A practitioner's guide to using mindfulness, acceptance, and values-based behavior change strategies.* Oakland, CA: New Harbinger Publications.

Eifert, G. H., McKay, M., & Forsyth, J. P. (2005). *ACT on life, not on anger: The new acceptance and commitment therapy guide to problem anger.* Oakland, CA: New Harbinger Publications.

Hayes, S. C., & Smith, S. (2005). *Get out of your mind and into your life: The new acceptance and commitment therapy.* Oakland, CA: New Harbinger Publications.

McKay, M., Forsyth, J. P., & Eifert, G. H. (2010). *Your life on purpose: How to find what matters and create the life you want.* Oakland, CA: New Harbinger Publications.

McKay, M., & Sutker, C. (2007). *Leave your mind behind: The everyday practice of finding stillness amid rushing thoughts.* Oakland, CA: New Harbinger Publications.

Nhat Hanh, T. (2001). *Anger: Wisdom for cooling the flames.* New York, NY: Riverhead Books, Penguin Putnam.

Rosenthal, N. E. (2011). *Transcendence: Healing and transformation through transcendental meditation.* New York, NY: Tarcher/Penguin.

Salzberg, S. (1995). *Loving-kindness: The revolutionary art of happiness.* Boston, MA: Shambhala Publications.

INTERNET RESOURCES

New Harbinger Publications

http://www.acceptanceandmindfulness.com

This website contains information on other New Harbinger Publications books, including some of our own, in which acceptance and mindfulness approaches are applied to many forms of human suffering.

The Association for Contextual Behavioral Science (ACBS)

http://www.contextualscience.org

This website is the hub for professionals and members of the public interested in acceptance and commitment therapy and other newer cognitive-behavioral therapies. It contains many useful resources for those interested in learning more about ACT as well as those actively engaged in ACT research and application. The website maintains a listserv for the public and offers a searchable database for those interested in finding an ACT therapist.

Georg H. Eifert

http://www.dreifert.com

This is Dr. Eifert's website. Here, you'll find information about Georg, his books, upcoming talks and workshops, and other resources.

John P. Forsyth

http://www.drjohnforsyth.com

This is Dr. Forsyth's website. Here, you'll find information about John, his upcoming talks and workshops, books, and resources. John also maintains a blog, where he shares wisdom and teachings about using ACT and other practices, and offers a variety of internet-based services (consultation, supervision, coaching, and therapy) related to ACT for mental health professionals and the general public.

Pema Chödrön

http://www.pemachodronfoundation.org

On this website, you will find information about Pema Chödrön's teachings, additional exercises, and forthcoming talks and books. Pema is a leading exponent of teachings on meditation and how they apply to everyday life. She is widely known for her humorous and down-to-earth interpretation of Tibetan Buddhism for Western audiences.

Transcendental Meditation

http://www.tm.org

Go to this website if you are interested in learning more about a very well-researched and easy-to-learn mantra meditation, transcendental meditation (TM), and how and where to learn it from a teacher. On this website you can also gain a wealth of information on the psychological and health benefits of TM for allowing your body to settle into a state of profound rest and relaxation and your mind to achieve a state of inner peace.

Tara Brach

http://www.tarabrach.com/talks-audio-video/

Dr. Tara Brach shares her wisdom and teachings on the practice of mindfulness and acceptance. Tara also offers a number of free audio exercises and videos of her teachings.

References

Allen, D. (2002). *Getting things done: The art of stress-free productivity.* New York, NY: Penguin Books.

American Psychiatric Association. (2013). *Diagnostic and statistical manual of mental disorders* (5th ed.). Washington, DC: Author.

Antony, M. M., & McCabe, R. E. (2004). *Ten simple solutions to panic.* Oakland, CA: New Harbinger Publications.

Arch, J., Eifert, G. H., Davies, C., Vilardaga, J. C., Rose, R. D., & Craske, M. G. (2012). Randomized clinical trial of cognitive behavioral therapy (CBT) versus acceptance and commitment therapy (ACT) for mixed anxiety disorders. *Journal of Consulting and Clinical Psychology, 80,* 750–765.

Assagioli, R. (1973). *The act of will.* New York, NY: Penguin Books.

Bandelow, B., Boerner, R., Kasper, S., Linden, M., Wittchen, H. U., & Möller, H. J. (2013). The diagnosis and treatment of generalized anxiety disorder. *Deutsches Ärzteblatt, 1110,* 300–310.

Barlow, D. H. (2004). *Anxiety and its disorders: The nature and treatment of anxiety and panic* (2nd ed.). New York, NY: Guilford Press.

Borkovec, T. D., Alcaine, O., & Behar, E. (2004). Avoidance theory of worry and generalized anxiety disorder. In R. G. Heimberg, C. L. Turk, & D. S. Mennin (Eds.), *Generalized anxiety disorder: Advances in research and practice* (pp. 77–108). New York, NY: Guilford Press.

Brach, T. (2004). *Radical acceptance: Embracing your life with the heart of a Buddha.* New York, NY: Bantam Books.

Brantley, J. (2003). *Calming your anxious mind: How mindfulness and compassion can free you from anxiety, fear, and panic*. Oakland, CA: New Harbinger Publications.

Chödrön, P. (2001). *The places that scare you: A guide to fearlessness in difficult times*. Boston, MA: Shambhala Publications.

Chopra, D. (2003). *The spontaneous fulfillment of desire*. New York, NY: Harmony Books.

Craske, M. G. (2003). *Origins of phobias and anxiety disorders: Why more women than men?* Oxford, UK: Elsevier.

Dahl, J. C., & Lundgren, T. L. (2006). *Living beyond your pain: Using acceptance and commitment therapy to ease chronic pain*. Oakland, CA: New Harbinger Publications.

Dalai Lama XIV [Tenzin Gyatso]. (1999). *The path to tranquility*. New York, NY: Penguin Putnam.

Doran, G. T. (1981). There's a S.M.A.R.T. way to write management's goals and objectives. *Management Review, 70*, 35–36.

Dr. Seuss. (1990). *Oh, the places you'll go!* New York, NY: Random House. (Original work published 1960.)

Dyer, W. (2012). *Wishes fulfilled: Mastering the art of manifesting*. New York, NY: Hay House.

Eifert, G. H., & Heffner, M. (2003). The effects of acceptance versus control contexts on avoidance of panic-related symptoms. *Journal of Behavior Therapy and Experimental Psychiatry, 34*, 293–312.

Eifert, G. H., McKay, M., & Forsyth, J. P. (2005). *ACT on life, not on anger: The new acceptance and commitment therapy guide to problem anger*. Oakland, CA: New Harbinger Publications.

Friedman, M. J., Keane, T. M., & Resick, P. A. (2014). *Handbook of PTSD: Science and practice*. New York, NY: Guilford Press.

Harris, R. (2008). *The happiness trap: How to stop struggling and start living*. Boston, MA: Trumpeter.

Hayes, S. C. (2004). Acceptance and commitment therapy, relational frame theory, and the third wave of behavioral and cognitive therapies. *Behavior Therapy, 35*, 639–665.

Hayes, S. C., Follette, V. M., & Linehan, M. M. (Eds.). (2004). *Mindfulness and acceptance: Expanding the cognitive-behavioral tradition*. New York, NY: Guilford Press.

Hayes, S. C., Luoma, J. B., Bond, F. W., Masuda, A., & Lillis, J. (2006). Acceptance and commitment therapy: Model, processes, and outcomes. *Behaviour Research and Therapy, 44*, 1–25.

Hayes, S. C., & Smith, S. (2005). *Get out of your mind and into your life: The new acceptance and commitment therapy.* Oakland, CA: New Harbinger Publications.

Hayes, S. C., Strosahl, K. D., & Wilson, K. G. (2012). *Acceptance and Commitment Therapy: The process and practice of mindful change* (2nd ed.). New York, NY: Guilford.

Hayes, S. C., Wilson, K. G., Gifford, E. V., Follette, V. M., & Strosahl, K. (1996). Experiential avoidance and behavioral disorders: A functional dimensional approach to diagnosis and treatment. *Journal of Consulting and Clinical Psychology, 64,* 1152–1168.

Hill, P. L., & Turiano, N. A. (2014). Purpose in life as a predictor of mortality across adulthood. *Psychological Science, 25,* 1482–1486.

Kabat-Zinn, J. (1994). *Wherever you go, there you are: Mindfulness meditation in everyday life.* New York, NY: Hyperion.

Kessler, R. C., Berglund, P., Demler, O., Jin, R., Merikangas, K. R., & Walters, E. E. (2005). Lifetime prevalence and age-of-onset distributions of DSM-IV disorders in the National Comorbidity Survey Replication. *Archives of General Psychiatry, 62,* 593–602.

Leonardo, E. D., & Hen, R. (2006). Genetics of affective and anxiety disorders. *Annual Review of Psychology, 57,* 117–137.

Lesser, E. (2008). *The seeker's guide: Making your life a spiritual adventure.* New York, NY: Ballantine Books.

Maraboli, S. (2014). *Life, the truth, and being free.* Port Washington, NY: A Better Today Publishing.

McKay, M., & Sutker, C. (2007). *Leave your mind behind: The everyday practice of finding stillness amid rushing thoughts.* Oakland, CA: New Harbinger Publications.

Nhat Hanh, T. (2001). *Anger: Wisdom for cooling the flames.* New York, NY: Riverhead Books, Penguin Putnam.

Ritzert, T., Forsyth, J. P., Berghoff, C. R., Boswell, J., & Eifert, G. H. (in press). Evaluating the effectiveness of ACT for anxiety disorders in a self-help context: Outcomes from a randomized wait-list controlled trial. *Behavior Therapy.*

Russo, A. R., Forsyth, J. P., Sheppard, S. C., & Promutico, R. (2009, November). *Evaluating the effectiveness of two self-help workbooks in the alleviation of anxious suffering: What processes are unique to ACT and CBT?* Paper presented at the 43rd annual meeting of the Association for Behavioral and Cognitive Therapies, New York, NY.

Salters-Pedneault, K., Tull, M. T., & Roemer, L. (2004). The role of avoidance of emotional material in the anxiety disorders. *Applied and Preventive Psychology, 11*, 95–114.

Sheppard, S. C., & Forsyth, J. P. (2009, November). Multiple mediators and the search for mechanisms of action: A clinical trial of ACT in the treatment of anxiety disorders. In S. C. Sheppard & J. P. Forsyth (Chairs), *Beyond the efficacy ceiling: Targeting universal processes across diverse problems in ACT clinical effectiveness trials.* Symposium presented at the 43rd annual meeting of the Association for Behavioral and Cognitive Therapies, New York, NY.

von Oech, R. (1998). *A whack on the side of the head: How you can be more creative.* New York, NY: Warner Business Books.

Wegner, D. M. (1994). Ironic processes of mental control. *Psychological Review, 101*, 34–52.

World Health Organization (2015). *Life expectancy data by country.* Retrieved from http://apps.who.int/gho/data/node.main.688.

Yadavaia, J. E., Hayes, S. C., & Vilardaga, R. (2014). Using acceptance and commitment therapy to increase self-compassion: A randomized controlled trial. *Journal of Contextual Behavioral Science, 3*, 248–257.

John P. Forsyth, PhD, is an internationally renowned author and speaker in the fields of acceptance and commitment therapy (ACT), mindfulness practices, and self-development and growth. For over twenty years, his writings, teachings, and research have focused on developing ACT and mindfulness practices to alleviate human suffering, awaken the human spirit, and nurture psychological health and vitality. His personal journey and experience, balanced with practical insights grounded in scientific evidence, offers hope to those wishing to find a path out of suffering and into wholeness.

He has coauthored several popular ACT books, including *Acceptance and Commitment Therapy for Anxiety Disorders* for mental health professionals, and three self-help books for the public: *The Mindfulness and Acceptance Workbook for Anxiety*, *ACT on Life Not on Anger*, and *Your Life on Purpose*.

Forsyth holds a doctorate in clinical psychology, and is professor of psychology and director of the Anxiety Disorders Research Program at the University at Albany, SUNY, in Upstate New York. He is a licensed clinical psychologist in New York, with expertise in the use and application of ACT for several forms of psychological and emotional suffering. He is also a widely sought-after ACT trainer and consultant, and serves as a senior editor of the ACT book series with New Harbinger Publications.

Forsyth regularly gives inspirational talks and practical workshops to the public and professionals in the United States and abroad, and offers ACT trainings at the Omega Institute for Holistic Studies in Rhinebeck, NY, where he serves as a member of the teaching faculty. He is known to infuse his teaching and trainings with energy, humility, and compassion, and his down-to-earth workshops are consistently praised for their clarity, depth, and utility. Collectively, Forsyth's work has helped foster growing interest in acceptance and mindfulness in psychology, mental health, medicine, and society.

Georg H. Eifert, PhD, is an internationally recognized author, scientist, speaker, and trainer in the use of acceptance and commitment therapy (ACT), an integrative approach balancing mindful acceptance, change, and compassion to foster psychological health and wellness. He is also professor emeritus of psychology at Chapman University in Orange County, CA, where he was previously department chair and associate dean of health sciences. He has won numerous awards for his research, teaching, and writing contributions. He is also a licensed clinical psychologist.

As an active developer, researcher, and practitioner of ACT and transcendental meditation (TM), Eifert is coauthor of several popular books, including the highly praised practitioner's treatment guide, *Acceptance and Commitment Therapy for Anxiety Disorders*, as well as several ACT books for the public: *ACT on Life Not on Anger*, *Your Life on Purpose*, and *The Anorexia Workbook*. He has also authored and coauthored several books in German.

Eifert regularly gives workshops and talks around the world, teaching ACT to both the public and professionals to help people end psychological suffering and lead more fulfilling lives. His workshops have been praised as inspiring, humorous, and empowering, and are renowned for their authenticity, clarity, and practical usefulness.

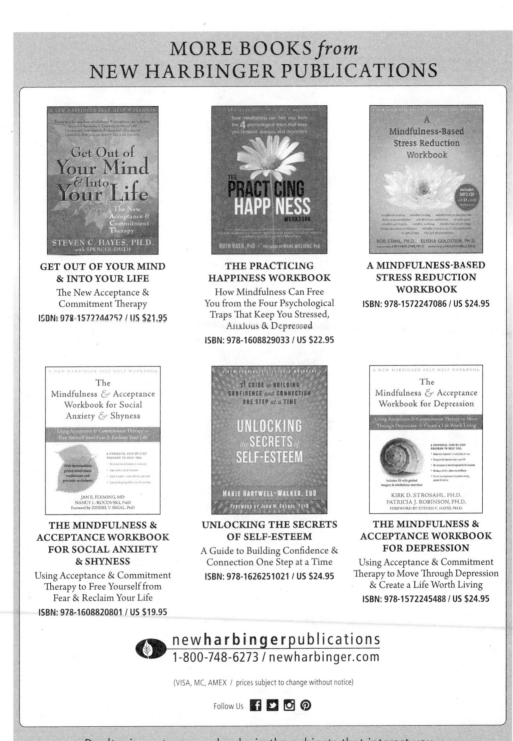